Microbiology for the Health Sciences

Gwendolyn R. W. Burton, Ph.D.

Professor
Division of Science
Front Range Community College
Denver, Colorado

Microbiology

for the
Health Sciences

Third edition

J. B. Lippincott Company   Philadelphia

London, Mexico City, New York,
St. Louis, São Paulo, Sydney

Acquisition/Sponsoring Editor: Patti Cleary
Developmental Editor: Eleanor Faven
Manuscript Editor: Lorraine Smith
Indexer: Maria Coughlin
Designer: William Boehm
Design Coordinator: Anita Curry/Anne O'Donnell
Production Manager: Kathleen P. Dunn
Production Coordinator: George V. Gordon
Compositor: Circle Graphics
Printer/Binder: R. R. Donnelley & Sons Company
Cover Design: Kevin Curry
Cover Printer: Philips Offset Company, Inc.

Third Edition

6

Library of Congress Cataloging in Publication Data

Burton, Gwendolyn R. W. (Gwendolyn R. Wilson)
  Microbiology for the health sciences.

  Bibliography: p.
  Includes index.
  1. Microbiology.   2. Medical microbiology.
I. Title.   [DNLM: 1. Allied Health Personnel.
2. Microbiology.   QW 4 B974m]
QR41.2.B88   1987   616'.01   87-3527
ISBN 0-397-54672-6

The author and publisher have exerted every effort to ensure that drug selection
and dosage set forth in this text are in accord with current recommendations
and practice at the time of publication. However, in view of ongoing research,
changes in government regulations, and the constant flow of information relating
to drug therapy and drug reactions, the reader is urged to check the package
insert for each drug for any change in indications and dosage and for added
warnings and precautions. This is particularly important when the recommended
agent is a new or infrequently employed drug.

For Cindy, Gary, Alan, Earl,
Robin, Penny, and Rae Lynn

Preface

Microbiology, the study of microbes, is a fascinating topic to those of us who feel its importance in our daily lives. Others find it necessary to learn the microbiological concepts and vocabulary in order to function well in their chosen vocations. For example, those who plan to work in any area of health care, such as prevention of disease or care and treatment of the diseased, must be aware of the principles of sterilization, disease causation, and disease prevention.

Microbiology for the Health Sciences will aid those who want to learn the basic microbiological concepts that apply to the health field. It is also intended for students who have little or no science background, and for mature students returning to school after several years' absence.

There is a need for a "simplified" microbiology text that presents the major concepts clearly and concisely for people entering the health occupations. This book is appropriate for use in a one-term allied health microbiology class or as one unit in a basic science class for health-oriented students.

Microbiology is an enormous and complex subject with many interrelated facets and hundreds of scientific terms. I have attempted a very fundamental approach to the subject matter by presenting at the beginning of each chapter the basic information necessary for understanding the more complex concepts with which the chapters conclude. Specialized vocabulary has been kept to a minimum. Key terms are in boldface type and are defined in the glossary at the beginning of each chapter for easy reference. A complete glossary can also be found in the back of the book. The glossaries also include aids to pronunciation. The objectives are clearly stated at the beginning of each chapter to enable the student to survey the topics to be covered. Questions for review are included at the end of each chapter.

Although this book is intended primarily for non-science majors, it is not an "easy" text, because microbiology is not an "easy" topic. As the student will discover, the concise nature of this text has made each sentence significant. Thus, the reader will be intellectually challenged to learn each new concept as it is presented. It is my hope that the students will enjoy their study of microbiology and be motivated to further explore this fascinating field, especially as it relates to their occupations. A student workbook has been prepared for use as a supplementary learning device. It closely follows the sequence of material in the textbook and can be used hand-in-hand while reading the text or as a review for further studying.

I am deeply indebted to those colleagues, friends, family members, and students who served as sources of illustrations, advice, and encouragement, especially Dr. Robert L. Taylor, Dr. Paul Engelkirk, Ursi Chappelle, and my husband and children. I particularly wish to acknowledge Patti Cleary, sponsoring editor, and Eleanor Faven, developmental editor in the health sciences division, J. B. Lippincott Company, for their editorial assistance in the preparation of this manuscript.

Gwendolyn R. W. Burton

Contents

Chapter 1

Introduction to Microbiology

Objectives

After studying this chapter, you should be able to
1. Define microbiology
2. List some important functions of microbes in the environment
3. State the relevance of microbiology to the health professions
4. List some areas of study in microbiology
5. List some contributions of Leeuwenhoek, Pasteur, and Koch to microbiology
6. State the germ theory of fermentation
7. State the germ theory of disease
8. List Koch's postulates and give some circumstances in which they do not apply
9. Describe the difference between light microscopes and electron microscopes and the applications of both
10. List the metric units used in microscopic measurements and indicate their relative sizes

New Words to Pronounce and Understand

Algae (al'-gee). Plants with chlorophyll (capable of producing their own food)

Bacteria (back-tier'-ee-uh). Procaryotic, mostly unicellular organisms; most primitive organisms

Fungi (fun'-ji). Microorganisms that are incapable of producing their own food and that live on decaying organic material

Immunology (im-mew-noll'-oh-gee). The science that deals with immunity from disease and the production of immunity

Microorganism (my'-kro-or'-gan-izm). Microscopic organisms, usually single cells, sometimes called microbes

Opportunist (op-poor-tune'-ist). A microbe that causes disease in susceptible persons with lowered resistance

Pathogen (path'-o-jen). Disease-causing microorganism

Protozoa (pro-toe-zoe'-uh). Single-celled microscopic animals found in water and soil; a few are pathogens

Tyndallization (tin-dull-uh-zay'-shun). A process of boiling and cooling in which spores are allowed to germinate and then are killed by boiling again

Virology (vi-rol'-oh-gee). The study of viruses and the diseases they cause

Virus (vi'-rus). An infective agent smaller than a bacterium

What is microbiology? *Micro-* means very small, anything so small that it must be viewed with a microscope; *-bio* means "living organisms"; and *-ology* means "the study of." Therefore, microbiology is the study of very small living organisms. These microorganisms include the bacteria, algae, protozoa, fungi, and viruses (Fig. 1-1). They are often called *microbes,* single-celled organisms, and germs.

You may never see any microorganisms or understand the effect they have on your daily life. Occasionally, you may realize they are alive and active in and on your body when a cut or a burn becomes infected or when you have a sore throat. Have you ever been very sick after a picnic, and wondered which of the foods you ate contained harmful germs? Most of us are aware of *pathogens,* or disease-causing microorganisms, only when we are affected by them. Actually, only a small percentage of microbes are pathogenic or able to cause disease (Fig. 1-2). The others are beneficial, harmless, or cause disease only if they accidentally get into the "wrong" place at the "right" time, when the person's resistance is low and the growth conditions are right. Normally, these *opportunists* are harmless microorganisms, the so-called normal flora, living on the skin, in the mouth, and in the intestine.

Microorganisms can be found nearly everywhere as normal inhabitants of the earth, and with few exceptions they contribute to the welfare of humans. The normal flora that live on and within our bodies actually inhibit the growth of pathogens in those areas by occupying the space, using the food supply, and secreting materials (waste products, toxins, antibiotics) that may prevent or reduce the growth of pathogens. Many nonpathogens enable us to produce yogurt, cheeses, raised bread, beer, wine, and many other foods and drinks.

Many bacteria and fungi are *saprophytes,* which help to fertilize the soil by returning the inorganic nutrients to the soil; they break down dead organic materials (plants and animals) into nitrates, phosphates, carbon dioxide, water, and other chemicals necessary for plant growth (Fig. 1-3). These saprophytes also destroy paper, feces, and other biodegradable substances, although they cannot recycle most plastics and glass. The nitrogen-fixing bacteria, which live with the plants called legumes (peas, peanuts, alfalfa, clover), are able to return nitrogen from the air to the soil in the form of nitrates for use by other plants. This knowledge is important to the farmer

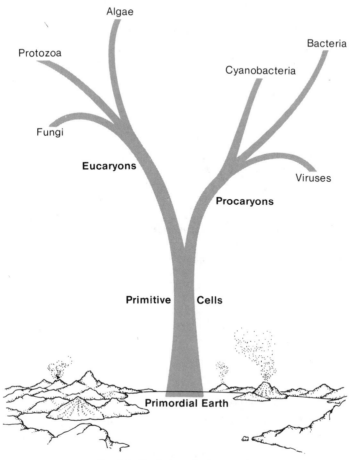

Fig. 1-1. Family tree of microorganisms.

who practices crop rotation to replenish his fields and to the gardener who keeps a compost pit as a source of natural fertilizer.

The purification of waste water is partially accomplished by bacteria in the holding tanks of sewage disposal plants, where feces, garbage, and other organic materials are collected and reduced to harmless waste. Some microorganisms such as the iron- and sulfur-using bacteria even break down metals and minerals. It is not difficult to observe the beneficial activities of the microbes because they are everywhere in our environment, in the land, water, and air.

Those who work in the health professions must be particularly aware of pathogens, their sources, and how they may be transmitted from one person to another. Physicians' assistants, dental assistants, nurses, laboratory technicians, respiratory therapists, orderlies, nurses' aides, and all others associated with patient care must take precautions to prevent the spread of pathogens. Harmful microorganisms may be transferred from health workers to patients; from patient to patient; from contaminated mechanical devices, instruments, and syringes to patients; from contaminated

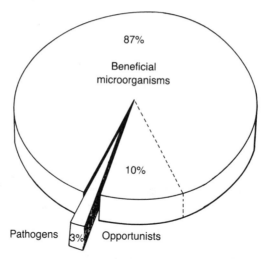

Fig. 1-2. Pathogens comprise about 3% of all the microorganisms. Another 10% are opportunistic microbes that
may cause disease if they land in the appropriate place.

bedding, clothes, dishes, and food to patients; and from patients to health workers
and other susceptible people.

The Scope of Microbiology

There are many fields of study within microbiology. One can specialize in any
of many different types of microorganisms. For example, the bacteriologist concen-
trates on *bacteriology,* the study of structure, functions, and activities of bacteria.
Phycology is the study of the various types of algae by scientists called phycologists.
Those who specialize in the study of fungi, *mycology,* are the mycologists. Proto-
zoologists explore the area of *protozoology,* the study of protozoa and their activities.

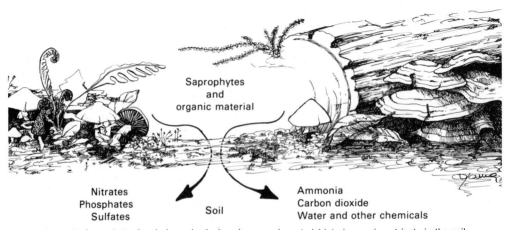

Fig. 1-3. Saprophytes break down dead, decaying organic material into inorganic nutrients in the soil.

Virology encompasses the study of viruses and their effects on living cells of all types. Virologists often become genetic engineers, manipulating the genetic material, DNA, from one cell to another.

Within the general field of microbiology there are many specialized areas in which the knowledge of all types of microorganisms and their applications is important. These areas include medical, veterinary, and agricultural microbiology, as well as applications in sewage disposal, industrial production, space research, and genetic engineering.

General Microbiology The study and classification of microorganisms and how they function is known as general microbiology. It encompasses all areas of microbiology.

Medical Microbiology The field of medical microbiology comprises the study of pathogens, the diseases caused by them, and the body's defenses against disease. It includes epidemiology, transmission of pathogens, prevention measures, aseptic techniques, treatment of infectious diseases, immunology, and the production of vaccines to protect against infectious diseases. The almost complete eradication of smallpox and diphtheria, the safety of modern surgery, and the treatment of AIDS victims are due to the many technological advances in this field.

Veterinary Microbiology The spread and control of diseases among animals is the concern of veterinary microbiologists. The production of food from livestock and other agriculturally important animals, the care of pets, and the transmission of diseases from animals to humans are areas of major importance in this field.

Agricultural Microbiology Included in the field of agricultural microbiology are studies of the beneficial and harmful roles of microbes in soil formation and fertility; in carbon, nitrogen, phosphorus, and sulfur cycles; in diseases of plants; in the digestive processes of cows and other ruminants; and in the production of crops and foods (Fig. 1-4). The *food microbiologist* is concerned with the production, processing, storage, cooking, and serving of food, as well as the prevention of food spoilage, food poisoning, and food toxicity. The *dairy microbiologist* oversees the grading, pasteurization, and processing of milk and cheeses to prevent contamination, spoilage, and transmission of diseases from environmental, animal, and human sources.

Sanitary Microbiology The field of *sanitary microbiology* includes the processing and disposal of garbage and sewage wastes, as well as the purification and processing of water supplies to ensure that no pathogens are carried to the consumer by the water. Sanitary microbiologists also inspect food processing installations and eating establishments to ensure the enforcement of proper food handling procedures.

Industrial Microbiology Many businesses and industries depend on the proper growth and maintenance of certain microbes to produce beer, wine, alcohol, and organic

Nitrogen gas in the air

Legumes

Nitrogen returns to air

Nitrates to replenish
the soil nutrients

Nitrogen-
fixing
bacteria

Fig. 1-4. Nitrogen fixation. The nitrogen-fixing bacteria that live on or near the roots of legumes convert free nitrogen from the air into nitrates to replenish the soil nutrients.

materials such as enzymes, vitamins, and antibiotics. *Industrial microbiologists* monitor and maintain the essential microorganisms for these commercial enterprises. *Applied microbiologists* conduct research aimed at producing new products and more effective antibiotics. The scope of microbiology, indeed, has broad, far-reaching effects on humans, on pathogens, and on their relationship to the environment.

Microbial Genetics   Research in microbial genetics has contributed greatly to a clearer understanding of the science of genetics in general. Genetic manipulation is much easier and faster with viruses and bacteria than with the more complex eucaryotic cells; thus, everyday organisms such as the intestinal *Escherichia coli* are invaluable tools in this study.

Space Microbiology   Sometimes called exobiology, space microbiology is a new area of microbiology begun when the first space vehicles were launched to probe outer space. It is concerned with the prevention of contamination of outer space with earth microbes and *vice versa*, and with the search for extraterrestrial life.

Environmental Microbiology   The field of environmental microbiology has become important because of increased concern about the environment. This field encompasses the areas of soil, air, water, sewage, food, and dairy microbiology, as well as the cycling of the elements (see Fig. 1-4) by microbial, environmental, and geochemical processes.

Some Milestones of Microbiology

Since before the beginning of humanity, parasites have lived on, or in, other living organisms. We know human pathogens were present because damage caused by them has been observed in the bones of mummies and early humans, indicating that diseases, such as osteomyelitis and syphilis, were present.

In ancient Egypt and China, the people kept clean by washing with water in an effort to prevent disease. They also knew that some diseases were easily transmitted from one person to another, and they learned to isolate the sick to prevent the spread of these diseases, which we recognize today as being contagious. The Egyptians were aware of the effectiveness of biological warfare. They often used the blood and bodies of their diseased dead to contaminate the water supplies of their enemies and to spread diseases among them.

The Book of Leviticus in the Bible was probably the first recording of laws concerning public health. The Hebrew people were told to practice personal hygiene by washing and keeping clean. They were also instructed to bury their waste material away from their camp sites, to isolate those who were sick, and to burn soiled dressings. They were prohibited from eating animals that had died of natural causes. The procedure for killing an animal was clearly described, and the edible parts were so designated.

Most of the knowledge about public sanitation and transmission of disease was lost in Europe during the Middle Ages when there was a general stagnation of culture and learning for almost a thousand years. However, during the Renaissance, widespread epidemics of smallpox, syphilis, rabies, and other diseases caused the physicians and alchemists of the day to look for reasons for the contraction and transfer of diseases. Most people believed that diseases were caused by curses of the gods, and as a result, many bizarre treatments (bleeding, drilling holes in the head, attaching leeches) were used to drive the devils or evil spirits away and relieve the symptoms.

An Italian physician, Girolamo Fracastorius, having observed the syphilis epidemic of the 1500s, indicated in 1546 that the agents of communicable diseases were living germs that could be transmitted by direct contact with humans and animals and indirectly by objects. Proof of these vague theories was long delayed because the agents of disease could not be observed and experimental evidence was lacking.

Until the development of magnifying lenses and microscopes that could sufficiently magnify the microorganisms for them to be seen, the discovery of disease-causing agents was impossible. Actually, it is not known who built the first microscope, but compound microscopes, using two lenses to increase the magnification, were developed by Johannes Janssen (1590), Galileo Galilei (1609), and Robert Hooke (1660). When Antony van Leeuwenhoek first described bacteria in 1667, he used a small, simple microscope with one lens the size of a large pinhead and observed the material placed on the point of a pin. Leeuwenhoek is called the "Father of Microbiology" because he described the three shapes of bacteria as well as protozoa, sperm, and blood cells when he observed pepper water, tooth scrapings, gutter water, semen, blood, urine, feces, and other materials. His letters to the Royal Society of London convinced the scientists of the late 17th century of the existence of microorganisms, which Leeuwenhoek called "animalcules." He did not speculate on the origin of these microbes or associate them with the cause of disease. These relationships were not established until the work of Louis Pasteur and Robert Koch in the late 19th century. Leeuwenhoek's fine art of grinding a single lens that would magnify an object to 300 times its size was lost at his death, for he had not taught this skill to anyone.

Detailed descriptions of microorganisms were delayed until the development of better microscopes in the 19th and 20th centuries. A discussion of modern microscopy can be found at the end of this chapter.

Although Leeuwenhoek was not concerned about the origin of microorganisms, many other scientists were searching for an explanation of the spontaneous appearance of living creatures in decaying meat, stagnating ponds, fermenting grain, and infected wounds. On the basis of observation, many of the so-called scientists of that time believed that life could develop spontaneously from decomposing nonliving materials. This is the theory of spontaneous generation or *abiogenesis*. For over two centuries, from 1650 to 1850, this theory was debated and tested. Following the work of many others, Pasteur and John Tyndall finally disproved the theory of spontaneous generation and proved that life must arise from preexisting life; this is called the theory of *biogenesis*.

The experiments devised by Louis Pasteur and other scientists in the mid-1800s resulted in several major advances in the field of microbiology: (1) the concept that life must arise from preexisting life; (2) sterilization and pasteurization techniques; (3) the germ theory of fermentation; (4) the germ theory of disease; and (5) the development of vaccines from killed bacteria for anthrax and from attenuated, or weakened, viruses for rabies.

The sterilization techniques used by Pasteur showed that boiled broth will remain sterile until it is contaminated by particles in the air. While repeating Pasteur's experiment, Tyndall found bacterial fragments, called endospores, that were not destroyed by the first boiling and that germinated into reproducing (vegetative) bacteria. This discovery led to the development of the fractional sterilization process, often called *tyndallization*, in which the endospores of bacteria are destroyed by boiling and cooling three times, allowing the spores to germinate between boilings.

When Pasteur was investigating the reasons for the spoilage of beer and wine, he developed the *germ theory of fermentation*, which states that a specific microbe produces a specific change in the substance on which it grows. Just as yeasts ferment sugar in grape juice to produce ethyl alcohol in wine, some contaminating bacteria, such as *Acetobacter*, may change the alcohol to acetic acid (vinegar), which, of course, ruins the taste of the wine. To eliminate the harmful contaminating bacteria from beer and wines, Pasteur heated them up to 50° to 60°C (122° to 140°F). This process, now called *pasteurization*, has been adapted to destroy the pathogens in milk by heating it to 63°C (145.4°F) for 30 minutes, or to 72°C (161.6°F) for 15 seconds.

By extending the germ theory of fermentation to animals and humans, Pasteur developed the *germ theory of disease*, which states that a specific disease is caused by a specific type of microorganism (Fig. 1-5). After isolating the causative pathogens of chicken cholera, anthrax, and rabies, he prepared vaccines against these diseases. He used the attenuated or weakened pathogen, which was no longer pathogenic but which made the injected animal immune to the disease. For example, Pasteur found the rabies virus in the brain and spinal cord of rabid dogs. He discovered that by transferring the virus from rabbit to rabbit many times, the virus became so weakened it no longer caused rabies in rabbits or dogs. It was this attenuated virus that he used to immunize animals and people against rabies.

For this work, Pasteur is known as the "Father of Immunology." However, the beginnings of immunology appeared in ancient China, where a type of vaccination against smallpox was practiced in which healthy people inhaled a powder made from the scabs of healing pustules of smallpox. Although many Chinese developed the disease as a result of this custom, others became immune. This method is called *variolation*, because the dying smallpox virus was used. In the late 1700s Edward Jenner used the cowpox virus to vaccinate people against smallpox after observing that milkmaids who caught cowpox, a mild disease, from cows were protected against smallpox, a far more serious disease.

Although Pasteur employed the technique of isolating a microorganism and growing it in a pure culture in nutrient media in the laboratory, Robert Koch, a German physician, is usually given credit for most pure-culture research methods in microbiology. He and his assistant, Julius Petri, developed the *petri dish,* which is still in use today, for microbial growth on solid media. Following a suggestion of an associate's wife, Frau Hesse, they used agar to solidify the growth medium so that

Fig. 1-5. *Bacillus anthracis,* from a 48-hr culture, showing endospores. This bacterium causes anthrax and was used by Pasteur and Koch in many experiments on disease causation (original magnification × 1200). (Burrows W: Textbook of Microbiology. Philadelphia, WB Saunders, 1963)

distinct colonies of bacteria could be observed. Agar is an extract from a marine seaweed used at that time to make jelly.

In addition, Robert Koch, in 1876, established an experimental procedure to prove the germ theory of disease; that is, a specific disease is caused by a specific pathogen. This scientific procedure is known as *Koch's postulates* (Fig. 1-6).

Koch's Postulates

1. The causative agent must be present in every case of the disease and must not be present in healthy animals.
2. The pathogen must be isolated from the diseased host animal and grown in pure culture.
3. The same disease must be produced when microbes from the pure culture are inoculated into healthy susceptible animals.

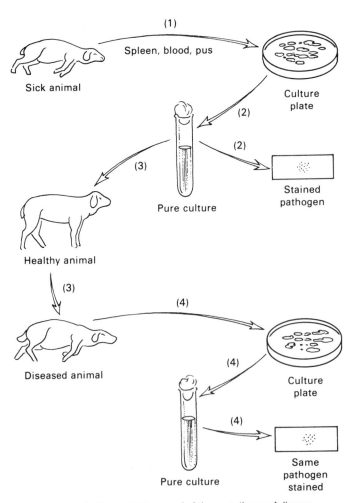

Fig. 1-6. Koch's postulates: proof of the germ theory of disease.

4. The same pathogen must be recoverable once again and grown in pure culture from this artificially infected host animal.

Koch's postulates not only proved the germ theory of disease but also gave a tremendous boost to the development of microbiology by stressing laboratory culture and identification of microorganisms. However, there are some circumstances in which these postulates may not be easy to apply, as outlined below:

Exceptions to Koch's Postulates

1. Many healthy people carry pathogens but do not exhibit symptoms of the disease. These "carriers" may transmit the pathogens to others who then may become diseased. This is usually the circumstance in epidemics of certain hospital (nosocomial) infections, gonorrhea, typhoid fever, diphtheria, pneumonia, and AIDS.

2. Some microbes are very difficult or impossible to grow in the laboratory in artificial media, such as the bacteria that cause leprosy and syphilis, and most viruses. Thus, pure cultures of those pathogens are difficult to obtain. However, many of these fastidious pathogens may now be grown in tissue cultures of living cells of various types, in egg embryos, or in certain animals. The leprosy pathogen thrives in armadillos, the spirochetes of syphilis grow well in the testes of rabbits and chimpanzees, and human immunodeficiency virus (HIV or AIDS virus) will proliferate in human lymphocyte cultures.

3. To induce a disease from a pure culture, the experimental animal must be susceptible to that pathogen. Many animals, such as rats, are very resistant to microbial infections. Many pathogens are species-specific, which means that they will grow in only one species of animal; for example, the pathogen that causes cholera in humans will not cause hog cholera, and *vice versa*. Because human volunteers are difficult to find and ethical reasons limit their use, the researcher may only be able to observe the changes caused by the pathogen in human cells that can be grown in tissue cultures in the laboratory.

4. Certain diseases develop only when an opportunistic pathogen invades a weakened host. These secondary invaders or opportunists cause disease in a weakened person who is ill or is recovering from another disease. Examples are pneumonia and ear infections, which may follow influenza. If researchers were looking for the influenza virus, they might be misled by isolating the bacteria that caused the pneumonia.

It is also important to remember that not all diseases are caused by microorganisms. Many, such as rickets and scurvy, result from diet deficiencies. Some are inherited or are caused by an abnormality in the chromosomes, as in sickle cell anemia. Other diseases, such as diabetes, result from malfunction of a body organ or system, and still others, such as cancer of the lungs and skin, are the result of environmental factors. The infectious diseases are caused by microorganisms.

The period of rapid development of microbiological techniques in the late 1800s is known as the "Golden Age of Microbiology." Efficient surgical techniques based on Pasteur's fermentation theories and sterilization techniques were developed. During this period Ignaz Semmelweis, a physician, showed that puerperal sepsis (infection following childbirth) was caused by infectious agents present in the mother and on the hands of doctors and midwives. He demonstrated that washing and disinfecting the hands greatly reduced the number of infections following childbirth. However, this work was not widely accepted. It was 30 years later that Joseph Lister showed there were few complications from infections following surgery and childbirth if the instruments were boiled and if the hands of the surgeon and the wound were disinfected with carbolic acid (phenol).

This technique of using disinfectants to prevent microorganisms from entering a surgical wound became known as *antiseptic surgery*. The application of antiseptic principles to surgery paved the way for many advances in surgical techniques, including *sterile techniques* and *aseptic techniques* (techniques that exclude pathogens), which now are practiced throughout the modern world in operating theaters and research laboratories.

Modern nursing techniques logically developed after the concepts of disease causation, transmission, and sterilization were explained. Florence Nightingale, an English nurse of the 19th century, developed modern principles of nursing, methods of training nurses, and procedures for organizing hospitals to reduce the spread of disease.

The Tools of Microbiology

Microscopes The cells of microorganisms are so small that they cannot be seen without the aid of powerful magnifying lenses or a microscope. Thus, the expansion of the field of microbiology beyond the 19th century depended upon the development of better microscopes so that the organisms could be properly observed and studied. Although submicroscopic infectious agents were known to exist, for example, the rabies and smallpox viruses, they could not be seen until the electron microscope was developed.

A single magnifying glass usually magnifies an object from about 3 to 20 times its actual size. The *light microscope* used today is a compound microscope with two lenses (Fig. 1-7). The eyepieces contain the ocular lens; the second lens is in the objective, near the object to be viewed.

The two-lens system of the compound microscope can magnify 40 to 1200 times. The magnification is usually indicated by a numeral followed by an $\times$, such as "1200$\times$," in which $\times$ means *times*. The total magnification of a compound microscope is obtained by multiplying the magnifying power of the ocular lens (usually 10$\times$) by the magnifying power of the objective lens (usually 10, 40, or 100$\times$). Thus, with the

Fig. 1-7. A modern light microscope. (Photograph courtesy Carl Zeiss, Inc.)

low-power objective, the total magnification is 10 times 10, or 100×. This objective is usually used to locate the microorganism to be studied. With the high-dry lens, the total magnification is 10 times 40, or 400×, which is used to study algae, protozoa, and other large microorganisms. With the oil-immersion objective (100×), a total magnification of 1000× is obtained, which is most useful for observing many characteristics of bacteria.

The oil-immersion objective must be used only with a drop of immersion oil between the slide and the objective lens; the oil reduces the scattering of light. For clear observation of the specimen, the light must be properly adjusted and focused. The condenser under the stage focuses the light on the specimen, adjusts the amount of light, and shapes the cone of light entering the objective. Generally, the higher the magnification, the more light that is needed.

Other light microscopes are built and adjusted for dark-field techniques, phase-contrast microscopy, and fluorescence. In dark-field microscopy, the light is directed toward the specimen from the side so that the only light to reach the objective is reflected from the bacteria or object to be studied. Thus, the microbe appears as a bright object on a dark background. This technique is frequently used to study very small bacteria like the spirochete *Treponema pallidum*, which causes syphilis. The phase-contrast microscope may be used to observe living microbes without staining because the light refracted by living cells is different from the surrounding medium, and thus they are more easily seen. The microscope used for fluorescence microscopy has an ultraviolet (UV) light source that illuminates the object but does not pass into the objective of the microscope. When UV light strikes certain dyes and pigments (*e.g.*, chlorophyll), they emit green, yellow, or orange light that can be seen in the microscope against a dark background. The UV light microscope is often used in immunology laboratories to show that antibodies stained with a fluorescent dye will combine with the specific antigens on bacteria. The fluorescent antibody technique is frequently used as a diagnostic test in medical bacteriology.

The *electron microscope* uses an electron beam instead of visible light and magnets instead of lenses to focus the beam. The electrons pass through the dry specimen, which is mounted in wax or plastic, and the image is seen on a fluorescent screen. The picture may then be photographed and enlarged to magnify the object several hundred thousand times, much more than with light microscopes. Thus, very tiny microbes and viruses may be observed. Also, by using thin sections of cells mounted in plastic, in the transmission microscope the internal structure of the cells can be studied. A recent modification of this scope is the scanning electron microscope, which is very useful for observing the surfaces and the three-dimensional image of an object. Figures 1-8, 1-9, and 1-10 show the difference in magnification and detail between electron and light photomicrographs.

Fig. 1-8. *Staphylococcus aureus*, as seen by light microscopy magnified 1000 times. (Photograph courtesy W. L. Wong)

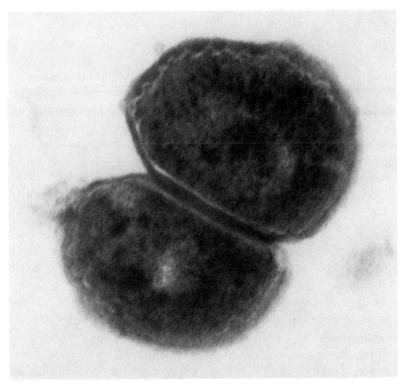

Fig. 1-9. *Staphylococcus aureus,* as seen by transmission electron microscopy magnified 40,000 times. (Photograph courtesy Ray Rupel)

Fig. 1-10. The three-dimensional qualities of scanning electron microscopy clearly reveal the corkscrew shape of cells of the syphilis-causing spirochete *Treponema pallidum,* attached here to rabbit testicular cells grown in culture (original magnification × 8000). (Volk WA, et al.: Essentials of Medical Microbiology, 3rd ed. Philadelphia, JB Lippincott, 1986)

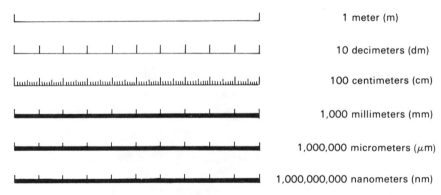

Fig. 1-11. Representation of some metric units.

Units of Measurement   In microbiology, several common metric units are used to describe the size of the microorganisms. The meter, the basic unit of the system, is equivalent to approximately 39 inches. It is divided into 10 decimeters, or 100 centimeters, or 1000 millimeters, or a million micrometers, or a billion nanometers, and so forth. The relationship among these units may be observed in Figure 1-11.

It should be noted that the old term *micron* (μ) has been replaced by the term *micrometer* (μm); the *millimicron* (mμ) is equivalent to the *nanometer* (nm); and the *Ångstrom* (Å) is 0.1 nanometer (0.1 nm), according to the International System adopted by scientists worldwide. On this scale, red blood cells are about 10 μm in diameter. Bacteria vary in width and length from about 0.2 μm to 5 μm, and viruses from about 0.05 μm to 0.15 μm. Some very large protozoa reach the length of 2000 μm, or 2 mm.

The sizes of microorganisms are calculated by using a microscope stage measuring device, called a micrometer, to determine the distance between the marks on the ocular micrometer (a small ruler on a glass disk), which is placed in the eyepiece of the microscope. This procedure is known as calibration. The ocular micrometer is then used to measure the length and width of the microbe on the specimen slide, using the same objective as was used during the calibration process.

Each type of microscope has its limits of visibility. The light microscope can be used for observation of cells larger than 0.2 μm, whereas the electron microscope can discern objects as small as 2 nm (0.002 μm) in diameter.

Problems and Questions

1. What does the study of microbiology include? What types of organisms?
2. Why is the study of microbiology important to people working in health occupations?
3. Why is Leeuwenhoek called the "Father of Microbiology"?
4. Why was there a controversy about spontaneous generation?
5. What contributions did Pasteur make to microbiology?

6. What did Pasteur do to save the wine industry in France?
7. What contributions to microbiology were made by Semmel-weis, Lister, Jenner, and Nightingale?
8. What did Koch's postulates prove?
9. List Koch's postulates and the circumstances under which they might not be applicable.
10. What types of microscopes are used to observe bacteria and viruses?
11. What units of measurement are used to describe the size of bacteria?

Chapter 2

Types of Microorganisms

New Words to Pronounce and Understand

Amphitrichous (am-fit'-ri-kus). Bacteria with flagella on both ends

Bacillus (bah-sill'-us), pl. *bacilli*. A rod-shaped bacterium; the genus *Bacillus* is made up of aerobic spore-forming rods

Centrosome (sen'-trow-soam). A eucaryotic cytoplasmic organelle containing two centrioles

Chromosomes (crow'-mow-soams). The genetic material carrying the genes of heredity, containing DNA

Clostridium (kloss-trid'-ee-um). A genus of anaerobic spore-forming rods

Coccus (cock'-us), pl. *cocci.* A spherical or ball-shaped bacterium

Cytology (sigh-tol'-oh-gee). The study of cells

Cytoplasm (sigh'-tow-plaz-um). The protoplasm outside the nucleus of the cell

DNA, deoxyribonucleic acid (dee-ox'-ee-rye'-bow-nu-clay'-ick). The genetic material in the chromosomes

Eucaryon (you-care'-ree-on). A cell with a true nucleus

Endoplasmic reticulum (end-oh-plaz'-mick re-tick'-you-lum). A eucaryotic cell organelle for transport and support

Flagella (fluh-gel'-uh). Protein strands used for movement

Golgi (goal'-gee). A eucaryotic cell organelle involved in secretion

Lipopolysaccharide (lip'-o-pol-ee-sack'-car-ride). A macromolecule of combined lipid and polysaccharide, often found in gram-negative bacterial cell walls

Lophotrichous (low-fot'-ri-kus). Bacteria with a tuft of flagella

Lysozyme (lie'-so-zime). The cellular digestive enzyme in lysosomes

Mesosome (me'so-soam). A procaryotic cell organelle involved in cellular respiration

Microtubules (my-crow-tube'-yules). Eucaryotic cell organelle involved in support and secretion

Mitochondria (my-tow-con'-dree-uh). Eucaryotic organelles involved in cellular respiration for the production of energy

Monotrichous (mon-ot'-ri-kus). Bacteria with one flagellum

Motile (mow'-till). The ability to move

Nucleoid (new'-klee-oid). The nuclear area of procaryotic cells

Nucleolus (new-klee'-oh-lus). The dense portion of the nucleus, containing RNA.

Nucleoplasm (new'-klee-oh-plaz'-um). The protoplasm inside the nucleus

Organelles (or-gan-ells'). Discrete structures inside the cell

Peptidoglycan (pep-tid'-o-gly'-can). The rigid component of bacterial cell walls, consisting of polysaccharide chains linked together by peptide chains

Peritrichous (pear-rit'-trick-us). Bacteria covered by flagella

Primordial (pry-more'-dee-al). Early or first in time

Procaryon (pro-kar'-ee-on). Primitive cells without a true nucleus

Protoplasm (pro'tow-plaz-um). The semifluid material inside cells

Ribosomes (rye'-bow-soams). Organelles necessary for protein
synthesis

RNA, ribonucleic acid (rye'-bow-new-clay'-ick). Nucleic acids
necessary for protein synthesis

Spirochetes (spy'-row-keets). Spiral-shaped bacteria

Taxonomy (tax-on'-oh-me). A systematic classification of
organisms

Teichoic acid (tie-ko'-ick). A chemical in the cell wall of
gram-positive bacteria

Vacuoles (vack'-you-oles). Membrane-bound storage spaces in
the cell

Cells: Eucaryons and Procaryons

In 1665, Robert Hooke, while peering through his crude microscope, observed
the small empty chambers in the structure of cork. He named them *cells* because they
reminded him of the bare rooms in a monastery. More than a century later, when
biologists had access to more advanced microscopes, they found that cells are not
empty, but rather contain a sticky (viscous) fluid. They learned that the chemical
material in the cell enables it to live and reproduce. They called this material *protoplasm,* meaning "the substance of life." Now we know the cell is composed of many
different substances and contains tiny particles called *organelles* that have important
functions. The living material of the cell is still occasionally called protoplasm. It
consists of two parts, the cytoplasm outside the nucleus and the nucleoplasm inside
the nucleus.

Two German biologists, Matthias Schleiden and Theodore Schwann, proposed
the cell theory in 1838. Their theory stated that all living things are composed of cells.
Rudolf Virchow completed this theory with the idea that cells must arise from preexisting cells. In other words, life must arise from life as it exists on the earth.

In biology, the cell is defined as the fundamental living unit of any organism
because, like the organism, the cell exhibits the basic characteristics of life. It obtains
food from the environment to produce energy and nutrients for metabolism (Fig. 2-1).
Metabolism is an inclusive term to describe all the chemical reactions by which food
is transformed for use by the cells. (See Chap. 4 for a detailed discussion of metabolism.) Through its metabolism, the cell can grow and reproduce. It can respond to
changes in its environment such as light, heat, cold, and the presence of chemicals.
It can mutate (change) as a result of accidental changes in its genetic material, the DNA
(deoxyribonucleic acid), which makes up the genes of the chromosomes, and thus
become better or less suited to its environment. As a result of these genetic changes,
the mutant organism may be better adapted for survival and development into a new
species of organism.

There is much evidence to indicate that almost 4 billion years ago the first bit
of life to appear on earth was a very primitive cell similar to the simple bacteria of
today. Bacterial cells exhibit all the characteristics of life, even though they do not have

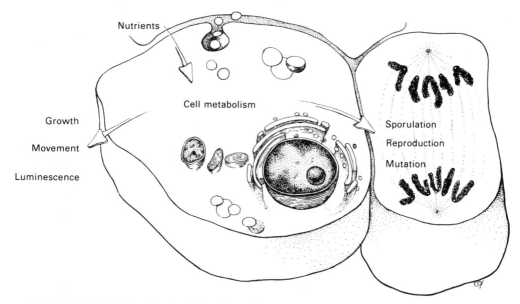

Nutrients

Cell metabolism

Growth

Movement

Luminescence

Sporulation

Reproduction

Mutation

Fig. 2-1. Cell metabolism. The metabolic cycles within the cell enable it to use nutrients for growth, movement, luminescence, sporulation, reproduction, and mutation.

the complex system of membranes and organelles found in the more advanced single-celled organisms. These less complex cells, which include bacteria and cyanobacteria (blue-green algae), are called *procaryons* or procaryotic cells (Fig. 2-2). The more complex cells, with a nucleus and many organelles, are called *eucaryons* or eucaryotic cells; these include such organisms as protozoa; fungi; green, brown, and red algae; and all plant and animal cells including those that make up the human body.

Viruses appear to be the result of regressive, or of what might be termed reverse, evolution, because they are composed of only a few genes protected by a protein coat, a few enzymes, and little other material. For viruses to live and reproduce, they must depend upon the energy and metabolic machinery of the host cell.

Cells

Procaryons
Bacteria
Cyanobacteria

Eucaryons
Plant
Animal
Protozoa
Fungi
Algae (green, brown, red)

Viruses

Fig. 2-2. Typical cells: procaryons, the less complex cells, and eucaryons, the more complex cells. Viruses are not true cells.

Therefore, because they are not truly viable cells, they are usually placed in a completely separate category and are not classified with the simple procaryotic cells.

It is important for the health professions student of microbiology to understand the structure of different types of cells, not only for purposes of classifying the microorganisms but also to understand the differences in their structure and metabolism. These factors must be known before we can determine or explain how the chemicals of modern chemotherapy destroy the pathogens and not the normal human cells.

The study of the structural makeup of cells, which is called cytology, has developed during the last 25 years with the aid of the electron microscope and sophisticated biochemical research. Because complete books have been written about the details of these tiny functional factories, only a brief discussion of their structure and activities is presented here.

Eucaryotic Cell Structure

Eucaryons (*eu* = true; *-karyo* = nut or nucleus) are so named because they have a true nucleus enclosed by a nuclear membrane. Figure 2-3 illustrates a typical eucaryotic animal cell. This illustration is a composite of most of the structures that might

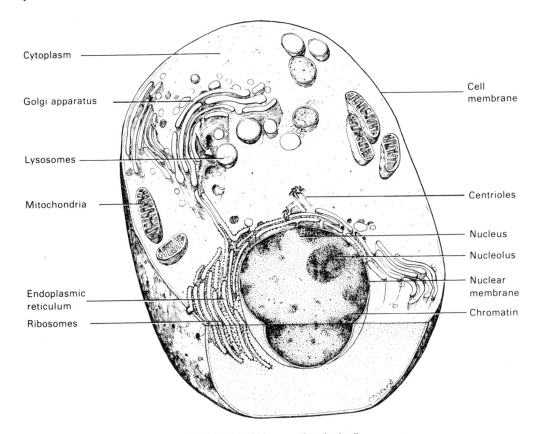

Fig. 2-3. A typical eucaryotic animal cell.

Fig. 2-4. Cross section through a yeast cell showing the nucleus (*N*) with pores (*P*), mitochondrion (*M*), and vacuole (*V*). The cell is surrounded by the cell membrane. The thick, outer portion is the cell wall. (Lechavalier HA, Pramer D: The Microbes. Philadelphia, JB Lippincott, 1970)

be found in the various types of human body cells. The electron photomicrograph in Figure 2-4 is of an actual yeast cell. A discussion of the functional parts of eucaryotic cells can be better understood by keeping the illustrated structures in mind.

Cell Membrane   The cell is enclosed and held intact by the outside cell membrane, also often called the plasma membrane or the cellular membrane. Structurally, it is a mosaic composed of the large molecules of proteins and phospholipids. These large molecules regulate the passage of nutrients, waste products, and secretions across the cellular membrane. Because only certain substances may enter and leave the cell, the plasma membrane has the property of *selective permeability*. This membrane is similar in structure and function to all the other membranes that are a part of the organelles of eucaryotic cells.

Nucleus   The organelle within the cell that unifies, controls, and integrates the functions of the entire cell is the nucleus, enclosed in the *nuclear membrane*. In this region the genetic control system lies within the *chromosomes*. The number of chromosomes and the number of genes on each chromosome are characteristic of the organism's species. Each different species will have a different number and size of chromosomes. Human cells have 46 chromosomes, each consisting of thousands of *genes*. The gene is the unit that codes for, or determines, the traits of an individual organism. When genes are broken apart chemically, they are found to be coiled strands of *deoxyribonucleic acid* (DNA) and proteins. It is the DNA that contains the genetic information for the production of essential proteins that will enable the cell to function properly. To understand more about how the base coding of the DNA can chemically control the entire organism, refer to Chapter 3 or to any general biology textbook.

Close observation of the nucleus of nondividing cells reveals the loosely wound strands of chromosomes, called the *chromatin material*, suspended in the nucleoplasm, which is the nutrient gelatinous matrix or base material. These chromatin strands will condense into tightly coiled chromosomes just before the cell divides. The very dense dark area of the nucleus is the *nucleolus*, where ribosomes are manufactured before they move to the cytoplasmic portion of the cell.

Cytoplasm   The part of the cell that does most of the normal work is the cytoplasm; it is controlled by information carried in the DNA of the nucleus. The cytoplasm is the cellular material outside the nucleus but enclosed by the cell membrane; it is composed of a semifluid gelatinous nutrient matrix and the cytoplasmic organelles, including the endoplasmic reticulum, ribosomes, Golgi apparatus, mitochondria, centrioles, microtubules, lysosomes, and other vacuoles. Each of these organelles has a highly specific function, and all of the functions are interrelated to maintain the cell and allow it to properly perform its activities.

The *endoplasmic reticulum* (ER) is a system of membranes that are interconnected and arranged to form a network of tubules connecting the outside of the cell to the nucleus. The ER transports nutrients to the nucleus and also provides some structural support for the cell. Much of the ER has a rough appearance and is designated as *rough endoplasmic reticulum* (RER). This rough appearance is due to the many *ribosomes* attached to the outer surface of the membranes. The ribosomes consist mainly of ribosomal RNA (*ribonucleic acid*) and play an important part in the synthesis (manufacture) of essential proteins for use by the cell and elsewhere in the organism.

The *Golgi apparatus*, or body, usually connects or communicates with the endoplasmic reticulum. This group of membranes completes the synthesis of secretory products and packages them into small sacs called vesicles for storage or export outside the cell.

The *lysosomes* are small sacs that originate from the Golgi apparatus. They contain *lysozyme* and other digestive enzymes to break down foreign material taken into the cell by *phagocytosis* (the engulfing of large particles by phagocytes). They also aid in breaking down worn out parts of the cell. These enzymes may destroy the entire cell by a process called *autolysis* if the cell is damaged or deteriorating.

The energy necessary for cellular function is provided by the formation of high-energy phosphate molecules such as adenosine triphosphate (ATP). The *mito-*

chondria are the "power plants" of the cell where most of the ATP molecules are formed by cellular respiration. In this process energy is released from glucose and other food nutrients so that the cell can function. The number of mitochondria in the cell varies greatly depending upon the activities required of that cell.

Two cylindrical organelles called the *centrioles* lie perpendicular to each other near the nucleus. The centrioles are involved in the formation of spindle fibers for eucaryotic cell division. This process, which results in two daughter cells with the same number of chromosomes as the parent cell, is called *mitosis*, "the dance of the chromosomes." Eucaryotic cilia and flagella also appear to arise from centriole material because their internal protein fibril configuration is very similar, even though it is quite complex.

Other structures that may be present in the cell include microfilaments, microtubules, granules, and vacuoles containing food, secretory products, and pigments. Always present in plant cells are the *chloroplasts* containing the chlorophyll required for photosynthesis. Photosynthesis is the process in which light energy is used to change carbon dioxide and water into carbohydrates and oxygen.

Cell Wall   A structure found on plant cells, algae, and fungi is the eucaryotic cell wall. It consists mainly of cellulose but may also contain pectin, lignin, chitin, and some mineral salts (usually found in algae). This eucaryotic cell wall is much simpler and different from the procaryotic bacterial cell wall. The cell wall provides rigidity and protection for these cells.

Procaryotic Cell Structure

The procaryons are structurally very simple cells when compared with the eucaryotic system of membranes, yet they are able to carry on the normal processes of life. In these cells, division is by binary fission—the simple division of the cell parts with formation of a separating membrane and a cell wall. A bacterium can be considered a "typical procaryotic cell"; this makes it easy to describe its parts.

Refer to the composite drawing (Fig. 2-5) of a "typical" gram-positive or gram-negative bacterial cell and to the electron micrograph in Figure 2-6, as we discuss this cell from internal to external structures. Within the cytoplasm, the nuclear material (nucleoid), mesosomes, polyribosomes, and other cytoplasmic particles can be seen. Note that these cells are not filled with internal membranes as are eucaryotic cells. The cytoplasm is surrounded by cell (plasma or cytoplasmic) membrane, cell wall, and sometimes a capsule or slime layer. These latter three structures make up the bacterial cell envelope. On some of these procaryons, flagella or pili, or both, may be observed outside the envelope, and spores may be seen inside, depending on the particular genus and species of the bacteria.

Nucleoid   The procaryotic nucleoid may be considered a primitive nucleus; it is not surrounded by a nuclear membrane, does not have a definite shape, and has little or no protein material. It usually consists of a single circular chromosome. The chromo-

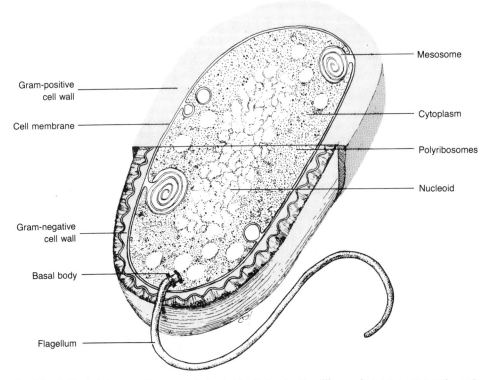

Fig. 2-5. An illustrated composite procaryotic bacterial cell showing the difference between gram-negative and gram-positive cell walls.

some is DNA, which serves as the control center of the bacterial cell, carrying the genetic information needed for producing several thousand enzymes and other proteins. It is capable of duplicating itself, of guiding cell division, and of directing cellular activities.

Cytoplasm Surrounding the nucleoid, and contained within the plasma membrane, is the semiliquid cytoplasm. The cytoplasm consists of water, enzymes, oxygen, waste products, essential nutrients, proteins, carbohydrates, and lipids—a complex mixture of all the materials required by the cell for its metabolic functions.

Cytoplasmic Particles Within the bacterial cytoplasm, many submicroscopic particles have been observed. Most of these particles are ribosomes, usually occurring in clusters called polyribosomes (*poly* = many). These ribosomes are smaller than eucaryotic ribosomes, but their function is the same: the synthesis of proteins.

Cytoplasmic granules occur in certain species of bacteria. These may be stained, by use of a suitable stain, and then identified microscopically. They may consist of starch, lipids, sulfur, iron, or other stored substances.

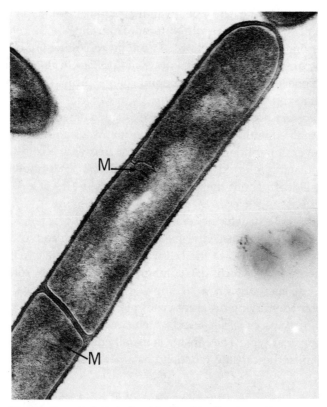

Fig. 2-6. Recently divided cells of *Bacillus licheniformis*, showing the light nuclear material and mesosomes *(M)*. (Lechavalier HA, Pramer D: The Microbes. Philadelphia, JB Lippincott, 1970)

Cell Membrane   Enclosing the cytoplasm is the plasma or cell membrane. This membrane is similar to the eucaryotic cell membrane. Chemically, the plasma membrane consists of proteins and phospholipids, which you will learn more about in Chapter 3. It is selectively permeable and controls which substances may enter and leave the cell. It is flexible and so thin it cannot be seen with a light microscope. However, it is frequently observed in electron micrographs of bacteria.

Many metabolic reactions take place on the cell membrane. The *mesosomes* are an inward folding of these membranes, and this is the area in bacteria where cellular respiration takes place. This process is similar to that occurring in the mitochondria of animal cells, in which the food nutrients are broken down to produce energy in the form of ATP molecules to be used in the cell's metabolic activities.

In photosynthetic bacteria and cyanobacteria, some internal membranes, which are derived from the cell membrane, contain chlorophyll and other pigments that serve to trap light energy for photosynthesis. However, bacteria do not have internal membrane systems similar to the endoplasmic reticulum and Golgi bodies of eucaryotic cells.

Bacterial Cell Wall The rigid exterior cell wall that defines the shape of bacterial cells is chemically complex. Thus, it is quite different from the simple cellulose plant cell wall, although serving the same functions. The main constituent of bacterial cell walls is a complex macromolecular polymer known as *peptidoglycan*, consisting of many polysaccharide chains linked together by peptide (small protein) chains. The thickness of this wall and its exact composition vary with the species of bacteria. Certain bacteria, grouped as gram-positive cells (to be explained later), have many layers of peptidoglycan combined with teichoic acid components. Gram-negative bacteria have a much thinner layer of peptidoglycan, but it is covered with a complex layer of lipid macromolecules, usually referred to as the *outer membrane,* as shown in Figure 2-7. Remember you will learn about these macromolecules in Chapter 3.

Capsules The outermost structure of some bacteria is the capsule, sometimes called the slime layer, a thick layer of slimy, gelatinous material produced by the plasma membrane and secreted outside of the cell wall. Capsules usually consist of complex sugars, or polysaccharides, which may combine with lipids and proteins, depending upon the species of microorganism. A knowledge of the chemical composition of capsules is useful in identifying different types of bacteria within a species; for example, the type A *Streptococcus pneumoniae,* which can cause pneumonia, is frequently identified by its capsular type. The capsule is usually detected by staining the cell and the surrounding area; the capsule remains unstained.

A   **B**

Fig. 2-7. (*A*) A portion of the gram-positive bacterium *Bacillus fastidiosus;* note the cell wall's thick peptidoglycan layer underlaid by the cytoplasmic membrane. (*B*) The gram-negative bacterium *Enterobacter aerogenes;* both the cytoplasmic membrane and the outer membrane are visible along some sections of the cell wall. (Volk WA, et al: Essentials of Medical Microbiology, 3rd ed. Philadelphia, JB Lippincott, 1986)

Encapsulated bacteria will usually produce colonies on nutrient agar that are smooth (S), mucoid, and glistening. Nonencapsulated bacteria tend to grow as dry, rough (R) colonies on nutrient agar growth medium. Capsules on bacteria may serve any of several functions. If it is a thin slime, the cells may be able to glide, slide, or move on the surface of solid material. Some capsules enable the bacterial species to attach to the mucous membranes and tooth surfaces so that they are not flushed away by body secretions. Frequently encapsulated bacteria are not easily digested by phagocytes (white blood cells).

Flagella   Many bacteria have flagella (singular: flagellum), which are threadlike protein appendages whose whiplike motion enables the bacteria to move or to be motile. Not all bacteria have flagella; however, for those that do, the number and arrangement of flagella is a characteristic of the species. Thus, the presence of flagella is used for classification purposes.

Those bacteria that have flagella over all of their surface (perimeter) are described as *peritrichous bacteria.* Those with a tuft of flagella in a single location are *lophotrichous,* those having flagella at both ends are *amphitrichous,* and those with a single polar flagellum are *monotrichous* bacteria (Fig. 2-8).

Some spirochetes have two flagellalike fibrils called *axial filaments,* one attached to each end of the bacterium. These axial filaments extend toward the other end of the bacterium, wrap around the organism between the layers of the cell wall, and overlap each other in the midsection. As a result, the spirochetes can move in a spiral, helical, or an inch-worm manner.

Bacterial flagella consist of three, four, or more threads of protein twisted like a rope, unlike the eucaryotic flagella and cilia, which have a complex arrangement of protein fibrils enclosed in a membrane. The flagella of bacteria arise from a basal body

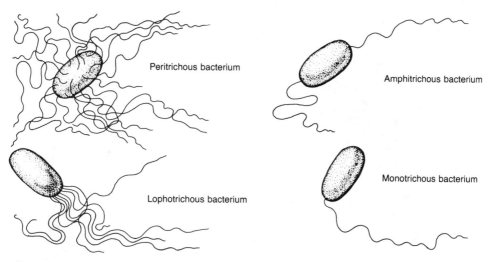

Fig. 2-8. The four basic types of flagellation on bacteria: peritrichous, flagella all over surface; lophotrichous, a tuft of flagella; amphitrichous, flagella at each end; and monotrichous, one flagellum.

in the cytoplasm and project outwardly through the plasma membrane, the cell wall, and the capsule, as shown in Figure 2-5.

Pili or Fimbriae   The fimbriae or pili (singular: pilus) are hairlike tubes frequently observed on enteric (intestinal) bacteria. They are much smaller than flagella, have a rigid structure, and are not associated with motility. These tiny appendages arise from the cytoplasm and extend through the plasma membrane, cell wall, and capsules. Their functions are many and varied, depending upon the bacterial species. They are believed to (1) enable the bacteria to attach to other bacteria or to other membrane surfaces such as the intestinal lining and red blood cells, (2) absorb additional oxygen and nutrients when the supply is low, (3) provide a site for the attachment of bacterial viruses, and (4) enable bacteria to transfer genetic material across a pilus bridge from one to another by a process known as conjugation, which is described in Chapter 4. The pili of *Escherichia coli* can be observed in Figure 2-9.

Spores or Endospores   A few genera of bacteria (*e.g.*, *Bacillus* and *Clostridium*) form endospores as a means of survival when their nutrient supply is low, a process called *sporulation*. During sporulation, the genetic material is enclosed in several protein coats that are resistant to heat, drying, and most chemicals. Spores have been shown to survive for many years on dust particles. When the dried spore lands on a moist, nutrient surface, it develops into a new vegetative bacterial cell. This germination of the spore may be compared with germination of a seed. However, spore formation is

Fig. 2-9. Piliated strain of *Escherichia coli*. Each cell possesses hundreds of pili. Some isolated, broken pili are also seen. A few flagella extend from the cells to the edge of the photograph. (Davis BD, et al.: Microbiology, 3rd ed. Philadelphia, Harper & Row, 1980)

Fig. 2-10. A bacillus with a well-defined endospore. (Lechavalier HA, Pramer D: The Microbes. Philadelphia, JB Lippincott, 1970)

related to the survival of the bacterial cell, not to reproduction because usually, only one spore is produced in a bacterial cell, and it germinates into only one bacterium. (Fig. 2-10).

Differences Between Procaryotic and Eucaryotic Cells

Eucaryotic cells are divided into plant and animal types because animal cells do not have a cell wall, whereas plant cells have a simple cell wall, usually consisting of cellulose. Procaryotic cells have a complex cell wall consisting of proteins, lipids, and polysaccharides. Note the other differences listed in Table 2-1.

Microbial Classification

Since Aristotle's time, naturalists have attempted to classify and name plants, animals, and microorganisms in a meaningful way, based on their appearance and behavior. Thus, the science of taxonomy (biological classification) was devised, based on the binomial system developed in the 18th century by the Swedish scientist Carolus Linnaeus. In the binomial system each organism is given two names (*e.g., Homo sapiens* for humans), the first of which is the genus and the second is the species.

Each organism is catagorized into larger groups based on their similarities and differences. According to the presently popular Whittaker classification scheme, all the living (and extinct) organisms can be placed in five kingdoms: **Plantae** for plants, **Animalia** for animals, **Fungi** for fungi, **Protista** for algae and protozoa, and **Monera** for cyanobacteria and bacteria. (However, microbiologists prefer Kingdom **Procaryotae** to **Monera,** thus, **Procaryotae** will be used in this book to include bacteria and cyanobacteria.) Viruses are usually not included because they are not truly living cells. Note that four of the kingdoms consist of eucaryotic organisms. Each kingdom consists of divisions or phyla divided into classes, orders, families, genera, and species. Additional subgroups are also frequently used. For an example, see Table 2-2.

Because written reference is often made to genera and species, biologists throughout the world have adopted a standard method of expressing these names that identify a specific organism. To express genus: capitalize the first letter of word, which is the genus name, and italicize the word—example: *Escherichia.* To express genus and species: capitalize the first letter of the genus name (the second word is the species name, which is not capitalized); then underline or italicize the entire name—example:

Table 2-1. Comparison between Eucaryotic and Procaryotic Cells

	Eucaryotic Cells		Procaryotic Cells
	Plant	*Animal*	
Biological distribution	All plants, fungi, and algae	All animals and protozoa	All bacteria and cyanobacteria
Nuclear membrane	Present	Present	Absent
Membranous structures other than cell membranes	Generally present	Generally present	Generally absent except mesosomes and photosynthetic membranes
Microtubules and centrioles	Present	Present	Absent
Ribosomes (weight)	80S	80S	70S
Chromosomes	Composed of DNA and proteins	Composed of DNA and proteins	Composed of DNA alone
Flagella or cilia	When present, have a complex structure similar to centrioles	When present, have a complex structure similar to centrioles	Flagella, when present, have simple protein structure; no cilia
Cell wall	When present, of simple chemical constitution, usually cellulose	Absent	In bacteria of complex chemical constitution containing peptidoglycan
Active cytoplasmic movements	Present	Present	Absent (not observed)
Photosynthesis (chlorophyll)	Present	Absent	Present in cyanobacteria and some bacteria

"The following section is devoted to *Escherichia coli.*" Frequently the genus is designated by an accepted abbreviation; in the example given, it would read *E. coli,* indicating the genus and species.

Table 2-2. Comparison of Human and Bacterial Classification

	Human	Syphilis Pathogen
Kingdom	Animalia	*Procaryotae*
Phylum/Division	Chordata	*Gracilicutes*
Class	Mammalia	*Scotobacteria*
Order	Primate	*Spirochaetales*
Family	Hominidae	*Spirochaetaceae*
Genus	*Homo sapiens*	*Treponema pallidum*
Species		

Bacteria

Characteristics

Bacteria were classified into 19 different categories in *Bergey's Manual of Determinative Bacteriology*, 8th ed. (1974), which was the standard reference of bacterial classification. In 1984 bacterial classification was redesigned because organism identification procedures have become more exact. The new comprehensive *Bergey's Manual of Systemic Bacteriology* is published in four volumes, indicating how the taxonomy of bacteria has expanded. An outline of these volumes can be found in Appendix A, and compared with the 8th edition of Bergey's Manual. Also, by using the computer, microbiologists have established numerical taxonomy systems that not only help to identify bacteria by their characteristics but also can help establish how closely related these organisms are by comparing the composition of the genetic material and other cell substances.

Many characteristics of bacteria are examined to provide data for identification and classification: (1) morphology, (2) staining, (3) motility, (4) growth, (5) nutritional requirements, (6) biochemical and metabolic activities, (7) pathogenicity, (8) amino acid sequencing of proteins, (9) genetic composition.

Morphology With the light microscope, the size, shape, and cell arrangement of the various bacteria are easily described. Bacteria vary widely in size, ranging from spheres that measure 0.5 μm in diameter to spirals 6 μm long. There are three basic shapes: spherical or coccoid—the cocci (singular: coccus); rods or bacilli (singular: bacillus); and spirals or spirilla (singular: spirillum), as shown in Figure 2-11. The cells of cocci are observed in many and various arrangements depending upon the species and how they divide (Table 2-3).

Bacilli (rods) may be short or long, thick or thin, pointed or with blunt ends; they may occur singly, in pairs (diplobacilli), or in chains (streptobacilli). Some rods resemble cocci, and are often called coccobacilli because they are very short, small bacilli, such as *E. coli*, a normal inhabitant of the intestine. Some bacilli stack up next to each other, side by side in a palisade arrangement, which is characteristic of diphtheroids and diphtheria organisms.

Spirilla usually occur singly, but some species may form chains. The different species of spirilla vary in size, length, rigidity, number, and amplitude of their coils. True spirilla have rigid cell walls that maintain the shape of a helix or coil. The spirochetes, *e.g.*, *Treponema pallidum*, the causative agent of syphilis, have a flexible cell wall enabling this coiled bacterium to move readily through tissues (refer back to Fig. 2-8). The vibros, such as *Vibrio cholerae*, which causes cholera, are rods with a small curve, like a comma.

Some bacteria may lose their characteristic shape because adverse growth conditions prevent the production of normal cell walls. These wall-deficient bacteria are called L-forms. Some will revert to their original shape when placed in favorable growth conditions, whereas others will not. Another group of very small bacteria, the

Fig. 2-11. Forms of bacteria. (*A*) Cocci. *Top: Streptococcus mutans*, demonstrating pairs and short chains (original magnification × 9400). *Bottom left:* Single cells and small clusters of *Staphylococcus epidermidis* (original magnification × 3000). *Bottom right:* Pairs, tetrads, and regular clusters of *Micrococcus luteus* (original magnification × 3000). (*B*) Bacilli. *Top:* Single cells and short chains of *Bacillus cereus* (original magnification × 1700). *Bottom:* Flagellated bacilli (unnamed) associated with periodontitis (original magnification × 3700). (*C*) *Top:* A cell of *Vibrio cholerae;* note curved cell and single flagellum (original magnification × 8470). *Bottom:* The spirillum *Aquaspirillum bengal;* note polar tufts of flagella (original magnification × 2870). (*D*) Variety of organisms in dental plaque after 3 days without brushing (original magnification × 1360). (Volk WA, et al: Essentials of Medical Microbiology, 3rd ed. Philadelphia, JB Lippincott, 1986)

genus *Mycoplasma*, characteristically produces little or no cell wall; thus, microscopically they appear in various pleomorphic shapes. These bacteria are not genetically related, but they have several properties in common: they have no rigid cell shape, they reproduce slowly, and they are relatively fragile, very susceptible to changes in osmotic pressure, and resistant to antibiotics that deter cell wall synthesis.

Table 2-3. Arrangement of Cocci

Arrangement	Description	Pathogenic Example	Disease
Diplococci	Pairs of cells	*Neisseria gonorrhoeae*	Gonorrhea
Streptococci	Cocci in chains	*Streptococcus pyogenes*	"Strep" sore throat
Staphylococci	Cocci in clusters	*Staphylococcus aureus*	Boils
Tetrads	Four cocci as in a box	*Micrococcus luteus*	Nonpathogenic
Octads	Eight cocci as in a box	*Sarcina ventriculi*	Nonpathogenic

Staining Various staining methods have been devised to examine bacteria that have been smeared and dried on a slide. Specific stains and techniques are used to observe bacterial morphology (shape, grouping, type of cell wall, nuclear material, capsules, flagella, spores, fat globules, and various types of granules).

The simple stain is sufficient to determine bacterial shape and grouping characteristics. For this method, as shown in Figure 2-12, crystal violet, safranin, carbol fuchsin, or methylene blue is applied to the dried smear on the slide, rinsed, dried, and examined with the oil immersion lens of the microscope. Dr. Hans Gram, in 1884, developed the Gram-staining technique, which bears his name, to differentiate between the gram-positive and gram-negative types of bacterial cell walls. The color retained by the bacteria after the staining process is dependent on the thickness and chemical composition of the cell wall. This staining process has four steps: (1) flood the smear with crystal violet for 1 minute; (2) rinse with water and cover the slide with Gram's iodine solution; (3) after 1 minute, wash off the iodine with water and decolorize with alcohol or acetone for 20 seconds; then (4) counterstain with safranin for 1 minute, rinse, dry, and examine under oil. The gram-positive bacteria will retain the purple color of the crystal violet. In the gram-negative cells, the purple color will be removed by the alcohol, so that the cells will be counterstained red by the safranin. Some strains of bacteria are neither consistently purple nor red following this procedure, hence they are called gram-variable bacteria. Most of these are members of the genus *Mycobacterium,* such as *M. tuberculosis* and *M. leprae.* They are more easily

Fig. 2-12. Bacterial staining techniques. (*A*) With a flamed loop, smear a loopful of bacteria suspended in broth or water on a slide. (*B*) Allow slide to air-dry. (*C*) Pass the slide through the flame to heat-fix the bacteria to the slide. (*D*) Flood the slide with the stain. (*E*) Rinse with water. (*F*) Blot dry with bibulous paper or paper towel. (*G*) Examine the slide with the 100 × microscope objective using a drop of immersion oil directly on the smear.

identified with the acid-fast stain. In this method, carbol fuchsin is driven into the bacterial cell wall with heat so that the acid–alcohol will not remove the red color from the mycobacteria. Most other bacteria will be decolorized by the acid–alcohol treatment, and the tuberculosis pathogens can be readily seen in a sputum smear from a tubercular patient as red organisms in a blue background.

The procedures for staining bacteria to observe capsules, spores, flagella, fat globules, granules, and nuclear material will be found in most microbiology laboratory manuals. Refer to Table 2-4 for the Gram-staining characteristics of certain pathogens.

Motility The ability of an organism to move by itself is called motility. Bacterial motility is usually associated with the presence of flagella or axial filaments. Most spiral bacteria and about half of the bacilli are motile, but cocci are generally nonmotile. Motility can be observed best in a young culture of organisms in a semisolid medium or by the hanging-drop technique. In the latter, motile bacteria suspended in a hanging drop of liquid can be seen darting about in every direction within the drop (Fig. 2-13). Some bacteria exhibit gliding motility on secreted slime on solid agar.

Growth The cultural characteristic of bacterial colonies of a single species will vary depending upon the type of nutrient agar medium, the nutrients, and the dyes present. The size, color, shape, and consistency of a colony growing on a particular agar medium will be characteristic of a given species of bacteria. In a liquid medium, the region in which the organism grows depends upon the oxygen needs of that particular species. The rate of growth is also an important characteristic to note.

Nutritional Requirements All bacteria need the elements carbon, hydrogen, oxygen, sulfur, phosphorus, and nitrogen in some form for growth. Special elements, such as potassium, calcium, iron, manganese, magnesium, cobalt, copper, zinc, and uranium, are needed by certain bacteria. Some have specific vitamin requirements; others need organic substances secreted by other living microorganisms during their growth. The nutritional needs are characteristic of the species of bacteria. These nutritional requirements are discussed in Chapter 4.

Fig. 2-13. Hanging drop preparation for study of living bacteria. (*A*) Depression slide. (*B*) Depression slide with coverglass over the depression area. (*C*) Side view of hanging drop preparation, showing the drop of culture hanging from the center of the coverglass above the depression. (Volk WA, Wheeler MF: Basic Microbiology, 3rd ed. Philadelphia, JB Lippincott, 1973)

Table 2-4. Some Important Pathogenic Bacteria

Bacterium	Diseases	Type	Gram-Stain Reaction[a]
Bacillus anthracis	Anthrax	Spore-forming rod	+
Bordetella pertussis	Whooping cough	Rod	−
Brucella abortus and B. melitensis	Brucellosis, undulant fever	Rod	−
Chlamydia trachomatis	Lymphogranuloma venereum, trachoma	Coccoid	−
Clostridium botulinum	Botulism (food poisoning) infections	Spore-forming rod	+
Clostridium perfringens	Gas gangrene, wound	Spore-forming rod	+
Clostridium tetani	Tetanus (lockjaw)	Spore-forming rod	+
Corynebacterium diphtheriae	Diphtheria	Rod	+
Escherichia coli	Urinary infections	Rod	−
Francisella tularensis	Tularemia	Rod	−
Haemophilus ducreyi	Chancroid	Rod	−
Haemophilus influenzae	Meningitis, pneumonia	Rod	−
Klebsiella pneumoniae	Pneumonia	Rod	−
Mycobacterium leprae	Leprosy	Rod	+ / −
Mycobacterium tuberculosis	Tuberculosis	Rod	+ / −
Mycoplasma pneumoniae	Atypical pneumonia	Pleomorphic	−
Neisseria gonorrhoeae	Gonorrhea	Diplococcus	−
Neisseria meningitidis	Nasopharyngitis, meningitis	Diplococcus	−
Proteus vulgaris and P. morgani	Gastroenteritis, urinary infections	Rod	−
Pseudomonas aeruginosa	Respiratory and urogenital infections	Rod	−
Rickettsia rickettsii	Rocky Mountain spotted fever	Rod	−
Salmonella typhi	Typhoid fever	Rod	−
Salmonella species	Gastroenteritis	Rod	−
Shigella species	Shigellosis (bacillary dysentery)	Rod	−
Staphylococcus aureus	Boils, carbuncles, pneumonia, septicemia	Cocci in clusters	+
Streptococcus pyogenes	Strep throat, scarlet fever, rheumatic fever, septicemia	Cocci in chains	+
Streptococcus pneumoniae	Pneumonia	Diplococcus	+
Treponema pallidum	Syphilis	Spirochete	−
Vibrio cholerae	Cholera	Curved/rod	−
Yersinia pestis	Plague	Rod	−

[a] + = gram-positive; − = gram-negative; +/− = gram-variable

Biochemical and Metabolic Activities   As bacteria grow, they produce many waste products and secretions, some of which are enzymes that enable them to invade their host and cause disease. The pathogenic strains of many bacteria, such as staphylococci and streptococci, can be tentatively identified by the enzymes they secrete. Also, in particular environments, certain bacteria are characterized by the production of carbon dioxide, hydrogen sulfide, oxygen, or methane.

Pathogenicity   The disease-producing abilities of pathogens are important. Many are able to cause disease because they have capsules or endotoxins (a part of the cell wall) or because they secrete toxins and enzymes that damage cells and tissues (see Chap. 7). Frequently, pathogenicity is tested by injecting the pathogen into mice. Some common pathogenic bacteria are listed in Table 2-4.

Amino Acid Sequencing   The proteins found within a bacterium are specific for that species. Thus, by comparing the amino acid sequence of certain bacterial proteins, the species and how closely related it is to other bacteria can be determined.

Genetic Composition   The composition of the genetic material (DNA) is unique to each species. Thus, by determining the base composition and by comparing the cytosine/guanine ratio with the total amount of bases, a numerical ratio can be calculated. Also, by identifying or hybridizing a sequence of bases in portions of DNA or RNA, the researcher can determine the degree of relationship between two bacteria, and perhaps the species, strain, or type of bacteria.

Some Lower Forms of Bacteria

The rickettsias, chlamydias, and mycoplasmas are bacteria, but they do not possess all of the attributes of typical bacterial cells. Because they are so small and difficult to isolate they were formerly classified as viruses.

Rickettsias and Chlamydias   This group includes both rickettsias and chlamydias. They are coccoid, rod-shaped, or pleomorphic (irregular) gram-negative bacteria with a bacterial-type cell wall; unlike viruses, they contain both DNA and RNA. Most known forms are intracellular parasites pathogenic to humans and other animals.

Most rickettsias are obligate intracellular parasites; because they appear to have leaky cell membranes, they must live inside another cell to retain all the necessary cellular substances. Hence, they are usually transmitted by arthropod vectors. An exception is *Coxiella burnetii,* the cause of Q fever, that may also be airborne or foodborne.

The one order of rickettsias includes parasites of arthropods (lice, fleas, ticks). These animals are frequently vectors (carriers) of rickettsial diseases because they transmit pathogens from one host to another by their bites or waste products. Diseases caused by arthropod-borne rickettsias include Rocky Mountain spotted fever and the typhus fevers.

The chlamydias are probably the most primitive of all bacteria because they

Fig. 2-14. Elementary bodies of chlamydia. (From S. Koester)

lack the enzymes to perform many essential metabolic activities, particularly the production of ATP. Thus, they are obligate intracellular parasites and must be transferred by direct contact between hosts, not by insects.

Chlamydias have two forms in their life cycle (Fig. 2-14). The infectious form, called the *elementary body*, attaches to the host cell. After it is engulfed by the host cell, the elementary body reorganizes into the larger, less infectious form, called the *reticulate body*. This form finally divides to produce many small infectious elementary bodies that will be released to spread and infect surrounding host cells or other individuals. Chlamydias are easily transmitted during sexual contact and cause many infections of the urethra (urethritis), bladder, (cystitis), fallopian tubes (PID), prostate (prostatitis), or other complications. They cause many diseases in vertebrate animals (cats, dogs, sheep, cattle, birds, humans), including trachoma (an eye disease), lymphogranuloma venereum (a venereal disease, LGV), and psittacosis (a respiratory infection in humans and birds, often called parrot fever).

Mycoplasmas The mycoplasmas are the smallest of the cellular microbes (Fig. 2-15). Because they lack cell walls, they assume many pleomorphic shapes, from coccoid to filamentous. Sometimes they are confused with L-forms of bacteria, but even in the most favorable growth media, they are not able to produce cell walls, which is not true for the L-forms. Mycoplasmas were formerly called pleuropneumonialike organisms (PPLO) because they were first isolated from cattle with lung infection. These organisms may be free-living or parasitic and are pathogenic to many animals and some plants. In humans, the pathogenic mycoplasmas cause primary atypical pneumonia and many secondary infections. Since they have no cell wall, they are resistant to treatment with penicillin and other antibiotics that work by inhibiting cell wall synthesis.

Viruses

The mature virus particles, the virions, are so small and simple in structure that they do not fit the living cell classification. They range in size from 0.02 μm to 0.3 μm in diameter. The smallest is about the size of the large hemoglobin molecule of red blood cells. Viruses have been found that produce diseases or genetic changes in animals, plants, algae, fungi, protozoa, and bacterial cells (Table 2-5).

Recently, virions have been described as having five specific properties that distinguish them from living cells: (1) they possess either DNA or RNA, never both; (2) their replication (duplication) is directed by the viral nucleic acid within a host cell; (3) they do not divide by binary fission or mitosis; (4) they lack the genes necessary for energy production; and (5) they depend upon the ribosomes and nutrients of the infected cells for protein production.

A typical virus particle has a core containing core protein and the genome of DNA or RNA surrounded by a capsid (protein coat), sometimes consisting of many small units called capsomeres (Fig. 2-16). Some virions have a protective envelope composed of fats and polysaccharides. The bacterial viruses may also have a tail and

Fig. 2-15. Scanning electron micrograph of *Mycoplasma pneumoniae;* note the coccoid structures within the filaments (original magnification × 10,000). (Volk WA, et al.: Essentials of Medical Microbiology, 3rd ed. Philadelphia, JB Lippincott, 1986)

Table 2-5. Relative Sizes and Shapes of Some Viral Particles (Virions)

Viruses	Nucleic Acid Type	Shape	Size Range (nm)
Animal Viruses			
Vaccinia	DNA	Complex	200 by 300
Mumps	RNA	Helical	150–250
Herpes simplex	DNA	Polyhedral	100–150
Influenza	RNA	Helical	80–120
Retroviruses	RNA	Helical	100–120
Adenoviruses	DNA	Polyhedral	60–90
Reoviruses	RNA	Polyhedral	60–80
Papovaviruses	DNA	Polyhedral	40–60
Polioviruses	RNA	Polyhedral	28
Plant Viruses			
Turnip yellow mosaic	RNA	Polyhedral	28
Wound tumor	RNA	Polyhedral	55–60
Alfalfa mosaic	RNA	Polyhedral	18 by 36–40
Tobacco mosaic	RNA	Helical	18 by 300
Bacteriophages			
T2	DNA	Complex	65 by 210
λ	DNA	Complex	54 by 194
φχ-174	DNA	Complex	25

tail fibers. There are no ribosomes for protein synthesis or sites of energy production, hence the virus must take over a functioning cell to produce new virus particles.

Viruses are classified by the following characteristics: (1) type of genetic material (either DNA or RNA); (2) shape of the capsid; (3) number of capsomeres; (4) size of capsid (particle); (5) presence or absence of an envelope; (6) host that it infects (plant, animal, or microorganism); and (7) the type of disease produced.

The genetic material of most viruses is either double-stranded DNA or single-stranded RNA, but a few have single-stranded DNA or double-stranded RNA. Viral genomes are usually circular molecules, but some are linear (with two ends). Capsids of viruses have various shapes and symmetry. They may be polyhedral (many sided), helical (coiled tubes), bullet shaped, spherical, or a complex combination of these shapes. Polyhedral capsids have 20 sides or facets, geometrically referred to as icosahedrons. Each facet consists of several capsomeres; thus, the size of the virus is determined by the size of each facet and the number of capsomeres in each. Frequently, the envelope around the capsid makes the virus appear spherical or irregular in shape when seen in electron micrographs. The envelope is usually acquired by certain animal viruses from the host nuclear or cellular membrane as the new virus particle leaves the cell. Apparently, viruses are able to alter these membranes and add protein fibers, spikes, and knobs that will enable the virus to recognize the next host cell to be invaded. A list of some of the viruses, their characteristics, and the diseases they cause is presented in Table 2-6.

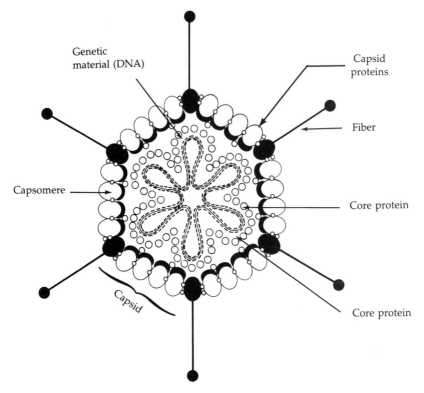

Genetic material (DNA)

Capsid proteins

Fiber

Capsomere

Core protein

Capsid

Core protein

Fig. 2-16. Model of an icosahedral virus: adenovirus. (Volk WA, et al.: Essentials of Medical Microbiology, 3rd ed. Philadelphia, JB Lippincott, 1986)

The virion usually infects a cell by injecting its DNA or RNA into the cell (Fig. 2-17) or by cellular phagocytosis (Fig. 2-18). The viral genetic material may remain latent or inactive in the cell and be transferred to each daughter cell when it divides. This is the *lysogenic cycle* of viral infection. However, the viral genetic material may be induced to take over the cell and make viruses by heat (fever), ultraviolet (UV) light, or certain chemical agents.

When the genetic material from the virus takes over the metabolic machinery of the cell to produce viruses, it has entered the *lytic cycle* of virus infection. It breaks up the cellular DNA and produces viral DNA or RNA. It then synthesizes viral protein capsids and assembles many new virus particles until the cell bursts (lysis has occurred) and releases the new viruses into the area to infect neighboring cells.

A good example of the lysogenic (latent) and lytic cycles is the ordinary "cold sore" caused by the herpes simplex virus. Those persons who get cold sores have the latent or temperate virus genetic material in the nearby nerve ganglion (after the initial infection) in the lysogenic cycle. When they develop a fever or are exposed to excess UV light of the sun, the viral genetic material may be stimulated to take over the cells to produce more viruses (lytic cycle) and the cold sore develops. Such viral

Table 2-6. Selected Important Groups of Viruses and Viral Diseases

Virus Type	Viral Characteristics	Virus	Disease
Poxviruses	Large, brick shape with envelope, double DNA	Poxvirus Poxvirus	Smallpox (variola) Cowpox (vaccinia)
Polyoma-Papilloma	Double DNA, polyhedral	Papillomavirus Polyomavirus	Warts Some tumors, some cancer
Herpesviruses	Polyhedral with envelope, double DNA	Herpes simplex I Herpes simplex II Herpes zoster Varicella	Cold sores or fever blisters Venereal herpes Shingles Chickenpox
Adenoviruses	Double DNA, icosa-hedral, no enve-lope		Respiratory infections, pneumonia, conjunc-tivitis, some tumors
Picornaviruses	Single RNA, tiny icosahedral, with envelope	Rhinovirus Poliovirus Hepatitis types A and B Coxsackievirus	Colds Poliomyelitis Hepatitis Respiratory infections, meningitis
Reoviruses	Double RNA, icosa-hedral with enve-lope	Enterovirus	Intestinal infections
Myxoviruses	RNA, helical with envelope	Orthomyxoviruses types A & B Myxovirus parotidis Paramyxovirus Rhabdovirus	Influenza Mumps Measles (rubeola) Rabies
Arbovirus	Arthropod-borne RNA, cubic	Mosquito-borne type B Mosquito-borne types A and B Tick-borne, corona-virus	Yellow fever Encephalitis (many types) Colorado tick fever
Retrovirus	Double RNA, helical with envelope	RNA tumor virus HTLV virus HIV (Human immuno-deficiency virus)	Tumors Leukemia AIDS

infections are usually limited by the body's defenses: the phagocytes and an antiviral protein called interferon that is produced by the infected cells.

Antibiotics are not effective against viral infections because these drugs work by inhibiting certain metabolic reactions within living pathogens. Because viruses are not independent metabolizing cells, agents that affect the synthesis of new virus particles may also cause damage to the host cell. For colds and influenza, antibiotics should be

Fig. 2-17. A partially lysed cell of *Vibrio cholerae* with attached virions of phage CP-T1. Note the empty capsids, the full head phage capsids, contracted tail sheaths, and base plates and spikes (original magnification × 257,000). (Courtesy of R. W. Taylor and J. E. Ogg, Colorado State University, Fort Collins, Colorado)

given only to prevent secondary bacterial infections that might occur following the virus infection.

Many tumors and cancers are apparently caused by viruses that change the genetic composition of the cell and cause uncontrolled growth of abnormal cells under certain environmental conditions. Some chemotherapeutic drugs used to treat cancer are chemicals that interfere with DNA and RNA synthesis in rapidly dividing cells, thus inhibiting or destroying these cells.

Fig. 2-18. Adsorption (*A*), penetration (*B–D*), and digestion of the capsid (*E–G*) of herpes simplex on HeLa cells, as deduced from electron micrographs of infected cell sections. The penetration involves local digestion of the viral and cellular membranes (*B,C*), resulting in fusion of the two membranes and release of the nucleocapsid into the cytoplasmic matrix (*D*). The naked nucleocapsid is intact in (*E*), is partially digested in (*F*), and has disappeared in (*G*), leaving a core containing DNA and protein. (Morgan C, et al: J Virol 2:507, 1968)

Remnants of viruses are often seen in infected cells and are used as a diagnostic tool to identify certain diseases. These are called *inclusion bodies,* and they may be found in the cytoplasm (cytoplasmic) or within the nucleus (intranuclear), depending upon the disease. In rabies, the cytoplasmic inclusion bodies are called Negri bodies. The inclusion bodies of AIDS and the Guarnieri bodies of smallpox are also cytoplasmic. The herpes and poliomyelitis viruses cause intranuclear inclusion bodies. In each case, the inclusion bodies may be merely aggregates or collections of viruses. Some important human viral diseases include the common cold, influenza, mumps, measles, chickenpox, smallpox, rabies, cold sores, venereal herpes, warts, poliomyelitis, encephalitis, and acquired immunodeficiency syndrome (AIDS).

Bacteriophages   The viruses that infect bacteria are called bacteriophages or simply phages. Those that infect the coliform (intestinal) bacteria, such as *E. coli,* are called coliphages. Most bacteriophages are species- and strain-specific. Refer to Figures 2-17 and 2-18 to observe the complexity of the phages. The tail plate, tail fibers, and spikes are used to attach to the bacteria, usually at the site of a *pilus,* and the phage DNA is injected into the bacteria much like water from a syringe (see Figure 2-19).

Viruses and Genetic Changes   Much research in genetics has been accomplished using bacteria and bacteriophages. Some pathogens are identified by the specific bacteriophages that will infect them. When bacteria are injected with the genetic material from a bacteriophage, the genetic constitution of those bacteria is changed by the addition of the phage genes. This process is called *phage conversion.* An example of such a conversion is the pathogenic diphtheria bacterium, which is pathogenic only when the phage genes are present. Evidently, the genes that enable diphtheria bacteria (*Corynebacterium diphtheriae*) to produce a lethal toxin are injected with the phage genes.

Fig. 2-19. (*A*) The bacterial virus T4 is an assembly of protein components. The head is a protein membrane with 20 facets, filled with deoxyribonucleic acid (DNA). It is attached to a tail consisting of a hollow core surrounded by a sheath and based on a spiked end-plate to which six fibers are attached. (*B*) The sheath contracts, driving the core through the wall, and viral DNA enters the cell. (Volk WA, Wheeler MF: Basic Microbiology, 4th ed. Philadelphia, JB Lippincott, 1980)

Other genetic changes produced in bacteria by bacteriophages are discussed in Chapter 4.

Protozoa

The protozoa are eucaryotic, single-celled, animal-like microorganisms, ranging in length from 3 μm to 100 μm. Most of them are free-living organisms found in soil and water. They have no chlorophyll so they cannot make their own foods by photosynthesis. Some ingest whole algae, yeasts, bacteria, and other smaller protozoans as their source of food (Fig. 2-20); others live on dead, decaying organic matter. The parasitic protozoa break down and absorb nutrients from the body of the host in which they live. A few parasitic protozoa are pathogens, such as those that cause malaria, giardiasis, and amebic dysentery (refer to Chap. 13). Other parasitic protozoa exist in a symbiotic (living together) relationship with the host animal, in which both organisms benefit. A typical example of symbiosis is the termite and its intestinal protozoa, which can digest the wood eaten by the termite; thus, both organisms absorb the nutrients necessary for life. Without the parasitic protozoa, the termite cannot digest wood, its main source of food, and thereby starves to death. Cattle and other animals also need protozoa in their stomachs to break down the cellulose in plants.

The protozoa are divided into groups according to their method of locomotion or the presence or absence of cilia (short, hairlike structures) and flagella (Table 2-7). The *amebas* (phylum Sarcodina), lacking cilia and flagella, move by pushing forward a bit of cytoplasm (a pseudopodium, or false foot) and slowly flowing into it; this process is called ameboid movement. The ameba also engulfs food by surrounding the particles and enclosing them into a membrane-bounded space called a digestive vacuole, there to be digested and used as a source of nutrients. *Phagocytosis* is the engulfment of large particles, whereas *pinocytosis* is the intake of smaller dissolved food particles. Some white blood cells move through tissues and ingest materials in the same manner. This process is further discussed in Chapter 10 under Phagocytosis. One important pathogenic ameba is *Entamoeba histolytica*, which causes amebic dysentery. This illness is difficult to treat because the pathogen forms resistant cysts deep within the intestinal lining where the amebas live and are protected.

The *flagellates* (phylum Mastigophora) move by means of one or many flagella. A few species are pathogenic: for example, *Trypanosoma gambiense* is carried by the tsetse fly and causes African sleeping sickness in humans; *Trichomonas vaginalis* causes persistent infections of the male and female genital tracts: and *Giardia lamblia* causes a persistent intestinal infection.

Ciliates (phylum Ciliata) move about as a result of large numbers of cilia on their surfaces. They are the most complex of all the protozoa. A pathogenic ciliate, *Balantidium coli*, causes a severe intestinal infection. In underdeveloped countries, it is usually transmitted to man from swine.

Fig. 2-20. Protozoa. (*A*) *Didinium nasutum* with partially ingested prey. (Lechavalier HA, Pramer D: The Microbe. Philadephia, JB Lippincott, 1970). (*B*) TEM cross section of *Giardia lamblia*. (From S. Koester and P. Engelkirk)

Table 2-7. Characteristics of Major Protozoa

Phylum	Means of Movement	Selected Differentiating Properties (Method of Reproduction)		Representatives
		Asexual	Sexual	
Ciliata	Cilia	Transverse fission	Conjugation	*Balantidium coli, Paramecium, Stentor, Tetrahymena, Vorticella*
Sarcodina	Pseudopodia (false feet)	Binary fission	When present, involves flagellated sex cells	*Amoeba, Difflugia, Entamoeba histolytica*
Mastigophora	Flagella	Binary fission	None	*Chlamydomonas, Giardia lamblia, Trichomonas, Trypanosoma*
Sporozoa	Generally nonmotile except for certain sex cells	Multiple fission	Involves flagellated sex cells	*Plasmodium, Toxoplasma gondii, Cryptosporidium, Pneumocystis carinii*

The nonmotile protozoa are classed as *Sporozoa*. The most important pathogens are those *Plasmodium* species that cause malaria in many areas throughout the world. One of these, *Plasmodium vivax,* causes a mild form of malaria in the United States. These pathogens are carried and transmitted by the female Anopheles mosquito. Two Sporozoa that have not previously been recognized as serious pathogens, *Pneumocystis carinii* and *Cryptosporidium,* cause severe secondary infections in immunosuppressed patients such as those with acquired immunodeficiency syndrome (AIDS). (See Chap. 13).

The protozoa differ from bacteria in that they are eucaryotic, much larger, and do not have a cell wall. They are distinguished from algae by their lack of chlorophyll and from the fungi by their lack of a cellulose or chitin cell wall, and protozoa have the ability to move.

Fungi

Fungi are found almost everywhere on earth, living on organic matter in water and soil, and on animals and plants. They may be harmful or beneficial. The fungi also live on many unlikely materials, causing deterioration of leather and plastics as well as jams, pickles, and many other foods. The beneficial fungi are important in the production of cheeses, yogurt, beer and wine, and other foods as well as certain drugs and antibiotics.

Characteristics

The fungi are eucaryotic organisms that include mushrooms, molds, and yeasts. As saprophytes, their main source of food is dead, decaying organic matter. Fungi are the "garbage disposers" of nature, the vultures of the microbial world. By secreting digestive enzymes into dead plant and animal matter, they decompose this material into absorbable nutrients for themselves and other living organisms. Imagine living in a world without saprophytes, stumbling through endless piles of decaying debris! Some fungi also live, parasitically, on living animals and plants.

Fungi are often referred to as plants only because they have cellulose or chitin cell walls. They differ from plants and algae in that they are not photosynthetic; they have no chlorophyll or other photosynthetic pigments. Although many fungi are unicellular during some phase of their life cycle (*e.g.*, yeasts), many species grow as filaments called *hyphae* (singular: hypha), which form a mass called the *mycelium* (plural: mycelia); thus, they are different from saprophytic bacteria. Remember, bacteria are procaryotic, whereas fungi are eucaryotic cells.

Reproduction and Spores Fungal cells can reproduce asexually by budding, by hyphal extension, or by the formation of asexual spores (Fig. 2-21). Sexual reproduction occurs in many fungi with the nuclear fusion of two gametes and subsequent division into many sexual spores. Some species of fungi produce both asexual and sexual

Fig. 2-21. Cross section of a budding yeast cell (original magnification × 15,500). (Lechavalier HA, Pramer D: The Microbes. Philadelphia, JB Lippincott, 1970)

spores or more than one type of asexual spore. Spores are named after the fungal class or the type of sporulating structure. Figure 2-22 is a representation of some typical fungi.

Spores of fungi are very resistant structures that are carried great distances by wind. They are resistant to heat, cold, acids, bases, and other chemicals.

Classification of True Fungi

The mycologists, those who study fungi, have separated the true fungi into five classes: Basidiomycetes, Oomycetes, Zygomycetes, Ascomycetes, and Deutero-mycetes. These classes are based on the mode of reproduction and the types of mycelia, spores, and gametes. The characteristics of each of these classes are shown in Table 2-8.

Mushrooms (Basidiomycetes) are a class of true fungi that consist of a network of filaments or strands, called the mycelium, that grow in the soil or in a rotting log, and the fruiting body (mushroom) that forms and releases spores. The spore is much like the seed of a plant and will germinate into a new organism. Many mushrooms are delicious to eat, but many that appear edible are extremely toxic and may cause permanent brain damage or death.

Molds are the filamentous fungi often seen in water and soil and on food. They

Fig. 2-22. Typical fungi. (*A*) *Penicillium* mold, blue-green spores arranged like a brush. (*B*) *Aspergillus*, blue-green with yellow areas. (*C*) *Rhizopus*, white to dark gray with root-like rhizoids. (*D*) *Saccharomyces cerevisiae*, a yeast.

Table 2-8. Selected Characteristics of the Major Classes of Fungi

Class	Type of Mycelium	Site of Spore Formation		Representative Groups
		Asexual	*Sexual*	
Ascomycetes	Septate	Tips of hyphae	Within sacs	Common antibiotic-producing fungi, penicillium, yeasts
Basidiomycetes	Septate	Tips of hyphae	Surface of basidium	Mushrooms, rusts
Deuteromy-cetes (fungi imperfecti)	Septate	Tips of hyphae	None present	Most human pathogenic molds and yeasts
Oomycetes	Aseptate	In sacs	Within a uni-cellular female sex organ (oogonium)	Some aquatic forms, mildew, plant blights, fish infections
Zygomycetes	Usually aseptate	In sacs	In mycelium	Bread mold (*Rhizopus nigricans*), aquatic species

grow in the form of filaments or hyphae that make up the mycelium of the mold. Reproduction is by spore formation, either sexually or asexually, on the reproductive hyphae. Various species of molds are found in each of the classes of fungi except Basidiomycetes (mushrooms). An interesting mold in class Oomycetes is *Phytophtera*, the potato blight mold that caused a famine in Ireland in the mid-19th century. The black bread mold *Rhizopus* is a zygomycete. Both of these groups are the more primitive molds with aseptate hyphae; this means the hyphae are not divided into individual cells. Although there may be many nuclei in aseptate hyphae, they are not separated by cell walls. Among the Ascomycetes and Deuteromycetes are found many antibiotic-producing molds, such as *Penicillium* and *Streptomyces*.

Molds have great commercial importance. They are the main source of antibiotics. Many new antibiotics are developed by growing soil cultures and isolating the molds that inhibit the growth of bacteria. The antibiotic penicillin was accidentally discovered when a *Penicillium notatum* mold contaminated an agar plate of staphylococcus and inhibited its growth. Today, antibiotics can be synthesized and chemically changed in the biochemistry laboratory, as has been done with the various penicillins. Some molds are also used to produce large quantities of enzymes, such as amylase, which converts starch to glucose, and citric acid and other organic acids that are used commercially. The flavor of cheeses such as bleu, roquefort, camembert, and limburger are the result of the molds grown on them.

Molds also can be harmful. The rusts and molds of crop plants, grains, corn, and potatoes not only destroy crops, but some are also toxic. The aflatoxin from the *Aspergillus* mold on peanuts and cottonseed and the ergot on rye and wheat are extremely toxic to humans and farm animals. Aflatoxins have been shown to be carcinogenic (cancer-causing) as well.

Yeasts are microscopic eucaryotic single-celled Ascomycetes or Deuteromycetes that lack mycelia. They usually reproduce by budding (see Fig. 2-21), occasionally by spore formation. Yeasts are found in soil and water and on the skins of many fruits and vegetables. People produced wine, beer, and alcoholic beverages for centuries before Pasteur discovered that yeasts, naturally occurring on the skin of grapes and other fruits and grains, were responsible for these fermentation processes. The common yeast *Saccharomyces cerevisiae* ferments sugar to alcohol under anaerobic conditions. In aerobic conditions, this yeast breaks down simple sugars to carbon dioxide and water; for this reason, it has long been used to leaven light bread. (See Chap. 4 for a description of aerobes and anaerobes.) Yeasts are also a good source of nutrients for humans because they produce many vitamins and proteins.

Dimorphism

A few fungi, usually pathogens, can live either as molds or as yeasts depending on growth conditions. When they are isolated from living tissues at body temperature (37° C), they appear in a unicellular parasitic form as yeasts. If they are grown at room temperature (20° C) or isolated from the soil or dust, they grow in the saprophytic form as a mold with hyphae and spores. *Histoplasma* (which causes histoplasmosis), *Sporothrix* (which causes sporotrichosis), *Coccidioides* (which causes coccidioidomycosis) and *Candida albicans* (which causes candidiasis) are examples of dimorphic fungi (Fig. 2-23).

Fungal Diseases

Considering the large number of fungal species, very few are pathogenic for humans, and most of those are found in Class Deuteromycetes, listed in Table 2-8. The diseases caused by fungi are categorized as superficial, deep-seated, or systemic mycotic infections. In some cases the infection may progress through all three of these categories.

Superficial Mycoses   Cutaneous and superficial fungal infections are caused by dermatophytes or other fungi that live on the skin or the mucous membranes of body openings. Dermatophytes (fungi living on or within the skin) cause athlete's foot, ringworm, and lesions of nails, scalp, and hair follicles.

A yeastlike fungus, *C. albicans* is an opportunist that normally lives harmlessly on the skin and mucous membranes of the mouth, intestine, and reproductive tract. When the chemical balance (homeostasis) is upset and the number of normal bacteria is reduced, this yeast flourishes to cause infections of the mouth (oral thrush), skin, and vagina (vaginal candidiasis). This type of local infection sometimes invades the bloodstream to become a generalized or systemic infection in many internal areas.

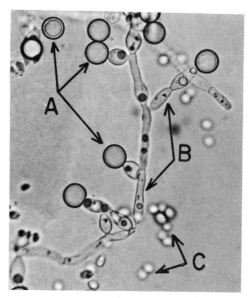

Fig. 2-23. Dimorphism shown in a culture of *C. albicans.* (*A*) Chlamydospores. (*B*) Pseudohyphae (elongated yeast cells, linked end to end). (*C*) Budding yeast cells (blastospores) (original magnification × 450). (Davis BD, et al.: Microbiology, 3rd ed. Philadelphia, Harper & Row, 1980)

Deep-seated and Systemic Mycoses The spores of some pathogenic fungi may be inhaled with dust from contaminated soil and from bird and bat feces, or they may enter through wounds of the hands and feet. If the spores are inhaled into the lungs they may germinate there to cause a respiratory infection similar to tuberculosis. This type of deep-seated pulmonary infection is caused by a species of *Coccidioides* (coccidioidomycosis), *Histoplasma* (histoplasmosis), *Blastomyces* (blastomycosis), and *Cryptococcus* (cryptococcosis). In each case the pathogens may invade further to cause systemic infections, especially in immunosuppressed individuals.

There are skin tests available for most of these infections, but the diseases are difficult to cure. Mycotic diseases are most effectively treated with nystatin, amphotericin B, or 5-fluorocytosine. These chemotherapeutic agents are toxic and are prescribed with due consideration and caution.

Algae

Algae are photosynthetic organisms that may be multicellular or unicellular. They are arranged in colonies or strands and are found in water and soil and on trees, plants, and rocks. Algae produce their energy by photosynthesis, using energy from the sun, carbon dioxide, water, and inorganic nutrients from the soil to build cellular material. However, a few species use organic nutrients, and others can survive with

Table 2-9. Characteristics of Algae (Major Groups)

Division	Common Name	General Structural Arrangement	Stored Materials
Chlorophyta	Green algae	Unicellular to multicellular	Starch, oils
Chrysophyta	Golden algae (includes diatoms)	Mainly unicellular	Oils
Euglenophyta	Euglena	Unicellular	Fats
Phaeophyta	Brown algae	Multicellular	Fats
Pyrrophyta	Dinoflagellates	Unicellular	Starch, oils
Rhodophyta	Red algae	Multicellular	Starch, oils

very little sunlight. The blue-green algae (cyanobacteria) are simple procaryotic cells, which are in the Kingdom *Procaryotae* with bacteria. The green, brown, and red algae are eucaryotic organisms in the Kingdom Protista with protozoa. Only one type of algae (*Prototheca*) is a true pathogen, although a few species secrete substances that are toxic to humans, fish, and other animals (Table 2-9).

It is easy to find algae. They comprise the large seaweed and the kelp found along the shores of the ocean, the green scum on ponds, and the slippery material on wet rocks. There are also many microscopic forms seen in pond water that differ from the colorless, motile protozoa in that they are photosynthetic, colored, and move very slowly.

Algae are an important source of food, iodine and other minerals, fertilizers, emulsifiers for pudding, and stabilizers for ice cream and salad dressings, and are used as a gelling agent for jams and nutrient media for bacterial growth. Damage to water systems is frequently caused by algae clogging the filters and pipes where many nutrients are present. Some typical algae are shown in Figure 2-24.

Problems and Questions

1. Which microbes are eucaryotic cells?
2. Which microorganisms are procaryons?
3. What function do the mitochondria and mesosomes have in common?

Fig. 2-24. Typical algae. (*A*) Vaucheria. (*B*) Diatom. (*C*) Navicula. (*D*) Oocystis. (*E*) Scenedesmus. (*F*) Spirogyra. ▶ (*G*) Nostoc. (*H*) Oscillatoria.

Motility	Method of Reproduction	Cell Wall Composition	Habitat
Mostly nonmotile	Asexual by multiple fission; spores sexual	Cellulose and pectin	Fresh water Salt water Soil Lichens
Unique movement in diatoms; others have flagella	Asexual and sexual	Pectin, some with silica or calcium	Fresh water Salt water Soil
Motile by means of flagella	Asexual only by binary fission	None	Fresh water
Motile	Asexual by motile zoospores; sexual by motile gametes	Cellulose, pectin, algin	Salt water (cool environment)
Motile	Asexual; sexual rare	Cellulose and pectin	Fresh water Salt water
Nonmotile	Asexual by spores; sexual by gametes	Cellulose, pectin, agar, carrageenan	Salt water (warm environment)

4. Where does protein synthesis occur in eucaryotic cells and in procaryotic cells?
5. Which microorganisms do not have a nuclear membrane?
6. List five differences between eucaryotic animal cells and procaryotic bacterial cells.
7. What is the difference between bacterial flagella and protozoan flagella?
8. Describe peritrichous, amphitrichous, lophotrichous, and monotrichous flagellation in bacteria.
9. List five properties of viruses that distinguish them from other living cells.
10. Describe the lytic and lysogenic cycles of viruses.
11. Describe a symbiotic relationship of a parasitic protozoan.
12. What is the role of fungi in recycling nutrients?
13. What are the differences between protozoa and green algae?

Chapter 3

Introduction to Chemistry of Life

Objectives

After studying this chapter, you should be able to

1. Differentiate among elements, atoms, molecules, and compounds
2. Describe an acid-plus-base reaction
3. Discuss the importance of water in biochemical reactions
4. List the characteristics of monosaccharides, disaccharides, and polysaccharides
5. Describe four main types of biochemical molecules
6. Distinguish between organic and inorganic compounds
7. Discuss the structure of carbohydrates, fats, proteins, and nucleic acids and their breakdown products
8. Describe the role of enzymes in metabolism
9. Discuss how DNA directs cellular activities

Key Words to Pronounce and Understand

Acids (a'-sids). Substances with sufficient hydrogen ions in solution to produce a *p*H above 0 but below 7.0

Adenosine triphosphate (ATP) (add-den'-o-sin tri'-fos-fate). High–energy-rich organic molecule

Atom (at'-um). Smallest unit of an element

Bases (base'-es). Substances with sufficient hydroxide ions in solution to produce a *p*H above 7.0 but below 14

Carbohydrates (car'-bow-high-drates). Organic compounds containing carbon, hydrogen, and oxygen in a ratio of 1:2:1

Compound (com'-pound). Chemical substance containing more than one kind of atom

Deoxyribonucleic acid (DNA) (dee-ox'-ee-rye'-bow-new-clay'-ick). Genetic macromolecule in chromosomes

Disaccharide (die'-sack'-car-ride). A carbohydrate with two sugar units

Electrolyte (ee-lect'-trow-light). A substance that exists as ions in a water solution

Element (ell'-e'-ment). General name given to a substance composed of identical atoms

Glycogen (gly'-ko-jen). Polysaccharide stored by animal cells

Hydrocarbons (high'-drow-car-buns). Organic compounds consisting of only hydrogen and carbon atoms.

Hydrolysis (high-drol'-e-sis). Reaction in which a compound is broken apart by the addition of water

Lipids (lip'-pids). Organic compounds containing carbon, hydrogen, and oxygen that are insoluble in water but soluble in fat solvents

Metabolite (met-tab'-bow-light). Substance that furnishes energy and building blocks for the vital processes of a cell

Monosaccharide (mon-oh-sack'-car-ride). A carbohydrate consisting of one sugar unit

Nucleic acids (new-clay'-ick). Polymers of DNA and RNA that carry the genetic information of a cell and direct protein synthesis

Nucleotides (new'-clee-o-tides). Basic subunits of the nucleic acids, each consisting of a purine or pyrimidine combined with a ribose sugar and a phosphate group.

Polymer (pol'-e-mer). Long-chain molecule consisting of repeated subunits

Polysaccharide (pol-ee-sack'-car-ride). Carbohydrate consisting of many sugar units

Protein (pro'-teen). Macromolecule consisting of one or more polypeptide chains of amino acids

Purine (pure'-reen). A nucleic acid base; adenine or guanine

Pyrimidine (perr-rim'-uh-dean). A nucleic acid base; thymine, cytosine, or uracil

Ribonucleic acid (RNA) (rye'-bow-new-clay'-ick). Nucleic acid necessary for protein synthesis; transcribed from DNA

Replication (rep-lee-kay'-shun). Duplication of DNA or chromosomes

Salt. Any solid ionic compound that forms ions other than hydrogen and hydroxide in solution

Transcription (trans-cript'-shun). Process involved in transcribing the genetic message from DNA to RNA

Translation (trans-lay'-shun). Process of translating the message carried by mRNA to synthesize proteins in the cell

The various ways in which microorganisms function and survive in their environment depend on their chemical makeup. To understand microbial cells and how they work, one must have a basic knowledge of the chemistry of atoms, molecules, and macromolecules. You remember that even procaryotic cells consist of very large macromolecules of DNA, RNA, proteins, lipids, polysaccharides, and many combinations of these that make up the capsule, cell wall, cell membrane, mesosomes, cytoplasm, and nuclear material. These macromolecules can be broken down into organic units or molecules of the nucleotides, amino acids, glycerol, fatty acids, monosaccharides, or simple sugars. Each of these molecules, in turn, may be broken down into inorganic molecules of water, carbon dioxide, ammonia, sulfides, and phosphates, and finally into the atoms of carbon, hydrogen, oxygen, nitrogen, sulfur, and phosphorus. Basic inorganic chemistry is introduced in this chapter and is followed by a discussion of the organic chemistry and biochemistry of the major macromolecules found in living cells.

Only when all of these units are in place and working together properly can the cell function like a well-managed industrial plant. As in industry, the cell must have the appropriate structures and parts, the regulatory molecules (enzymes) to control its activities, the fuel (nutrients) to provide energy, and raw materials for manufacturing the end products.

Basic Chemistry

Atoms, Molecules, Elements, Compounds

All substances, whether gas, liquid, or solid, have certain fundamental characteristics in common. If one could break down any substance into particles, into its smallest elemental units, it would be composed of *atoms*. Although it is difficult to observe atomic structure, atoms are known to consist of a mass of positively charged protons, neutral neutrons, minute negatively charged electrons, and other even smaller subparticles. The protons and neutrons are found in a central nucleus, and the electrons float around the nucleus, like negatively charged satellites attracted to a positively charged planet. Figure 3-1 illustrates an oxygen atom. When a multitude of atoms, with identical numbers of electrons and protons and the same chemical properties, exist together, the substance is known as an *element*; for example, carbon (C), hydrogen (H), oxygen (O), nitrogen (N), sulfur (S).

The atoms of each element have their own special weight (or mass) called *atomic weight*, which is the total mass of the number of protons and neutrons (electrons are negligible in weight). The atomic weight of a specific element is an average of the weights of all isotopes of that element as they occur in nature. *Isotopes* are atoms of the same element, with identical chemical characteristics but with different atomic weights because they have various numbers of neutrons within the atoms. For example, carbon-12 has six protons and six neutrons for a weight of 12, whereas carbon-14 has six protons and eight neutrons for a weight of 14; both are isotopes of the element,

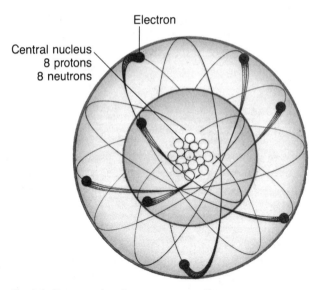

Fig. 3-1. Representation of an oxygen atom. Eight protons and eight neutrons are tightly bound in the central nucleus, around which the electrons revolve. (Rosdahl CB: Textbook of Basic Nursing, 4th ed. Philadelphia, JB Lippincott, 1985)

carbon. The weight of the six negatively charged electrons is negligible. Elements are also identified by a number that indicates the number of positive charges, or protons, in the nucleus. This is called the *atomic number*. Thus the atomic number of carbon is 6. Atomic weights and numbers can be found in a periodic table of the elements in any chemistry book; some are shown in Table 3-1.

If two or more atoms of the same or different elements combine together into a single stable unit, that unit is called a *molecule*; examples include carbon dioxide (CO_2), water (H_2O), or sulfur dioxide (SO_2). When many molecules exist together in a substance that can be seen or weighed, the substance is called a *compound, e.g.,* carbon dioxide gas (CO_2). Although there are only 105 known elements, the number of compounds that are known is already in the millions, and new ones are being created and discovered each year. The component parts of living cells and systems are composed of many large and complex molecules (macromolecules) that act, react, and interact to produce and maintain life. You will learn about many of these macromolecules, such as the polysaccharides, structural proteins, regulatory enzymes, and genetic DNA, although many of the most complex still remain to be fully identified.

Chemical Bonding

In general, atoms form molecules by gaining or losing electrons (forming ionic bonds) or by sharing electrons (forming covalent bonds). An *ionic bond* holds together molecules, such as sodium chloride (NaCl, common table salt) and many others, that ionize in water. When sodium chloride dissolves in water, the sodium atom (Na) loses a negative electron and assumes a positive charge, thus becoming a positive ion (Na^+)

Table 3-1 The First 20 Elements

Element	Symbol	Atomic Number	Atomic Weight
Hydrogen	H	1	1
Helium	He	2	4
Lithium	Li	3	6.9
Beryllium	Be	4	9
Boron	B	5	10.8
Carbon	C	6	12
Nitrogen	N	7	14
Oxygen	O	8	16
Fluorine	F	9	19
Neon	Ne	10	20.1
Sodium	Na	11	23
Magnesium	Mg	12	24.3
Aluminum	Al	13	27
Silicon	Si	14	28.1
Phosphorus	P	15	31
Sulfur	S	16	32.1
Chlorine	Cl	17	35.5
Argon	Ar	18	40
Potassium	K	19	39.1
Calcium	Ca	20	40.1

in solution. Likewise, the chlorine atom (Cl) accepts one electron from the donor sodium atom (Na) to become a chloride ion (Cl^-). The ionic bonds between sodium and chlorine atoms are easily broken, and they re-form in solution because the unlike charges are attracted to each other. They may temporarily form NaCl molelcules, and then dissociate into ions again (Fig. 3-2). Positively charged ions are called *cations*, and negatively charged ions are *anions*.

Other molecules, especially those in carbon compounds, are held together by covalent bonds. A *covalent bond* is formed by atoms sharing one or more pairs of electrons. In the example, methane (CH_4), the hydrogen atoms each share two electrons with the carbon atom (Fig. 3-3). This is a much stronger bond than an ionic bond; thus, the molecule is much more stable. All of organic chemistry is based on the stable, covalently bonded carbon molecules and how they react with other molecules. Biochemistry, the chemistry of living cells and systems, is a study of the large macromolecules composed of covalently bonded carbon, hydrogen, oxygen, nitrogen, phosphorus, and sulfur atoms. The loosely bound electrons on the surface of the macromolecules enable them to react and bind with other molecules in living organisms. Peptide bonds (which hold amino acids together in a protein) and glycosidic bonds (which bind the sugar groups of polysaccharides together) are also covalent bonds.

Hydrogen bonding occurs when a hydrogen atom that is covalently bonded to an oxygen or nitrogen atom is attracted to another oxygen or nitrogen atom on a different molecule or group, as seen in the α-helix of DNA and protein structure.

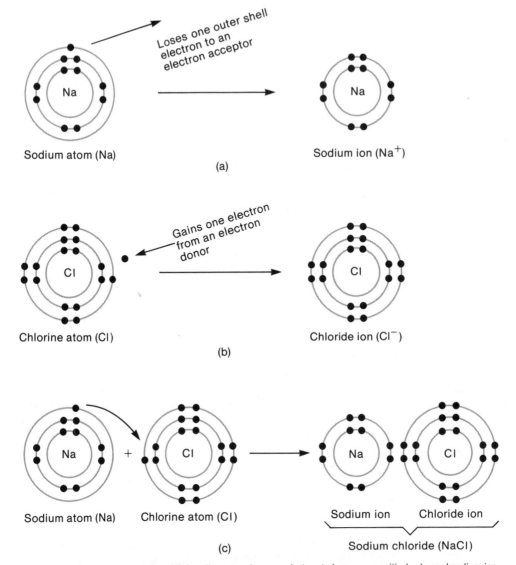

Fig. 3-2. Ionic bond formation. (*A*) A sodium atom loses an electron to become a positively charged sodium ion (Na$^+$). (*B*) A chlorine atom gains an electron to become a negatively charged chloride ion (Cl$^-$). (*C*) The positive sodium ion is attracted to the negative chloride ion to form the sodium chloride molecule, held together by a weak ionic bond.

Importance of Water in Living Cells and Systems

Water is the most abundant molecule in living cells; it is absolutely essential for living cells to function. The molecule, consisting of two hydrogen atoms on one side of an oxygen atom, gives the molecule polarity; that is, water molecules have positive and negative ends (Fig. 3-4). This characteristic makes water an ideal solvent, or

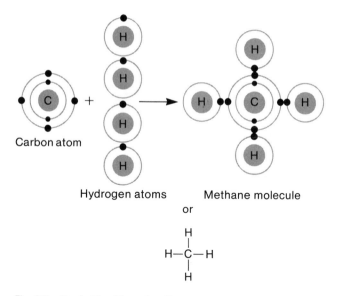

Carbon atom

Hydrogen atoms   Methane molecule

or

$$H-\underset{\overset{\displaystyle |}{H}}{\overset{\overset{\displaystyle H}{|}}{C}}-H$$

Fig. 3-3. Covalent bond formation. The methane molecule with four hydrogen atoms sharing electrons with a carbon atom, forming four covalent bonds.

suspending medium, for other ionic or charged molecules. The hydrogen bonding, or attraction between water molecules, is called *polar bonding*.

This polarity of water accounts for four major characteristics that make it an essential part of living cells.

1. Water is an excellent solvent (a liquid in which some other chemical, called the solute, is dissolved, thus forming a solution). The nutrients and waste

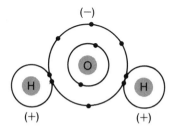

Fig. 3-4. A water molecule, showing two hydrogen atoms covalently bonded to an oxygen atom. The arrangement gives the molecule a more positive charge near the hydrogen protons and a negative charge near the oxygen electrons, thus providing an attraction between water molecules (polar bonding).

materials may move in and out of a cell, across the cell membrane, because they are dissolved in water.

2. Its polarity makes the molecules adhere, producing surface tension and capillary action, hence, water can move within and among cells and tissues.

3. It also serves as an excellent buffer against heat changes to protect the cell from fluctuation in temperature, because it can absorb and hold large amounts of heat.

4. Water enters into *hydrolysis* reactions (digestion of large macromolecules by breaking apart the molecular units) and *dehydrolysis* reactions (in which the macromolecules are synthesized with the removal of a water molecule).

Solutions, Acids, Bases, Salts, *p*H

Solutions of various types are the result of the mixing of elements with elements, elements with compounds, or compounds with compounds. It is these homogeneous mixtures, called solutions, that form almost all existing substances. The most common solutions are those in which a compound is dissolved in the solvent, water. Other solvents, such as alcohol, are more commonly used with organic compounds. There are some compounds that have characteristics that set them distinctly apart from others; these are acids and bases. One interesting feature of these two groups is that any acid will react with any base, almost without exception. This is not so with other classes of compounds. It is also relatively easy to measure the acidity or alkalinity of solutions of acids and bases.

Acids   The sour taste of lemons, grapefruit, and vinegar is a familiar sensation. Acids can be recognized by this sour taste; however, with many acids this is *not* a safe method of identification because they may be poisonous or very destructive to human tissues. Acids are identified by a more reliable, safer technique using chemical indicators or dyes that exhibit a distinct color in an acid solution. Some common acids are shown in Table 3-2.

All acids behave in a similar way, so there must be a feature that is common to each; this is the ability to produce hydrogen when in solution. An acid molecule will

Table 3-2 A Few Common Acids and Their Formulas

Acid	Formula	Location or Use
Hydrochloric acid	HCl	Acid in stomach
Sulfuric acid	H_2SO_4	Industrial mineral acid and battery acid
Boric acid	H_3BO_3	Eye wash
Nitric acid	HNO_3	Industrial oxidizing acid
Acetic acid	$HC_2H_3O_2$	Acid in vinegar
Formic acid	$HCHO_2$	Acid in some insect bites
Carbonic acid	H_2CO_3	Acid in carbonated drinks

$$HCl \quad + \quad H_2O \quad \longrightarrow \quad H^+ \; + \; Cl^- \quad + \quad H_2O$$

Hydrogen chloride molecule + Water molecule   Hydrogen ion + Chloride ion + Water molecule

Fig. 3-5. Hydrochloric acid.

have at least one hydrogen atom. As an illustration, consider hydrogen chloride or hydrochloric acid, which has the formula HCl. Hydrochloric acid in pure form is a gas, but when bubbled into water it reacts, and frees its hydrogen ion (H^+) and gives an electron to the chloride (Cl^-) particle. The result is a cation (the positively charged hydrogen) and an anion (the negatively charged chloride), as illustrated in the reaction equation (Fig. 3-5).

Notice that the HCl is an electrolyte; that is, it is a substance with charged particles that can conduct electricity. All acids produce hydrogen ions, which are the particles that contribute to the sour taste of acids and also affect the color of indicators. Indicator dyes are acidic or basic compounds that have distinctive color when in acid or base solutions.

Bases If you have had the misfortune to taste soap, you know what bases taste like. However, this is not a wise method to use for identification of a base. These substances have a hydroxide ion as their common feature. When dissolved in water, they release the hydroxide ion and a cation, and become electrolytes. Table 3-3 lists some common bases. Notice the hydroxide ion (OH^-) in their formulas.

As mentioned before, all acids will react with all bases. When they react they form one common product, water (H_2O). To illustrate, three reactions between different acids and bases are listed in Fig. 3-6.

Acid–base reactions can be summarized by a general statement: *An acid plus a base produces a salt and water.*

Salts Salts are another general class of electrolytic compounds. Chemical formulas are often written in a manner to assist in determining whether a substance is acid, base, or salt. For example, acids are written with an H or Hs at the left, as in HCl and H_2SO_4. Bases have an OH at the right, such as NaOH and $Mg(OH)_2$. The formulas for salts have neither an H at the left nor an OH at the right. Sodium chloride, NaCl, and sodium hydrogen carbonate, $NaHCO_3$, are examples.

Table 3-3 Some Common Bases

Base	Formula	Location or Use
Sodium hydroxide	NaOH	Caustic soda
Potassium hydroxide	KOH	Caustic potash
Ammonium hydroxide	NH_4OH	Household cleaners
Calcium hydroxide	$Ca(OH)_2$	Limewater
Magnesium hydroxide	$Mg(OH)_2$	Antacid drug

$$HCl + NaOH \longrightarrow NaCl + H_2O$$
$$H_2SO_4 + Mg(OH)_2 \longrightarrow MgSO_4 + 2\ H_2O$$
$$H_2CO_3 + NaOH \longrightarrow NaHCO_3 + H_2O$$

Fig. 3-6. General equation: "acid" + "base" $\longrightarrow$ "salt" + "water."

It is important, not only for human cells, tissues, and organs, but also for all microorganisms to have and maintain the appropriate acid, base, and salt balance to metabolize and function properly. When a nutrient medium is prepared for growing microbial cells in the laboratory, the correct acid–base–salt balance is as important as the availability of the necessary nutrients.

pH   pH is a measure of acidity. Acids have the property of being acidic, and bases are basic or alkaline in nature. The pH scale used to indicate acidic or alkaline character ranges from 0 to 14, with 7 as the neutral point (Fig. 3-7). Pure water has a pH of 7. If an acid is added to the water, the pH will decrease to between 0 and 7. Adding a base gives a pH between 7 and 14. Table 3-4 is a list of some common substances and their pH.

The pH of substances can be measured with a pH meter, with indicator solutions, or with chemically treated papers that turn a definite color at certain pH ranges. These papers are called indicator papers. In the human body the pH of various fluids (blood, lymph) must remain within very narrow ranges to keep the delicately balanced metabolic process working properly; as with microbial cells, if the pH varies too far from optimum, metabolism is disrupted and death may result.

Basic Organic Chemistry

Organic chemistry is that branch of the science of chemistry that deals primarily with the element carbon and its covalent bond. This definition makes organic chemistry a broad and an important branch of the science of chemistry.

Carbon Bonds

In our current understanding of life, carbon is the primary requisite for all living systems. The element carbon exists in three forms: diamond, graphite, and carbon or carbon black. These three forms of the element have dramatically different physical

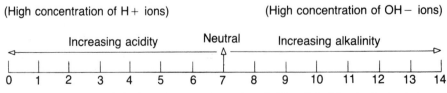

Fig. 3-7. The pH scale is derived by using a complex mathematical formula to determine the free hydrogen ion (H^+) concentration. (Rosdahl CB: Textbook of Basic Nursing, 4th ed. Philadelpia, JB Lippincott, 1985)

Table 3-4 The pH of Some Common Substances

Substance	pH
Household ammonia cleaner	11.9
Blood (human)	7.35–7.45
Pure H_2O	7
Milk	6.9
Black coffee	5
Orange juice	2.9
Gastric juice (stomach acid)	1.5

properties, and it is difficult to believe that they are truly the same substance. In addition to these unique physical differences, carbon has a valence of 4, which means that its atoms will bond to four other atoms. For convenience, the carbon atom will be illustrated with the symbol C and four bonds, as shown:

$$-\overset{|}{\underset{|}{C}}-$$

The uniqueness of carbon lies in the ability of its atoms to bond to each other to form an unbelievable number of compounds. The variety of carbon compounds increases dramatically when atoms of other elements also attach in different ways to the carbon atom.

When two carbon atoms bond together there are three types of resulting covalent bonds: *single bonds, double bonds,* and *triple bonds.* Each line represents a bond between the carbon atoms, which is formed from a pair of shared electrons.

$$-\overset{|}{\underset{|}{C}}-\overset{|}{\underset{|}{C}}- \qquad \overset{\diagdown}{\diagup}C{=}C\overset{\diagup}{\diagdown} \qquad -C{\equiv}C-$$

Single bond   Double bond   Triple bond

When atoms of other elements attach to additional available bonds of the carbon atom, stable compounds are formed. For example, if hydrogens are bonded to the available bonds, compounds called *hydrocarbons* are formed. Just a few of the many hydrocarbon compounds are shown in Figure 3-8.

$$H-\overset{H}{\underset{H}{C}}-H \qquad \overset{H}{\diagdown}C{=}C\overset{H}{\diagup} \qquad H-C{\equiv}C-H$$

Methane   Ethylene   Acetylene

Fig. 3-8. Simple hydrocarbons.

Fig. 3-9. The benzene ring.

When more than two carbons are linked together, longer molecules are formed. Many carbon atoms bonded together is logically called a *chain*. The long-chain hydrocarbons are usually liquid or solid; the short-chain hydrocarbons, such as the ones in Figure 3-8, are gases.

"Ring" Compounds

Carbon atoms that link to carbon atoms may close the chain, forming ring or cyclic compounds. An example is benzene, which has six carbons and six hydrogens bonded, as shown in Figure 3-9.

Biochemistry

Biochemistry is the study of living matter and its biochemical changes or metabolism. The large biochemical molecules, called macromolecules, are present in every cell in animals, plants, and microorganisms. These macromolecules are of many different types and are classified as carbohydrates, lipids, proteins, and nucleic acids. The vitamins, enzymes, hormones, and energy-carrying molecules, such as adenosine triphosphate (ATP), are also included among these biochemicals.

Humans obtain their nutrients from the foods they eat. The carbohydrates, fats, and proteins contained in these foods are digested, and their components are absorbed by the blood and carried to every cell in the body. In the body cells, the components from the food biochemicals are absorbed and rearranged. In this way, the proper compounds necessary for cell structure and function are synthesized. Microorganisms also absorb their essential nutrients into the cell by various means to be described in Chapter 5. These nutrients are then utilized in metabolic reactions as sources of energy and building blocks for enzymes and structural macromolecules.

Carbohydrates

Carbohydrates are composed of carbon (C), hydrogen (H), and oxygen (O) in the ratio of $1:2:1$, or simply CH_2O.

Fig. 3-10. Glucose. The straight-chain and alpha and beta forms may all exist in equilibrium in solution.

Monosaccharides The simplest carbohydrates are sugars; the smallest molecule of sugar is the monosaccharide (Gr. *mono* = one; *sakcharon* = sugar). The most important monosaccharide in nature is *glucose* ($C_6H_{12}O_6$), which may occur in the chain or alpha or beta ring configurations, as shown in Figure 3-10.

The main source of energy for body cells, glucose (dextrose), is found in most sweet fruits and in blood sugar. The glucose carried in the blood to the cells is oxidized to produce the high-energy molecule ATP with its high-energy phosphate bonds. This ATP molecule is the main source of energy used to drive most metabolic reactions. Other monosaccharides, with the aldehyde group on the first carbon, are galactose and ribose (a five-carbon sugar). An important monosaccharide that has a ketone group on the second carbon is *fructose* (Fig. 3-11). Fructose, the sweetest of the monosaccharides, is found in fruits and honey.

Fig. 3-11. Fructose in straight-chain form. (Fructose may also exist in the ring form as shown in Fig. 3-12.)

Fig. 3-12. The dehydration synthesis and hydrolysis of sucrose.

Disaccharides Disaccharides are sugars that result from the combination of two monosaccharides. Sucrose (or table sugar) is a sweet *disaccharide* made up of a glucose molecule and a fructose molecule (Fig. 3-12).

Disaccharides react with water in a process called hydrolysis. This causes them to break down into two monosaccharides:

$$\text{maltose} + H_2O \rightleftharpoons \text{glucose} + \text{glucose}$$
$$\text{lactose} + H_2O \rightleftharpoons \text{glucose} + \text{galactose}$$
$$\text{sucrose} + H_2O \rightleftharpoons \text{glucose} + \text{fructose}$$
$$\text{disaccharides} \rightleftharpoons 2 \text{ monosaccharides}$$

Maltose is the sugar in malt. Lactose is the sugar found in milk. Sucrose comes from sugar cane, sugar beets, and maple sugar. The synthesis of disaccharides from two monosaccharides with the removal of water is called *dehydration synthesis* or *dehydrolysis* (see Fig. 3-12).

Polysaccharides Polysaccharides, such as starch, cellulose, and glycogen, are essentially polymers made up of hundreds of glucose units or long chains of the monosaccharide, glucose, held together by glycosidic bonds. *Polymer* means "many parts", these large polysaccharide molecules are made of many saccharide molecules. Some of these molecules are so large that they are insoluble in water. In the presence of the proper enzymes or acids, polysaccharides may be hydrolyzed or broken down into disaccharides and then finally into monosaccharides (Fig. 3-13).

1 starch (polysaccharide)

2 maltose (disaccharide)

4 glucose (monosaccharide)

Fig. 3-13. The hydrolysis of starch.

β (beta) linkage (alternating "up and down") in cellulose

α (alpha) linkage (no alternation) in starch

Fig. 3-14. The difference between cellulose and starch.

Polysaccharides serve two main functions. One is to store energy that can be used when the food supply is low. The common storage molecule in animals is *glycogen*, which is found in the liver and in muscles. In plants, glucose is stored as *starch* and is found in potatoes and other vegetables and seeds. Some algae store starch; and bacteria contain glycogen granules as reserve nutrient supply.

The other function of polysaccharides is to provide a "tough" molecule for structural support and protection. Many bacteria secrete polysaccharide capsules for protection against drying and phagocytosis. Plant and algae cells have cellulose cell walls to provide support and shape, as well as protection against the environment.

Cellulose is insoluble in water and indigestible for humans and most animals. Some protozoa, fungi, and bacteria have enzymes that will break the β-glycosidic bonds linking the glucose units in cellulose. These are the microorganisms that are able to disintegrate dead plants in the soil and that live in the digestive organs of herbivores (plant eaters). Starch and glycogen are easily digested by animals because they have the digestive enzyme to hydrolyze the α-glycosidic bonds that link the glucose units into long, loose, helical or branched polymers (Fig. 3-14).

Fibers of cellulose extracted from certain plants are used to make paper, cotton, linen, and rope. These fibers are relatively rigid, strong, and insoluble because they consist of 100 to 200 parallel strands of cellulose.

When polysaccharides are combined with other chemical groups (amines, lipids, and amino acids), extremely complex macromolecules are formed that serve specific purposes. Glucosamine and galactosamine (amine derivatives of glucose and galactose, respectively) are important constituents of the supporting polysaccharides in connective tissue fibers, cartilage, and chitin. Chitin is the main component of the hard outer covering of insects, spiders, crabs, and fungi. The main portion of the rigid cell wall of bacteria consists of aminosugars and short polypeptide chains that combine to form the peptidoglycan layer.

Lipids

Lipids are a class of biochemical compounds composed mainly of fats and oils. Most of them are insoluble in water but soluble in fat solvents such as ether, chloroform, and benzene. Lipids are essential constituents of almost all living cells. They may be classified into the following categories:

1. Simple lipids (contain C, H, O)
   a. Fats and oils (butter, vegetable oils)
   b. Waxes (beeswax, lanolin)
2. Compound lipids (contain C, H, O, N, and P)
   a. Phospholipids (in cell membranes)
   b. Glycolipids (in nerve cells)
3. Derived lipids (contain C, H, O)
   a. Steroids (sex hormones, cholesterol)
   b. Fat-soluble vitamins A, D, E, K

The simple lipids (*fats* and *oils*) consist of one molecule of glycerol and three fatty acid molecules joined together by the removal of three molecules of water (dehydrolysis), which produces a triglyceride fat or oil (Fig. 3-15).

If the hydrocarbon side chains have no double bonds between carbons, it is called a *saturated fatty acid* because every carbon atom is saturated with hydrogen. When there are double bonds between the carbons ($C = C$), it is an *unsaturated fatty acid*. Sources of unsaturated fats are peanut, olive, corn, soybean, and cottonseed oils. Fats are liquids or low-melting solids at room temperature, depending on the relative composition of the fatty acids. Unsaturated fatty acids with short carbon chains are usually liquids. Many people are on low-saturated fat diets to help prevent lipid cholesterol deposits in their hearts and arteries.

A nutritious human diet should include at least the two essential fatty acids because the body cannot synthesize them. These are linoleic acid ($C_{17}H_{31}COOH$), from fish liver oils and vegetable oils, and arachiedonic acid ($C_{19}H_{31}COOH$) from egg yolk, liver, kidney tissues, and fish liver oils. However, different fatty acids are produced by and are necessary for the growth of bacteria and other microorganisms depending on the species of the organism.

Saponification is the hydrolysis of a fat into glycerol (glycerin) and its three fatty acids. When NaOH or KOH (strong alkalis) are used to hydrolyze fats, the results are sodium or potassium salts of the fatty acids, which are soaps. Detergents, bile salts, and fat-digestive enzymes also saponify fats.

glycerol + 3 butyric acids
(a fatty acid)
$\xrightarrow{-3H_2O}$
tributyrin
(a triglyceride fat)

Fig. 3-15. The synthesis of a fat.

Waxes   Waxes are chemically different from fats because they are long-chain or complex alcohols, other than glycerol, with fatty acids attached. Waxes are semisolid substances that serve as a protective coating on the surfaces of leaves, stems, fruits, insects, and some bacteria.

Compound Lipids   Compound lipids include the phospholipids of cell membranes and the glycolipids of nerve and brain cells. Even when an organism is starving, the amount of these nonfat lipids in the cells does not vary.

Derived Lipids   Derived lipids are classified as lipids because they are also soluble in fat solvents. These steroids are complex molecules of four interlocking carbon rings. Many steroid anti-inflammatory medications are produced by fungi and bacteria and are used in the treatment of arthritis and cancer patients. Other examples of steroids include cholesterol, male and female hormones, adrenal cortex hormones, and vitamin D. Vitamin A, E, and K are *not* steroids but are fat-soluble vitamins.

Cholesterol is a necessary body metabolite. It is found in most eucaryotic membranes and in nervous tissues and aids in fatty acid adsorption. It is also essential for the production of sex hormones, vitamin D, and adrenal cortex hormones. However, an excess of cholesterol may be deposited in the arteries and cause heart disease, or in the gallbladder and become gallstones.

Vitamin D helps maintain the calcium and phosphorus balance in the body. Good sources of vitamin D are fish oils and sunlight. Vitamin A can be obtained from liver, eggs, butter, cheese, carrots, and green leafy vegetables; a lack of this vitamin can lead to night blindness or hardening of the mucous membranes.

Vitamin E (from plant oils, leafy vegetables, and eggs) reduces sterility in animals and the wasting effects of aging. Vitamin K, which is synthesized in the body, is necessary for normal blood clotting.

Proteins

Proteins are among the most essential chemicals in all living cells. Some are the structural components of membranes, cells, and tissues, whereas others are enzymes and hormones that chemically control the metabolic balance within the cell and the individual organism. All proteins are polymers of amino acids; however, they vary widely in the number of amino acids, in the sequence of amino acids, and in their size, configuration, and functions.

Proteins are synthesized by plants, algae, and bacteria from carbon dioxide, water, nitrates, and sulfates, through the process called photosynthesis. In this process, the chemicals combine with the aid of the sun's energy. Humans can synthesize proteins, but they must ingest eight essential amino acids to synthesize the others necessary in the building of proteins. Nonphotosynthetic microorganisms also must absorb their essential amino acids that are not synthesized or stored in living cells. All the amino acids (ingested and synthesized) must be present during the protein syn-

$$\text{Basic amine group} \qquad H-\overset{\displaystyle H}{\underset{\displaystyle |}{N}}-\overset{\displaystyle H}{\underset{\displaystyle |}{\underset{\displaystyle |}{\underset{\displaystyle R}{C}}}}-\overset{\displaystyle O}{\underset{}{\overset{\displaystyle ||}{C}}}-OH \qquad \text{Acid carboxyl group}$$

Fig. 3-16. The basic structure of amino acids.

thesis process in the cells. Any excess can be used to produce energy or eliminated with the soluble wastes.

Amino Acid Structure There are 20 different amino acids. Each is composed of carbon, hydrogen, oxygen, and nitrogen; three also have sulfur atoms in the molecule. The general formula for amino acids is shown in Figure 3-16.

The "R" group represents any of the 20 groups that may be substituted into that position to build the various amino acids. For instance, —H in place of the —R represents glycine, and —CH_3 in that position results in a structural formula representing alanine.

The thousands of different proteins in the body are composed of a great variety of amino acids in various arrangements and amounts. The number of proteins that can be synthesized is unlimited, for all practical purposes. They are not limited by the number of different amino acids, just as the number of words in the written language is not limited by the number of letters in the alphabet. The actual number of proteins produced by an organism and the amino acid sequence of those proteins are determined by the particular genes present on the chromosomes.

Protein Structure When water is removed, by dehydrolysis, the amino acids are linked together by a peptide bond as shown in Figure 3-17. A *dipeptide* is formed by bonding two amino acids; three linked together form a tripeptide. A long chain or polymer of amino acids is referred to as a *polypeptide*. Polypeptides are said to have *primary protein structure*, a sequence of amino acids in a chain, (Fig. 3-18). Some fibrous proteins are made of strands of polypeptides bonded to each other by hydrogen bonds and wound together into a helix. Collagen, found in connective tissue, scars, and tendons is such a fibrous protein, consisting of three polypeptides in a triple helix, forming a very strong structure.

Most polypeptide chains naturally twist into spirals or helices as a result of the

amino acid₁ + amino acid₂ ⟶ dipeptide

Fig. 3-17. The formation of a dipeptide (R = any amino acid side-chain group).

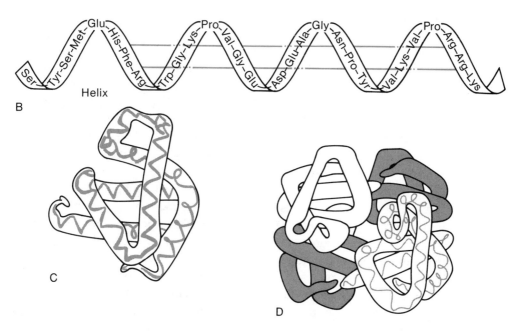

Ser—Tyr—Ser—Met—Glu—His—Phe—Arg—Trp—Gly—Lys—Pro—Val—Gly—Lys

A

Helix

B

C

D

Fig. 3-18. Basic protein structure. (*A*) Primary sequence of amino acids. (*B*) Secondary helix. (*C*) Tertiary globular structure. (*D*) Quarternary structure with four polypeptide chains.

charged side chains protruding from the carbon–nitrogen backbone of the molecule. This helical configuration is refered to as *secondary protein structure,* and is found in fibrous proteins such as the keratin fibers of hair, nails, and skin, and the microtubules and microfilaments of cells.

Because a long coil can become entwined by folding back on itself, a polypeptide helix becomes globular (see Fig. 3-18). In some areas the helix is retained, but other areas curve randomly. This gobular, *tertiary protein structure* is stabilized, not only by hydrogen bonding but also by disulfide bond cross-links between two sulfur groups (S—S). This three-dimensional configuration is characteristic of enzymes, which work by fitting on and into specific molecules.

When two or more polypeptide chains are bonded together by hydrogen and disulfide bonds, the resulting structure is referred to as *quaternary protein structure* (see Fig. 3-18). For instance, hemoglobin consists of four globular-shaped myoglobins. The size, shape, and configuration of a protein is specific for the function it must perform. If the amino acid sequence and, thus, the configuration of hemoglobin in red blood cells is not perfect, the red blood cells may become distorted and assume a sickle shape (as in sickle cell anemia). In this state they are unable to carry oxygen, which is necessary for cellular metabolism. Myoglobin, the oxygen-binding protein found in skeletal muscles, was the first protein to have its primary, secondary, and tertiary structure defined.

Enzymes   *Enzymes* are protein molecules produced by living cells as "ordered" by the DNA or genes on the chromosomes. Enzymes are essential as catalysts in the biochemical reactions of metabolism; in other words, they speed up these reactions. Almost every reaction in the cell requires the presence of a specific enzyme. All enzymes are proteins; many consist of protein only, whereas some require a non-protein *cofactor*, such as metal ions (Ca^{2+}, Fe^{2+}, Mg^{2+}, Cu^{2+}) or organic compounds such as vitamin C. Although enzymes influence the direction of the reaction and increase its rate, they do not provide the energy needed to activate the reaction.

Enzymes are usually named by adding the ending *-ase* to the word indicating the substrate upon which the enzyme functions. For example, a protease catalyzes the breakdown of proteins, whereas a lipase catalyzes the breakdown of lipids.

Poisons and toxins usually cause damage to the body by interfering with the action of certain necessary enzymes. For example, cyanide poison binds to the iron and copper ions in the cytochrome systems of the mitochondria of cells. As a result, the cells cannot use oxygen to synthesize ATP for energy, and they soon die.

Proteins, including enzymes, may be denatured by heat or certain chemicals. In a denatured protein, the bonds that hold the molecule in a tertiary structure are broken. With the bonds broken, the protein is no longer functional. Enzymes are also discussed in Chapter 4.

Nucleic Acids

The fourth major group of macromolecules in living cells are the nucleic acids: deoxyribonucleic acid (DNA) and ribonucleic acid (RNA). DNA is the macromolecule that makes up the major portion of the chromosomes. Its important task is to carry the genetic information for each cell of an organism. The information from the DNA must be carried to the rest of the cell for it to function properly; this is accomplished by RNA. Thus, RNA is found not only in the nucleus but in the cytoplasm as well.

Function   Nucleic acids have two very important functions. First, the nucleic acids determine precisely which proteins are synthesized and the protein enzymes control the metabolism of the organism. Also, the genetic information must be passed from one generation to the next, from each parent cell to each daughter cell. This is the second role of DNA: it is the genetic "molecular blueprint of life."

Structure   In addition to carbon, hydrogen, oxygen, and nitrogen, DNA and RNA contain the element phosphorus, whereas the proteins contain sulfur. The building blocks of these nucleic acid polymers are the *nucleotides*. These are more complex

Fig. 3-19. Two nucleotides consisting of a nitrogen base, a five-carbon sugar, and a phosphate group.

monomers than the amino acids, the building blocks of proteins. The nucleotides consist of three subunits: a nitrogen-containing base, a five-carbon sugar, and a phosphate group joined together, as shown in Figure 3-19.

As previously stated, there are two kinds of nucleic acids in cells: DNA and RNA. DNA contains deoxyribose as its five-carbon sugar (a pentose), whereas RNA has ribose sugar. There are three types of RNA, which are named for the function they serve: messenger RNA (mRNA), ribosomal RNA (rRNA), and transfer RNA (tRNA). The five most important nitrogen-containing bases are adenine (A), guanine (G), thymine (T), cytosine (C), and uracil (U). Thymine occurs in DNA and uracil in RNA. The other bases occur in both DNA and RNA.

The nucleotides join between their sugar and phosphate groups to form very long polymers, 100,000 or more monomers long, as shown in Figure 3-20.

DNA Structure In 1953, James Watson and Francis Crick proposed a double-stranded helical structure for DNA to indicate how it could copy itself exactly (replicate) to pass the genetic information to each daughter cell. For a double-stranded DNA to form, the bases must bond together. It was found that adenine always bonds with thymine (with two hydrogen bonds) and guanine with cytosine (with three hydrogen bonds) because of the size and bonding attraction between the molecules. The bonding forces of the

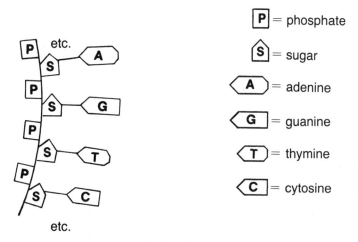

Fig. 3-20. Nucleic acid polymer.

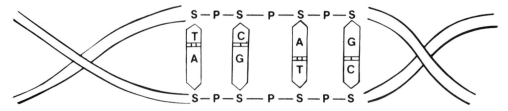

Fig. 3-21. The DNA double helix.

double-stranded polymer cause it to assume the shape of a double α-helix, which is similar to a right-handed staircase (Fig. 3-21).

Replication   When a cell is preparing to divide, all of the DNA molecules in the chromosomes of that cell must duplicate, thereby ensuring that the same genetic information will be passed to each daughter cell. This process is called DNA replication. It occurs by the separation of the DNA strands and the building of complementary strands by the addition of the correct nucleotides, as indicated in Figure 3-22. The duplicated DNA of the chromosomes can then be separated during ordinary cell division so that the same number of chromosomes, the same genes, and the same amount of DNA as in the parent cell are found in each daughter cell (except during meiosis, the reduction division to produce egg and sperm cells).

Protein Synthesis   In a normally functioning living cell, the DNA of the chromosomes controls all the metabolic activities. It accomplishes this by directing the synthesis of the protein enzymes that regulate the chemical reactions occurring in normal metabolism.

The translation and interpretation of the information carried by the DNA molecule to produce the proper proteins is a complex procedure. It is the sequence and order of the four nitrogen-containing bases (A, T, C, and G) that determine or carry

Fig. 3-22. Replication of DNA before cell division.

the code for the amino acid sequences of the protein to be synthesized in the cytoplasm of the cell. A diagrammatic representation of this process is shown in Figure 3-23.

You should remember that the *chromosomes* in the nuclear region of the cell consist of many *genes* that carry the genetic information for the inherited traits of the organism. Each gene consists of several *cistrons,* which are the portions of the DNA of the chromosome that code for *one* particular protein or enzyme.

When a cell is stimulated (by need) to produce a particular protein, such as insulin, the DNA of the appropriate cistron is activated to unwind temporarily from its helical configuration. This unwinding exposes the bases, which then attract the bases of free nucleotides, and a *messenger RNA* (mRNA) begins to build on one strand, the activated strand, of the opened DNA. Thus, the DNA has served as a *template,* or pattern, and has coded for a complementary mirror image of its structure in the RNA. This procedure is called *transcription* because the message from the DNA is transcribed onto the mRNA. After the mRNA has been synthesized over the length of the cistron,

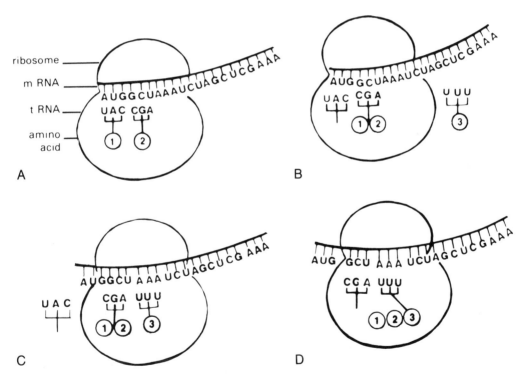

Fig. 3-23. Outline of protein synthesis. (*A*) Messenger RNA bound to ribosome. Amino acids 1 and 2 are bonded to their transfer RNAs. The t-RNA-amino acid 1 is bound to the peptidyl binding site. The t-RNA-amino acid 2 is bound to the amino acid binding site. (*B*) Amino acid 1 is released from its t-RNA and is joined to amino acid 2 through a peptide bond. (*C*) The ribosome moves along the m-RNA, and t-RNA 1 leaves the peptidyl binding site. The t-RNA 2 with the attached dipeptide moves to the peptidyl site and t-RNA amino acid 3 binds to the amino acid binding site. (*D*) Amino acid 2 is bonded to amino acid 3 as in step *B*. The process repeats until the protein is completed.

it is freed from the active DNA strand to carry the message to the cytoplasm to direct the synthesis of that particular protein (here, insulin).

The freed mRNA passes through the pores of the nuclear membrane into the cytoplasm and takes its position on the protein "assembly line": the ribosomes containing ribosomal RNA (rRNA), which attracts the mRNA. The ribosomes usually reside on the endoplasmic reticulum membranes in eucaryotic cells.

The base sequence of the mRNA is read or interpreted by the rRNA in groups of three bases, called *codons*. The sequence of the three bases of the codon codes for, or determines, which amino acid goes in that position in the protein being synthesized. The amino acids must be transferred or carried by an activated *transfer RNA* (tRNA) from the cytoplasmic matrix to the site of protein assembly. The three-base sequence of the codon determines which tRNA will bring its specific amino acid to the ribosome, because the RNA has an *anticodon*, three-base sequence, which is complementary to, or will be attracted to, the codon of the mRNA. For example, the tRNA with the anticodon base sequence UUU carries the amino acid lysine to the mRNA codon AAA. Similarly, the mRNA codon CCG codes for the tRNA anticodon GGC, which carries the amino acid proline at the opposite end of the tRNA molecule. This code system is called the *genetic code*. A chart can be prepared to show which sequence of three bases in the DNA codes for a particular codon in mRNA, which calls a particular anticodon on the tRNA carrying a specific amino acid.

The process of translating the message carried by the mRNA and decoded by the rRNA, which calls the particular tRNAs to bring the amino acids to be bound together in the proper sequence to make a specific protein (*e.g.*, insulin), is called *translation*. This process is summarized in Figure 3-23. It should be noted that the living cell is constantly producing mRNA in its nucleus, which will direct the synthesis of all the proteins, including metabolic enzymes necessary for the normal functions of that specific type of cell. Also, the mRNA and tRNA are short-lived nucleic acids that may be reused many times, then destroyed and resynthesized in the nucleus. The rRNA is made in the dense portion of the nucleus called the nucleolus; the ribosomes last longer in the cell than the mRNA.

As the tRNA molecules attach to mRNA while it is sliding over the ribosomes, they bring the correct activated amino acids into contact with each other so that peptide bonds are made and a polypeptide is formed. As the polypeptide grows and becomes a protein, it folds into the unique shape determined by the amino acid sequence. This characteristic shape allows the protein to perform its specific function. If one DNA cistron base is out of sequence, the amino acid sequence will not be correct and the protein configuration will not allow the protein to function properly. For instance, some diabetics may not produce insulin properly because a mutation in the DNA of their chromosomes caused a rearrangement of the bases in the cistron that codes for insulin. This is the basis for most genetic and inherited diseases, such as phenylketonuria (PKU), sickle cell anemia, cerebral palsy, cystic fibrosis, cleft lip, clubfoot, extra fingers, albinism, and many other birth defects resulting from DNA errors. Likewise, nonpathogenic microbes may mutate to become pathogens, and pathogens may lose the ability to cause disease by mutation, or change in the DNA sequence.

A new science, genetic engineering, that attempts to repair the genetic damage in some diseases has developed. As yet, the morality of manipulation of human genes has not been resolved by society. However, many genetically changed microbes are able to produce substances, such as human insulin, interferon, growth hormones, new pharmaceutical agents, and vaccines, that will have a substantial effect on the medical treatment of humans.

Problems and Questions

1. Describe the relationship between electrolyte, solvent, solute, and solution.
2. Differentiate between acids and bases, and give some examples of each.
3. If nutrient growth medium is too acidic or too basic, might a bacterial culture die? Why?
4. Why is it possible for humans to digest starch but not cellulose and chitin? Which microorganisms can digest cellulose?
5. Is the peptidoglycan layer of bacterial cell wall a polymer? If so, provide reasons to support this claim.
6. Are the fat-soluble vitamins lipids? Why? Where would lipids be found in bacterial cells?
7. What are the differences between structural proteins and enzyme proteins in a cell? Describe the primary, secondary, tertiary, and quaternary structure of proteins. How does an enzyme function?
8. Draw a hypothetical bacterium and indicate the types of macromolelcules found in its various parts.
9. Explain the chemical characteristics of polymers, carbohydrates, polysaccharides, sugars, cellulose, starch, lipids, proteins, fats, waxes, enzymes, peptides, and nucleic acids.
10. Differentiate between DNA, mRNA, rRNA, and tRNA. Which four bases are found in DNA? In RNA?

Chapter 4

Physiology of Microorganisms

New Words to Pronounce and Understand

Anabolism (an-ab'-bow-liz-em). Metabolic reactions that result in the biosynthesis of complex cellular materials

Autotrophs (awe'-toe-trophs). Organisms that obtain carbon from inorganic sources, as from carbon dioxide

Catabolism (ca-tab'-bow-liz-em). Metabolic reactions that break down organic materials into simple molecules

Catalyst (cat'-uh-list). A chemical agent that speeds up a reaction

Catalyze (cat'-uh-lyz). To speed up a reaction

Chemolithotrophs (key-moe-lith'-oh-trophs). Organisms that use a chemical source of energy and an inorganic source of nutrients

Chemoorganotrophs (key-moe-or-gan'-oh-trophs). Organisms that use a chemical source of energy and an organic source of nutrients

Chemotrophs (key'-moe-trophs). Organisms that obtain their energy from chemical sources

Corynebacterium diphtheriae (co-ri'-knee-back-tear-ee-um diff-theer'-ee-ee). Species of bacteria that causes diphtheria

Enzyme (en'-zime). A protein molecule that catalyzes biochemical reactions

Escherichia coli (es-ur-eek'-ee-uh co'-lie). A normal intestinal bacterium

Filamentous (fil-uh-men'-tus). Having many threads or filaments

Gene (jean). A portion of a chromosome, carrying genetic information for one polypeptide

Glycolysis (gly-col'-eh-sis). The anaerobic breakdown of glucose to pyruvic acid or lactic acid with the production of energy

Heterotrophs (het'-ter-oh-trophs). Organisms that obtain carbon from organic sources

Logarithm (log'-uh-rhy-thm). Mathematically, the power to which a number must be raised to produce a given number

Metabolism (muh-tab'-bow-liz-em). The sum of all the chemical reactions in living cells

Mutagenic (mew-tuh-jen'-ick). Producing mutations or genetic changes in organisms

Mutation (mew-tay'-shun). An inheritable change in a gene

Mutant (mew'-tant). An organism that has survived mutation

Mycobacterium tuberculosis (my-co-back-tear'-ee-um tu-bur-cue-low'-sis). Species of bacteria that causes tuberculosis

Photolithotrophs (foe-toe-lith'-oh-trophs). Organisms that use light for energy and inorganic chemicals for nutrients

Photoorganotrophs (foe-toe-or-gan'-oh-trophs). Organisms that use light for energy and organic chemicals for nutrients

Phototrophs (foe'-toe-trophs). Organisms that use light as their source of energy

Protoplasm (pro'-toe-plaz-um). The substance inside a cell

Protoplast (pro'-toe-plast). A bacterial cell with no cell wall

Pseudomonas (sue-doe-moan'-us). A genus of soil bacillus; may cause wound or lung infections

Saprophyte (sap'-row-fight). Organism that obtains its nutrients from dead, decaying organic matter

Staphylococci (staff-ill-oh-coc'-sigh). Cocci occurring in clusters; some may cause "staph" infections

> **Streptococci** (strep-toe-coc'-sigh). Cocci in chains; some may cause "strep" infections
>
> **Vibrio cholerae** (vib'-ree-oh col'-lar-ree). A species of bacteria that causes cholera

Microorganisms are perhaps the best organisms to use in our study of the basic metabolic processes of life. Species of bacteria can be found that represent each of the nutritional types of organisms on earth. We can learn much about ourselves by studying the nutritional needs of bacteria, their metabolic cycles, and why under certain conditions they grow or die. The population growth cycles of bacteria illustrate the growth phases of any population of a species of organism including humans.

Each tiny single-celled bacterium strives to produce more cells like itself, and it often does so at a rate that is alarming, as long as water and the nutrient supply are available. Under favorable conditions, in 24 hours, the offspring of a single *Escherichia coli* bacterium would outnumber the entire human population of the earth!

Bacteria are easy to find, to grow, and to maintain in the laboratory. Their morphology, their nutritional needs, and some of their metabolic reactions are easily observable, so that when these normal characteristics change in a pure culture, the resultant mutant (a genetically changed organism) can be quickly identified. Because some bacteria, molds, and viruses produce generation after generation so rapidly and easily, they have been used extensively in genetic studies. In fact, most of the genetic knowledge of today was and is being obtained from the study of these microorganisms.

Nutrition

The study of bacterial nutrition and other phases of microbial physiology helps one to understand the vital chemical processes of every living cell, including those of the human body.

Nutritional Requirements

All living protoplasm consists of six major chemical elements: carbon, hydrogen, oxygen, nitrogen, phosphorus, and sulfur. Other elements usually necessary in lesser amounts include sodium, potassium, chlorine, magnesium, calcium, iron, iodine, and some trace elements. The combinations of all of these elements make up the vital macromolecules of life, including carbohydrates, fats, proteins, and nucleic acids (DNA and RNA).

Each organism must have a source of energy and nutrient chemicals to build the necessary cellular materials of life. Those materials that organisms cannot synthesize in building the macromolecules of protoplasm are termed *essential nutritional requirements*. These are the nutrients that must be continually supplied to every organism for it to live. Essential nutrients will be variable from species to species.

The majority of microbes are *aerobes*, which means that they grow best in an atmosphere that contains oxygen. *Anaerobes* are those microbes that prefer to live without oxygen. *Facultative* anaerobes can survive in an atmosphere containing oxygen, whereas *obligate* anaerobes die if exposed to oxygen.

Nutritional Types

Because microorganisms have evolved from the beginning of life on earth, there are microbes representing each of the nutritional types.

Heterotrophs are organisms that obtain carbon from organic materials. All animals, including humans, and most microorganisms, including the pathogens, are heterotrophic organisms. Even the saprophytic fungi and bacteria that live on dead, decaying animal and plant material are heterotrophs.

Autotrophs are organisms that use inorganic carbon compounds, usually carbon dioxide (CO_2) as their basic carbon source. Plants, algae, and many bacteria are autotrophic organisms.

Heterotrophs and autotrophs may be further divided into *chemotrophs* and *phototrophs* according to their sources of energy. Chemotrophs are those organisms that use chemical substances as a source of energy, whereas phototrophs are those that use light for their energy source.

Descriptive terms have been developed to indicate the sources of energy and chemical nutrients for each type of microorganism by combining the words chemotroph and phototroph with terms indicating the sources of chemical nutrients. *Organo-* indicates the organic nutrients derived from living material such as carbohydrates, fats, proteins, and nucleic acids; *litho-* indicates inorganic sources of nutrients such as water, carbon dioxide, nitrates, phosphates, and sulfates. Thus, the first part of the words *chemoorganotroph*, *chemolithotroph*, *photoorganotroph*, and *photolithotroph* indicates the source of energy, and the middle portion of the word identifies the source of nutrients for the living organism (*-troph*). Another group of terms often used instead of these four are, respectively, *chemoheterotroph*, *chemoautotroph*, *photoheterotroph*, and *photoautotroph*. These relationships are further explained in the following outline:

I. Heterotrophic organisms (those using an organic carbon nutrient source)
   A. Chemoorganotrophs (chemoheterotrophs) are those chemotrophs that have a chemical source of energy and use organic materials as a source of nutrients. All animals, protozoa, fungi, and most bacteria fall into this subdivision.
   B. Photoorganotrophs (photoheterotrophs) include those phototrophs that use the ultraviolet rays of the sun as a source of energy and organic matter for nutrients. A few bacteria and a few types of algae are of this nutritional type.
II. Autotrophic organisms (those using an inorganic carbon nutrient source)
   A. Chemolithotrophs (chemoautotrophs) are chemotrophs that use inorganic chemicals such as iron, sulfur, water, carbon dioxide, nitrates,

and phosphates as sources of energy and nutrients. This nutritional type includes only a few groups of bacteria—those that oxidize nitrogen, iron, sulfur, uranium, methane, and carbon monoxide—but they are very important in the environmental cycles of these compounds.

B. Photolithotrophs (photoautotrophs) are phototrophs that trap the sun's ultraviolet energy source and use inorganic materials, such as water, carbon dioxide, nitrates, and phosphates, as sources of food nutrients. Most plants, algae, and the photosynthetic bacteria are photolithotrophic organisms. They contribute energy to the ecosystem by trapping energy from the sun and using it to build organic compounds (carbohydrates, fats, nucleic acids, and proteins) from the inorganic materials in the soil, water, and air. The ecosystem consists of the interaction between the living organisms and the nonliving environment. In photosynthesis, oxygen also is released for respiration by animals.

The interrelationships among these nutritional types are of prime importance in the functioning of the ecosystem. The photolithotrophs (plants) are the producers of food and oxygen for the chemoorganotrophs (animals). Both of these would clutter the earth with debris when they died if the chemoorganotrophic saprophytic decomposers (fungi and bacteria) did not break down the dead organic matter into the inorganic compounds (carbon dioxide, nitrates, phosphates) of the soil and air to be recyled by the photolithotrophs.

Enzymes, Metabolism, and Energy

Microorganisms are able to grow only if they obtain the proper raw materials for nutrients and for the manufacture of enzymes they need to promote metabolic reactions. These processes are similar to those in our own body cells. The term *metabolism* designates all chemical reactions that occur within any cell. These metabolic reactions are enhanced and regulated by the enzymes present.

Enzymes

Metabolic Enzymes   Enzymes are organic catalysts; that is, they are organic molecules that accelerate the rate of a biochemical reaction at certain temperatures without being used up in those reactions. These reactions would occur at the same temperature without enzymes but at a much slower rate. A *substrate* is a compound on which an enzyme exerts its effect. The enzyme must fit the combining site of the substrate as a key fits a lock. Usually, an enzyme is specific, that is, it works on only one type of substrate, but occasionally it can attach to different substrates because the shapes of the combining sites on the substrate molecules are similar (Fig. 4-1).

All enzymes are protein molecules; the three-dimensional shape of the protein

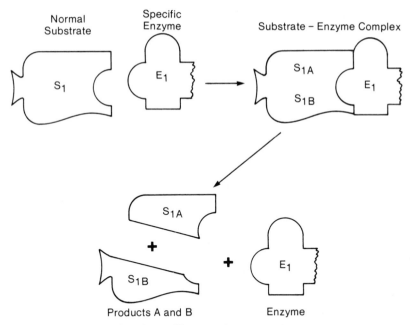

Fig. 4-1. Action of a specific enzyme breaking a substrate molecule.

enables it to attach to a substrate or substrates and accelerate a very slow reaction, without changing the enzyme in the process. The enzyme continues to move from substrate molecule to substrate molecule at a rate of several hundred each second, producing a supply of the end product, as long as this particular end product is needed by the cell. However, enzymes do not last indefinitely; they finally degenerate and lose their activity. Therefore, the cell must synthesize and replace these important proteins. Because there are hundreds of metabolic reactions continually occurring in the cell, there must be thousands of enzymes available to control and direct the essential metabolic pathways. At any particular time, all of the required enzymes need not be present; this situation is controlled by the genes on the chromosomes and the needs of the cell, which are determined by the internal and external environment. Those enzymes found inside the cell are called *endoenzymes,* and those secreted outside the cell to perform extracellular functions are *exoenzymes.* The digestive enzymes are good examples of endoenzymes. Exoenzymes are the enzymes secreted by saprophytes, which are then able to digest materials outside the organism. These nutrients digested outside are then absorbed into the organism.

Some enzymes require *cofactors* to activate them to perform their intended functions because they normally exist in the cell in an inactive state. These cofactors are usually mineral ions such as magnesium, calcium, or iron. Other enzymes function only in the presence of a *coenzyme* that acts as a carrier of small chemical groups (such as H_2) that are removed from the substrate. These coenzymes are small organic vitamin-type molecules such as flavin-adenine dinucleotide (FAD) and nicotinamide-adenine dinucleotide (NAD). The activity of these coenzymes is easily recognized in the citric acid cycle for the production of energy from glucose; these reactions are discussed later in this chapter. Coenzymes, like enzymes, do not have to be present in large amounts because they are recycled through many reactions. However, the lack of certain vitamins from which the coenzymes are synthesized will halt all those reactions involving that particular coenzyme–enzyme complex.

Enzymes are usually named by adding the suffix -ase to the name of the substrate or type of substrates with which they bind. Proteases, carbohydrases, and lipases are enzymes specific for proteins, carbohydrates, and lipids, respectively. These particular enzymes also may be called hydrolases because they break down macromolecules by the addition of water in a process called hydrolysis. These hydrolytic processes enable saprophytes to break apart such complex materials as leather, wax, cork, wood, rubber, hair, some plastics, and even mechanical equipment. Some of the enzymes involved in the formation of large polymers, DNA, and RNA, are called polymerases. These polymerases are active each time the DNA of a cell is replicated, and during the synthesis of RNA molecules.

Inhibition of Enzymes   Many factors affect the activity of enzymes (see Fig. 4-1). Any physical or chemical change may diminish or completely stop enzyme activity, because these protein molecules function properly only under optimum conditions. Optimum conditions for enzyme activity include a relatively limited range of pH (acidity) and temperature, and the appropriate concentration of enzyme and substrate. Extremes in heat and acidity can denature (or alter) enzymes by breaking the bonds responsible for their three-dimensional shape, resulting in the loss of enzymatic activity. This explains why bacteria grow best at certain temperatures and pH, characteristic for each species of organism.

Although the mineral ions, calcium, magnesium, and iron, enhance the activity of enzymes by serving as cofactors, other heavy metal ions such as lead, zinc, mercury, and arsenic usually act as poisons to the cell. These toxic ions will inhibit enzyme activity by replacing the cofactors, or sometimes replacing only hydrogen, at the combining site of the enzyme, thus inhibiting normal metabolic processes. Some disinfectants containing mineral ions are effective in inhibiting the growth of bacteria by this means.

Sometimes, a similar substrate can be used as an inhibitor to deliberately interfere with a particular metabolic pathway. It binds with the enzyme; thus the end product is not produced. For example, a chemotherapeutic agent, such as a sulfonamide drug, may bind with certain enzymes to prevent essential metabolites from being formed and thereby inhibits the growth of a pathogen.

Cellular Metabolism

Because metabolism is the total of all the chemical reactions in the cell, it includes the production of energy and intermediate products (metabolites) as well as the end products. Furthermore, these reactions must proceed in many directions simultaneously, breaking down some materials to provide energy and raw materials for the synthesis of other compounds. Thus, most metabolic reactions can be divided into two types: catabolism and anabolism. *Catabolism* is the metabolic degradation (breakdown) of organic compounds with the production of energy and smaller molecules. *Anabolism* refers to those biosynthetic processes that use energy for the synthesis of protoplasmic materials needed for growth, maintenance, and other cellular functions. In this manner, the cell works much like a factory. It gathers and produces raw materials to be used in the production of macromolecules for building, maintenance, and repair. It must also have fuel or energy available to run this metabolic machinery. This energy may be trapped from the rays of the sun (as in photosynthesis), or it may be produced by certain catabolic reactions. Then the energy is bound into high-energy bonds in special molecules, usually adenosine triphosphate (ATP). These high-energy molecules serve as the fuel, just as coal is used to fire the furnaces in the production of steel and other important alloys.

The most important high-energy compound found within the cell is ATP, but it is not the only one. It is found in all cells because it is used to transfer energy from energy-yielding molecules, like glucose, to an energy-using reaction. Thus, ATP is a temporary, intermediate molecule. If ATP is not used shortly after it is formed it is soon hydrolyzed to adenosine diphosphate (ADP), a more stable molecule, and adenosine monophosphate (AMP) in catabolic reactions. ADP can also be used as an emergency energy source by the removal of another phosphate group to produce AMP (a catabolic reaction; Fig. 4-2). Both AMP and ADP bind with high-energy phosphate groups to produce ATP when the energy is removed from energy-yielding reactions.

Although the metabolic pathways require the production of much energy, energy must also be available to the organism for growth, reproduction, sporulation, and movement. Some organisms even use energy for bioluminescence, such as the

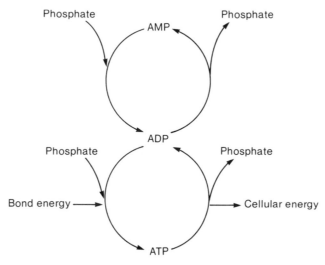

Fig. 4-2. Conversion of bond energy to cellular energy.

plankton which glow in the darkness of the ocean. Much energy of any system is lost in the form of heat.

Energy Production (Catabolism)

Cellular Respiration of Glucose   The complete catabolism of glucose takes place in three phases: (1) glycolysis, (2) the citric acid cycle, and (3) the electron transport system. The first phase is anaerobic, and the last two require aerobic conditions (Fig. 4-3).

  Glycolysis. Glycolysis is the term for the stepwise breakdown of glucose into pyruvic acid in the absence of oxygen. It is the basic set of reactions in the anaerobic phase of cellular respiration. Somewhere in the metabolism of almost all cells, glycolysis, or the degradation of glucose, takes place to produce small amounts of ATP. Heterotrophs can degrade starch and glycogen to provide glucose for these glycolytic reactions. Other sugars, such as fructose, can also be used in these reactions. Auto-

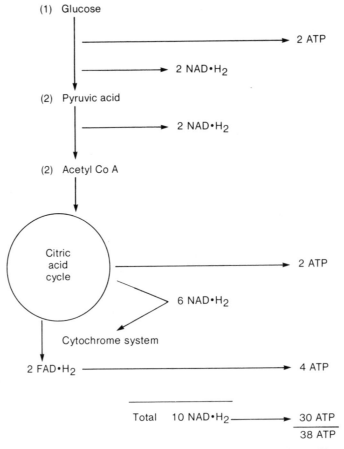

Fig. 4-3. Summary tabulation of high-energy molecules produced by aerobic cellular respiration of one molecule of glucose.

trophs synthesize glucose during photosynthesis so they can derive energy from the glucose to drive other metabolic reactions. The amount of energy (ATP) derived from a glucose molecule depends on whether or not the cell has oxygen available to bond with the hydrogen atoms released during the aerobic phase of cellular respiration. It should be noted that the aerobes and facultative anaerobes are much more efficient in energy production than the obligate anaerobes because they have oxygen available to aid in the production of much more ATP.

Citric Acid Cycle and Electron Transport System. In the aerobic phases of cellular respiration, oxygen is used as the final hydrogen acceptor following a long series of molecular reactions controlled by specific enzymes. Aerobic microorganisms and facultative anaerobes use pyruvic acid to produce about nine times more energy than obligate anaerobes can produce by the fermentation of glucose and the other sugars. Even in the presence of oxygen, obligate anaerobes do not have the appropriate enzymes and coenzymes to catalyze this metabolic pathway.

The citric acid cycle is also known as the tricarboxylic acid cycle (TCA), and is often called the Krebs cycle after the scientist who defined this phase of aerobic cellular respiration. As indicated in Figure 4-3, the citric acid cycle involves a series of reactions, controlled by specific enzymes yielding the end products carbon dioxide and hydrogen atoms. These activated hydrogen atoms are temporarily bound to NAD and FAD and transferred to the electron transport system, where the cytochromes aid in the oxidative phosphorylation of ADP to ATP, and the hydrogen bonds with the oxygen to form water (cellular water).

The complete process of cellular respiration of one molecule of glucose yields 38 ATP molecules. Two ATP molecules are gained from the glycolysis phase and two from the citric acid cycle; the other 34 result from oxidative phosphorylation in the electron transport system. The chemical equation representing this highly efficient catabolic reaction is

$$C_6H_{12}O_6 + 6\ O_2 + 38\ ADP + 38\ \textcircled{P} \rightarrow 6\ H_2O + CO_2 + 38\ ATP$$

where $\textcircled{P}$ indicates activated phosphate groups.

Although the metabolic pathway and amount of energy that can be produced from cellular respiration of glucose has been shown as an illustration, one must be aware that there are many variations to this pathway depending on the individual organism and its available nutrient and energy resources. Some bacteria degrade glucose to pyruvic acid by other metabolic pathways. Also, glycerol, fatty acids from lipids, and amino acids from protein digestion may be fed into the citric acid cycle to produce energy for the cell when necessary, that is, when there are insufficient carbohydrates available (Fig. 4-4).

Anaerobic Fermentation When the hydrogen atoms released from the breakdown of sugars are bound to organic molecules instead of oxygen, the glycolytic process is referred to as *fermentation*. Pyruvic acid will usually accept the hydrogen atoms to produce lactic acid or ethanol (ethyl alcohol), but other end products may be formed.

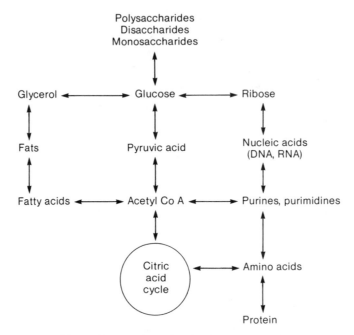

Fig. 4-4. Other nutrients entering and exiting from the metabolism of glucose.

The products produced depend on the species of the organism and, also, on the sugar used as the source of carbohydrate. In human muscle cells, the lack of oxygen during extreme exertion results in pyruvic acid being converted to lactic acid. This compound, existing in the muscle tissue, is the cause of the soreness that develops in exhausted muscles. There are some bacteria (*Lactobacillus* and *Streptococcus*) that also produce lactic acid during the fermentation process. These organisms are found in the mouth where the presence of lactic acid can enhance tooth decay, and their presence in milk causes the normal souring of milk into curd and whey. The yeasts, *Saccharomyces*, will ferment grain and fruit sugars into ethanol, the alcohol found in beer, wines, and liquors. Acetic acid bacteria (*Acetobacter*) are able to oxidize ethanol to acetic acid and spoil the beer and wine by changing them to vinegar. These and other various end products of fermentation have many industrial applications.

Aerobic Oxidation by Chemolithotrophs   Certain autotrophs, the chemolithotrophs, are able to perform respiration reactions by oxidizing hydrogen (H_2) to water (H_2O), carbon (C) and carbon monoxide (CO) to carbon dioxide (CO_2), ammonia (NH_3) and nitrite (NO_2^-) to nitrate ions (NO_3^-), hydrogen sulfide (H_2S) and free sulfur (S) to sulfates (SO_4^{2-}), and iron to iron oxides. As one can imagine, these microorganisms (usually soil and water bacteria) are very important in recycling the elements and some compounds into forms more usable by plants and other microorganisms. They also must be acknowledged as major factors in the destruction of iron parts of machinery, promoting rust.

Anaerobic Respiration by Chemotrophs   In the absence of oxygen, some oxidation–reduction reactions occur, biologically, in certain anaerobes. The electron donor usually is an organic compound such as glucose, but it may be inorganic iron or sulfur compounds (as used by *Thiobacillus*). Inorganic compounds (nitrates, sulfates, and carbonates) serve as the final electron (hydrogen) acceptors in place of oxygen. Some facultative anaerobes convert nitrates (NO_3^-) to nitrites (NO_2^-) and free atmospheric nitrogen gas (N_2). Others reduce carbonates (CO_3^{2-}) to carbon dioxide (CO_2) and to methane (CH_4). Some obligate anaerobes convert sulfate (SO_4^{2-}) to free sulfur (S) or to hydrogen sulfide gas (H_2S). These bacteria are found in the soil, sea water, marine mud, fresh water, acid mine waters, sewage, and sulfur springs. Obviously, they are unable to produce as much as ATP from their energy sources as heterotrophic organisms because their nutrients do not contain as much bound chemical energy.

Metabolic Biosynthesis (Anabolism)

Energy Conversion   In general, chemoheterotrophs produce energy from organic compounds by fermentation, anaerobic respiration, and aerobic respiration, as previously discussed. However, all of the phototrophs (algae, cyanobacteria, photosynthetic bacteria, and plants) must derive their energy from light, usually the sun, by *photosynthesis*. This process provides energy to the greatest mass of organisms, not only all of the photosynthetic organisms but heterotrophs as well, because the heterotrophs consume phototrophs.

Energy Use   The biosynthesis of organic compounds requiring the use of energy is called *anabolism*, or an anabolic reaction. In living cells this biosynthetic metabolism may be one of two types: *photosynthesis* by photolithotrophs or photoorganotrophs, or *chemosynthesis* by chemolithotrophs or chemoorganotrophs.

In photosynthesis, light energy is converted to chemical bond energy to be used to synthesize organic biochemicals. Those phototrophic organisms using inorganic raw materials (CO_2, H_2O, H_2S, S) for biosynthesis are the photolithotrophs (photoautotrophs). Those phototrophs using small organic molecules, such as acids and alcohols, to build carbohydrates, fats, proteins, nucleic acids, and other important biochemicals are the photoorganotrophs (photoheterotrophs).

Photosynthesis   The goal of photosynthetic processes is to trap and convert the radiant energy of light into chemical bond energy in ATP and carbohydrates, particularly glucose, which can then be converted into more molecules of ATP via the respiratory pathways. The general overall photosynthesis reaction is

$$6\ CO_2 + 12\ H_2O \xrightarrow[ATP]{light} (CH_2O)_6 + 6\ O_2 + 6\ H_2O + ADP + \textcircled{P}$$

Notice that this reaction is almost the reverse of the oxidative respiration reaction, and it is nature's way of balancing substrates in the environment.

The photosynthetic process may be considered as two major reactions, the light phase and the dark phase. During the *light phase*, chlorophyll or other photosynthetic pigments absorb light and are activated by the radiant energy to release electrons into a series of reactions resulting in the formation of ATP. Simultaneously, hydrogen from H_2O is bound to the coenzyme NADP as $NADP \cdot H_2$, releasing oxygen. In the *dark phase* of photosynthesis, ATP, $NADP \cdot H_2$, and CO_2 are combined to synthesize carbohydrates, usually in the form of glucose and starch. These compounds can then be used in the glycolytic production of ATP or for maintenance and growth of the organism.

Photosynthesis does not necessarily require the presence of oxygen; in other words, it can take place anaerobically, as occurs in the purple and green bacteria (obligate anaerobic photoautotrophs). These bacteria do not use H_2O but instead use H_2 or H_2S gas or other hydrogen donor molecules produced by other bacteria in soil or mud. The overall reaction of anaerobic bacterial photosynthesis then becomes

$$6\ CO_2 + 12\ H_2S \xrightarrow{\text{light}} (CH_2O)_6 + 6\ H_2O + 12\ S$$

or

$$6\ CO_2 + 12\ H_2 \xrightarrow{\text{light}} (CH_2O)_6 + 6\ H_2O$$

The bacterial photosynthetic pigments use shorter wave lengths of light, which penetrate deep within a pond or into mud where it appears to be dark.

In the absence of any light, some photolithotrophic organisms may survive anaerobically by the fermentation process alone. Other phototrophic bacteria also have a limited ability to use simple organic molecules in photosynthetic reactions; thus, they become photoorganotrophic organisms under certain conditions. A few species of cyanobacteria have also been found to exist as facultative phototrophs and facultative autotrophs, meaning that in certain environments they become photoheterotrophs. In other words, they have backup metabolic systems.

Chemosynthesis The chemosynthetic process involves a chemical source of energy and raw materials to synthesize the necessary metabolites and macromolecules for growth and functioning of the organisms. These chemotrophic organisms may be either autotrophs or heterotrophs.

The chemoautotrophs are the same chemolithotrophic bacteria, previously discussed, that obtain energy by aerobic oxidation of inorganic compounds or by anaerobic respiration of inorganic substances. These are the only organisms that do not depend on the radiant energy from the sun. They are considered among the most primitive bacteria and are frequently found near volcanoes deep within the ocean.

The chemoorganotrophs have been defined as those organisms that derive both their energy and nutrients from organic materials. Most bacteria, as well as protozoa, fungi, and all animals belong to this group. Although they vary greatly in the details of their metabolism, they all use carbohydrates, lipids, and proteins to synthesize their own carbohydrates, lipids, proteins, nucleic acids, and high-energy molecules such as ATP. These metabolic pathways may be carried on with or without oxygen by aerobic or anaerobic respiration, fermentation, and other biodegradation and biosynthetic reactions.

Microbial Growth

Growth in bacteria is represented by an increase in the number of organisms rather than in their size. When each bacterial cell reaches its optimum size it divides by binary fission (*bi* = two) into two daughter cells. Binary fission means that each bacterium simply splits into two similar cells. These in turn will divide, and as a result a viable, healthy colony of cells is maintained as long as the nutrient supply, water, and space allow. This process continues until the waste products from cells build up to a toxic level, or until the nutrients are depleted. The actual division of staphylococci by binary fission is shown in the electron micrograph in Figure 4-5.

The growth of microorganisms in nature (*in vivo*) as well as in laboratory (*in vitro*) is greatly influenced by temperature, *p*H (acidity), moisture content, available nutrients, and the character of other organisms present. Therefore, the number of

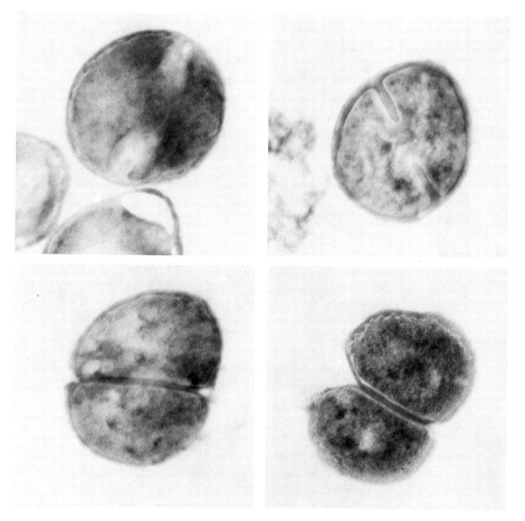

Fig. 4-5. Binary fission of staphylococci (original magnification × 30,000). (Photograph courtesy Ray Rupel)

bacteria in nature fluctuates unpredictably because these factors vary with the seasons, rainfall, temperature, and time of day.

In the laboratory, however, a pure culture of a single species of bacteria can usually be grown if the appropriate growth medium and environmental conditions are provided. The temperature, pH, and amount of oxygen are quite easily controlled to provide optimum conditions for growth. Then the appropriate nutrients must be provided in the growth medium. Some bacteria are so fastidious (having complex nutritional requirements) they will not grow outside of living cells; thus, they must be cultured in living animals or tissue cultures.

Culture Media

Basically, there are two types of media for culturing bacteria: (1) a chemically defined synthetic medium and (2) a rich, natural, complex medium containing digested extracts from meats, fish, and plants providing the nutrients, vitamins, and minerals necessary. These media can be used in liquid or broth form, available in tubes, or they may be solidified by the addition of agar and poured into tubes or petri dishes so the bacteria can be grown within or on the surface of the agar.

An *enriched medium* is a broth or solid medium containing a rich supply of special nutrients for the growth of a particular fastidious organism, but not for other microorganisms that might be present. Thus, the desired species would grow best and predominate the culture, and a pure culture could easily be obtained from a mixed specimen. A good example of this is Thayer-Martin agar for the growth of *Neisseria* species.

A *differential medium* is used to grow several species of bacteria, but each will have a distinctive appearance. Eosin methylene blue (EMB) agar is frequently used to separate and identify gram-negative organisms in fecal specimens.

A *selective medium* has added inhibitors to discourage the growth of certain organisms but not inhibit the one sought. For example, mannitol salt agar encourages the growth of staphylococci but inhibits other gram-positive bacteria. It is also a differential agar because the colonies of various species of *Staphylococcus* have a different appearance on mannitol salt medium.

Population Counts

Once the desired species of bacteria has been separated from other organisms in a specimen, it can be grown as a pure culture under the best possible conditions. The changes in an isolated bacterial population over an extended period will follow a definite predictable pattern that can be shown by plotting the population growth curve on a graph (Fig. 4-6).

Often microbiologists need to know the rate of bacterial growth and how many bacteria are present at any one time. This information is particularly important in determining the degree of bacterial contamination in drinking water and in milk and food. The number can be determined by counting the total number of bacterial cells,

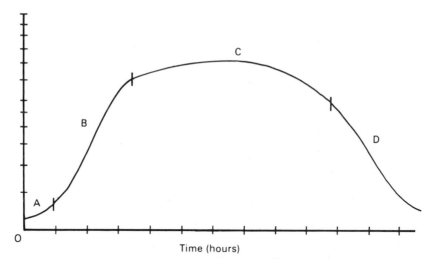

Fig. 4-6. Population growth curve of living organisms. The logarithm of the number of bacteria per milliliter of medium is plotted against time. (*A*) Lag phase. (*B*) Logarithmic growth phase. (*C*) Stationary phase. (*D*) Death phase.

living and dead, in 1 ml of solution, or by counting only the viable or living bacteria present. A total count is easier and faster but less accurate because it includes both living and dead cells, but if the 1-ml sample is taken when the microorganisms are growing and dividing rapidly in the growth phase, few dead cells will be present. In many hospitals, electronic cell counters are incorporated into the autoanalyzers used in blood, urine, and spinal fluid analysis. Many research laboratories use spectrophotometers, which determine the number of organisms present by measuring the turbidity of the solution due to the number of organisms. Chemical analyses of nitrogen or carbon content also can be used to determine the number of bacteria present by chemically destroying them.

The *viable plate count* is the most accurate method for determining the number of living bacteria in a milliliter of liquid, which may be milk, water, diluted food, or broth. In this procedure, as shown in Figure 4-7, 1 ml of solution is diluted to 100 ml three times, and samples are taken from each dilution. These 1-ml samples are grown in nutrient agar. The number of colonies observed growing on the nutrient agar plates the following day indicates the number of viable bacteria present at that particular dilution. This number multiplied by the dilution factor indicates the number of living bacteria in the original culture at the time the sample was taken. Thus, if 220 colonies were counted on an agar plate grown from a 1-ml sample from the second dilution bottle (1:10,000 dilution), there were 220 x 10,000 = 2,200,000 bacteria in 1 ml of the original material at the time the dilutions were made and cultured. For the count to be statistically significant and most accurately representative of the number of living microorganisms in the solution, the number used in the calculations should be taken from the agar plate that has between 30 and 300 colonies.

Fig. 4-7. The viable plate count technique. One milliliter of the original culture is successively diluted and cultured on agar plates.

A similar technique has been developed to count viruses. The diluted viruses are grown on a "lawn" of bacteria or layer of tissue culture cells. Each cell lysed by a virus causes a clear zone (plaque) in the culture of cells following incubation. Thus, the number of plaques represents the number of viruses in 1 ml of the diluted solution. This number must then be multiplied by the dilution factor.

A method of approximating the number and type of bacteria in urine involves streaking a known volume of urine from a calibrated inoculation loop onto various appropriate differential media. The color and number of colonies enables a micro-biologist to determine the presence of large numbers of certain bacteria that often cause urinary infections, including species of *Staphylococcus, Streptococcus,* and partic-ularly *E. coli* and other coliforms.

Population Growth Curve

The population growth curve for any particular species of bacteria may be determined by growing the organism in pure culture (a culture of only one organism) at a constant temperature. The graph in Figure 4-6 is constructed by plotting the logarithm of the number of bacteria against the incubation time.

The first stage of the growth curve is the *lag phase* (*A* in Fig. 4-6), during which the bacteria absorb nutrients, synthesize enzymes, and prepare for reproduction. In the *logarithmic group phase* (exponential growth phase; *B* in Fig. 4-6), the bacteria multiply so rapidly that the population number doubles during each generation time. The generation time, which is the time between the formation of a new bacterium and its division into two daughter cells, varies with the species of bacteria. *Escherichia coli* from the intestine, *Vibrio cholerae* (which causes cholera), *Staphylococcus,* and *Strep-tococcus* all have a generation time of about 20 minutes, whereas *Pseudomonas,* from the soil, may divide every 10 minutes, and *Mycobacterium tuberculosis* may divide only once in 18 hours. The logarithmic growth phase is always brief unless the rapidly dividing culture is maintained by constant addition of nutrients and oxygen and frequent removal of the waste products and excess microorganisms. Many industrial and re-search procedures depend on the maintenance of an essential species of micro-organism. These are continuously cultured in a controlled environment called a *chemo-stat* (Fig. 4-8), which regulates the supply of nutrients and the removal of waste products and excess microorganisms. Chemostats are used in industries where yeast is grown to produce beer and wine, where fungi and bacteria are cultivated to produce antibiotics, where *E. coli* are grown for genetic research, and in any other process needing a constant source of microorganisms.

As the nutrients and oxygen in the culture tube are used up and waste products from the metabolizing bacteria build up and change the pH of the culture medium, the rate of division slows, such that the number of bacteria dividing equals the number dying. The result is the *stationary phase* (*C* in Fig. 4-6). It is during this phase that the culture reaches its greatest population density.

As overcrowding occurs, the toxic waste products increase and the nutrient supply decreases. The microorganisms then die at a rapid rate; this is the *death phase* (*D* in Fig. 4-6). The culture may die completely or a few microorganisms may continue to survive for months. If the bacterial species is a spore-former it will form spores to survive beyond this phase. When the cells are observed in old cultures of bacteria in the death phase, some of them may look different from the healthy organisms seen in the growth phase. As a result of the unfavorable conditions, morphological changes in the cells may appear. Some bacteria become long, multinucleated, filamentous rods, or branching or globular forms. Some develop without a cell wall (protoplasts)

Fig. 4-8. Chemostat used for continuous cultures. Rate of growth can be controlled either by controlling the rate at which new medium enters the growth chamber or by limiting a required growth factor in the medium. (Volk WA, et al.: Essentials of Medical Microbiology, 3rd ed. Philadelphia, JB Lippincott, 1986)

and others take an L shape because they have very little cell wall (L-forms). When these involuted forms are inoculated into a fresh nutrient medium, they usually revert to the original shape of the healthy bacteria.

A population growth curve may be plotted for all organisms, including humans. At present, the human population is in the logarithmic growth phase with a generation time of 35 years. No population of organisms is known to continue in this phase forever without careful control of the food supply, numbers of individuals, and proper disposal of waste products. Eventually the forces of nature (food shortages, epidemics, wars, toxic waste products) will probably cause the world population to stabilize in the stationary growth phase and, we hope, not proceed beyond to the terminal death phase.

Bacterial Genetics

The nucleoid region of bacteria usually consists of only one DNA type of chromosome with no protein on the outside as is found in eucaryotic chromosomes. This chromosome is a circular strand of genes linked together. Genes are the fundamental units of heredity that carry the information needed for the special characteristics of each different species of bacteria. Thus, the genes direct all functions of the cell, providing it with its own particular traits and individuality. Because there is only one chromosome that replicates just before cell division, identical traits of a species are passed from the parent bacterium to the daughter cells following binary fission.

The DNA molecule that makes up any gene on the chromosome is subject to

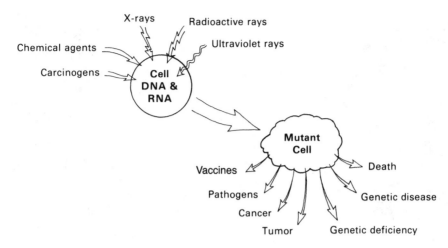

Fig. 4-9. Agents that may cause mutagenic changes.

accidental alteration, which changes the trait controlled by that gene. If the change in the gene alters or deletes (eliminates) a trait in such a way that the cell does not die or become incapable of division, the altered trait will be transmitted to the daughter cells of each succeeding generation. A change in the characteristics of a cell caused by a change in the DNA molecule (genetic alteration) that is transmissible to the offspring is called a *mutation*. A lethal mutation is one that causes the cell to die because an essential functional gene is missing. Spontaneous mutations usually occur about once in every 10 million cell divisions. The mutation rate can be increased by exposing the cells to physical or chemical agents that affect the DNA molecule. These agents are called *mutagens*. In the research laboratory, x-rays, ultraviolet light, and radioactive substances, as well as certain chemical agents, are used to induce more frequent mutations (Fig. 4-9). These mutants are used in genetic and medical research and in the development of vaccines. The types of mutagenic changes frequently observed in bacteria involve color, colony appearance, cell shape, biochemical activities, nutritional needs, antigenic sites, virulence, pathogenicity, and drug resistance. The nonpathogenic living virus vaccines, such as the Sabin vaccine for polio, are examples of laboratory-induced mutations of pathogenic microorganisms.

Changes in Bacterial Genetic Constitution

There are at least four ways, other than mutation, that the genetic constitution of bacteria can be changed: phage conversion, transduction, transformation, and conjugation. These types of gene transfers result in extra genetic material in the recipient cell. If this extra bit of DNA remains in the cytoplasm of the cell, it is called a *plasmid* (Fig. 4-10). Some plasmids contain many extra chromosomal genes, others only a few, but the cell is changed by the addition of those genetic components. Plasmids may simultaneously replicate themselves with the replication of chromosomal DNA or at various other times. When a plasmid becomes incorporated into the

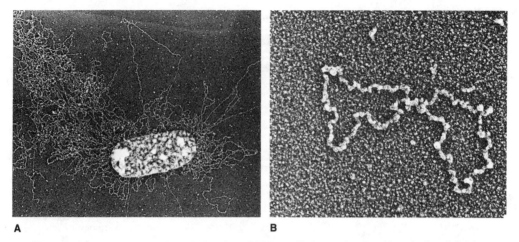

Fig. 4-10. (*A*) Disrupted cell of *Escherichia coli;* the DNA has spilled out and a plasmid can be found slightly to the left of top center. (*B*) Enlargement of a plasmid (about 1 μm from side to side). (Volk WA, et al: Essentials of Medical Microbiology, 3rd ed. Philadelphia, JB Lippincott, 1986)

chromosome, it is referred to as an episome, although some geneticists prefer to continue to call it a plasmid. Some plasmid genes can be expressed as extra-chromosomal genes, but others must become chromosomal episomes before the genes become functional.

Phage Conversion The genetic change of phage conversion occurs when a temperate bacteriophage (bacterial virus) infects a lysogenic bacterium (Fig. 4-11) by injecting its DNA into the cytoplasm of the bacterium. The number of genes in the bacterium is thus increased by the number of genes injected by the phage. For example, the diphtheria bacterium (*Corynebacterium diphtheriae*) is pathogenic only when it has been infected by a bacteriophage that enables it to produce the toxin that causes diphtheria.

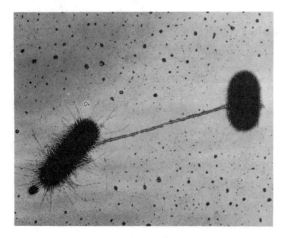

Fig. 4-11. Initiation of conjugating in *Escherichia coli*. The donor cell (with numerous short pili) is connected to the recipient bacterium by an F pilus, as described in the text (original magnification × 3000). (Anderson TF: Cold Spring Harbor Symp Quant Biol 18:197)

Transduction Transduction means "to carry across." Some cellular genetic material may be carried across from one bacterial cell to another by a bacterial virus. This phenomenon may occur when a temperate bacteriophage infects a bacterial cell by injecting its DNA. The viral DNA then combines with the bacterial chromosome as a prophage. If a stimulating chemical, heat, or ultraviolet light activates the prophage, it begins to produce new viruses by the production of phage DNA and proteins. Because the viral DNA has actually been a part of the bacterial chromosome, as the entire chromosome disintegrates, small pieces of bacterial DNA may remain attached to the maturing phage DNA. During the assembly of the virus particles, one or more bacterial genes may be incorporated into some of the mature bacteriophages. When all the phages are freed by cell lysis, they will proceed to infect other cells, injecting bacterial genetic material as well as viral genes. Thus, cellular genes that are attached to the phage DNA are carried to new cells by the virus.

There are two types of transduction: specialized and generalized. The explanation in the previous paragraph describes specialized transduction in which the infecting phage must be lysogenic so that it can integrate into the bacterial chromosome or a plasmid. As the virus genome breaks away to replicate and produce more viruses, it carries a few identifiable bacterial genes with it. These genes are then carried to the newly infected cell by the virus. In this way genetic capabilities involving the fermentation of certain sugars, antibiotic resistance, and other phenotypic characteristics can be transduced to other bacteria. This process has been shown in the laboratory to occur in species of *Bacillus, Pseudomonas, Haemophilus, Salmonella,* and *Escherichia,* and it is assumed to occur in nature.

In generalized transduction, the bacteriophage is a virulent lytic phage that does not incorporate into the bacterial genome or plasmid. Rather, it picks up fragments of bacterial DNA during the assembly of new virus particles and carries these genes to other cells that the new viruses infect. This generalized transduction has been observed in species of *Streptococcus, Staphylococcus,* and *Salmonella,* and in *Vibrio cholerae.*

Only small segments of DNA are transferred from cell to cell by transduction compared with the amount that can be transferred by transformation and conjugation.

Transformation In the transformation process, a recipient bacterial cell is genetically transformed by the addition of DNA fragments from another strain of bacteria with at least one different observable characteristic. The first experiments in transformation proved that DNA is, indeed, the genetic material. When a DNA extract from encapsulated pathogenic *Streptococcus pneumoniae* type 1 was added to a growing culture of nonencapsulated, nonpathogenic *S. pneumoniae* type 1, the resulting culture showed the presence of living encapsulated type 2 *S. pneumoniae.* Thus, the nonencapsulated streptococci must have been transformed by the genes coding for capsule that were incorporated into the cells. Although this type of genetic recombination is not widespread, it has been demonstrated in several genera including *Bacillus, Escherichia, Haemophilus, Staphylococcus,* and *Neisseria.* Transformations have even been shown to occur between *Staphylococcus, Streptococcus,* and others.

Large DNA molecules from a donor cell can penetrate the cell wall and cell membrane of a *competent* recipient cell only, that is, one capable of receiving the DNA molecule. Recipient bacteria usually become competent during the late logarithmic growth phase when the cell secretes a protein competence factor that increases its permeability to DNA.

Some competent bacterial cells have incorporated DNA fragments from certain animal viruses (*e.g.*, cowpox), retaining the latent virus genes for long periods. This knowledge may have some importance in the study of viruses that remain latent in humans for many years before they finally cause disease, as may be the case in Parkinson's disease. These human virus genes may hide in the normal flora bacteria until they are released to cause disease.

Conjugation Conjugation occurs when two bacteria attach to each other, usually by a pilus bridge, and some genetic material is transferred from the donor cell to the recipient. Many biologists compare this transfer of genetic material to the sexual process in animals, labeling the donor "male" and the recipient, "female." This type of genetic recombination occurs mostly among the species and among some genera of the enteric bacteria, but is has been reported within species of *Pseudomonas* and *Streptococcus* as well. In electron micrographs, microbiologists have noted sex pili that are larger than other pili. The donor sex pilus attaches to the recipient cell, which is usually nonpiliated, to form the pilus bridge. Genetic material from a plasmid or from the chromosomes is then transferred across the pilus bridge from donor to recipient cell (Fig. 4-12, Conjugation). Although many genes may be transferred by conjugation, the ones most frequently noted include those coding for antibiotic resistance, colicin (a protein that kills certain enteric bacteria), and the fertility factor (F^+, HFr^+). Bacteria with the F^+ or HFr^+ genes have the ability to produce pili, including sex pili, so those bacteria may become donor cells. If the fertility factor is on a plasmid, it is an F^+ gene, but if it is incorporated within the chromosome it is referred to as the HFr^+ gene. A complete copy of the plasmid (with F^+) usually moves to the recipient (F^-) cell, and thus it usually becomes F^+. However, the recipient (F^-) cell usually receives only a portion of the chromosome from an HFr^+ cell, not including the HFr^+ gene; thus, the recipient remains HFr^- in that circumstance, does not produce pili, and cannot become a donor cell.

Transduction, transformation, and conjugation are excellent tools for mapping bacterial chromosomes and for studying bacterial and viral genetics. Although each of them is frequently used in the laboratory, it is believed that they occur in natural environments under certain circumstances.

Genetic Engineering

An array of techniques has been developed to transfer eucaryotic genes, particularly human, into other easily cultured cells to facilitate the large-scale production of important proteins. Bacteria, yeasts, human leukocytes, macrophages, and fibroblasts have been used as manufacturing plants for proteins, such as the human growth hormone, insulin, and interferon. In the near future, perhaps the genes themselves will be implanted into people with genetic deficiencies. This work is not conducted without some risk to mankind. The greatest fear is that genes may be introduced into bacteria to produce toxins or diseases, yet unknown, that will destroy the human race. With this in mind, extreme care and caution is exercised during genetic manipulation experiments.

Many industrial and medical benefits may be derived from genetic engineering research. There is a potential for incorporating nitrogen-fixing capabilities into more of the soil microorganisms, for making animal proteins for food and medicines, for increasing the production of antibiotics, for synthesizing important enzymes and hormones for treatment of inherited disease, and for making portions of viruses and bacterial pathogens to be used as vaccines. Such vaccines would contain only part of the pathogen (for instance, the capsid of the smallpox virus) to which the person would form protective antibodies without the possibility of the presence of complete virulent pathogens.

Problems and Questions

1. What factors influence the growth of microorganisms in nature?
2. What factors are kept constant to produce a population growth curve in the laboratory?
3. What factors contribute to the death of a pure culture of bacteria in a tube of nutrient broth?
4. What are the major elements found in living cells? What other elements are also necessary for the metabolic functions of the cell?
5. Distinguish between (a) heterotrophs and autotrophs; (b) chemotrophs and phototrophs; (c) chemoorganotrophs and chemolithotrophs; (d) photoorganotrophs and photolithotrophs.
6. Why are saprophytic decomposers necessary for ecological balance?
7. Describe catabolism, anabolism, respiration, fermentation, and photosynthesis.
8. Describe five ways by which the genetic constitution of bacteria may be altered.
9. What is a plasmid? an episome?
10. Describe the process of genetic engineering and give an example.

Chapter 5

Human and Microbial Interactions

New Words to Pronounce and Understand

Antibiosis (an-tee-buy-oh'-sis). An antagonistic relationship

Bacillus (buh-sil'-lus). A rod-shaped bacterium

Commensalism (co-men'-sal-is-um). A relationship in which one member benefits and the other is unaffected in any way

Infection (in-feck'-shun). The growth of parasitic microorganisms in a host

Mutualism (mew'-chew-al-is-um). A relationship in which both organisms benefit

Parasitism (par'-uh-sit-is-um). A relationship in which an organism benefits at the expense of the host organism

Pathogen (path'-o-jen). A microorganism that produces disease in the host

Spirochete (spy'-row-keet). A spiral-shaped bacterium

Symbionts (sim'-bee-yonts). Organisms living together

Symbiosis (sim'-bee-oh'-sis). A constant relationship between two or more unlike species of organisms

Synergism (sin'-er-jiz-um). A mutualistic relationship in which organisms accomplish together what neither could do alone

Normal Flora of Humans

The normal flora of a person includes all the microbes that normally are found on or within the human body. These microorganisms include bacteria, fungi, protozoans, and viruses. A fetus has no normal flora. During and after delivery a newborn is exposed to many microorganisms, from the mother, in food, in the air it breathes, and on everything it touches. Both harmless and helpful microbes take up residence on the skin, at all the body openings, and in the mucous membranes that line the digestive tract (mouth to anus) and the urogenital tract. In these areas the moist, warm environment provides excellent conditions for growth. The conditions for proper growth (moisture, pH, temperature, oxygen supply, nutrients) vary throughout the body; thus, the types of resident normal flora differ from one part to another. See Table 5-1 for a list of the normal flora frequently found within and on the human body.

Only a few types of microbes establish themselves as normal flora because most of the organisms in our external environment do not find the body to be a suitable host. In addition to the resident normal flora, there are *transient* normal flora that take up temporary residence in humans. The body is constantly exposed to the flow of microorganisms from the outside, and these *transient* microbes frequently are attracted to the moist body areas. These microbes are temporary "guests" for many reasons: they may be washed from the external areas by bathing; they may not be able to compete with the *resident* flora; they may fail to survive in the acid or alkaline environment of the area; or they may be flushed out in excretions such as urine, feces, tears, and perspiration.

Destruction of the resident normal flora will disturb the balance established between the host and its microorganisms. Prolonged therapy with certain antibiotics often destroys the normal intestinal flora; diarrhea is usually the result of such an imbalance which, in turn, leaves the body more susceptible to secondary invaders. When the number of normal resident microbes is greatly reduced, opportunistic invaders may establish themselves within those areas. One important opportunist usually found in small numbers near the body openings is the yeast *Candida albicans* which, in the absence of sufficient numbers of other normal flora, may grow unchecked in the mouth, vagina, or lower intestine, causing the disease candidiasis (also known as thrush or moniliasis; see Fig. 2-23).

Flora of the Skin

The resident flora of the skin consists primarily of bacteria and fungi. The number and species of microorganisms present depends on many factors. Moist, warm conditions in hairy areas where there are many sweat and oil glands, such as under the arms and in the groin, stimulate the growth of staphylococci, streptococci, diphtheroids, aerobic spore-forming bacilli, nonpathogenic mycobacteria, gram-negative enteric bacilli (*Escherichia coli*), as well as the fungi *Candida albicans* and *Cryptococcus*. Dry, calloused areas of skin have few bacteria, whereas the moist folds between the toes and fingers support many bacteria and fungi. The surface of the skin

Table 5-1 Locations of Microorganisms Normally Found in Humans

Normal Flora	Skin	Eye	Ear	Mouth	Nose	Respiratory Tract	Intestine	Urogenital Tract
Bacteria								
Bacillus spp.	+	–	–	+	–	–	+	–
Bacteroides	+	–	–	+	+	+	+	+
Borrelia spp.	–	–	–	+	–	–	–	+
Clostridium spp.	–	–	–	–	–	–	+	+
Coliforms	+	–	–	–	–	+	+	+
Escherichia coli	–	–	–	–	–	+	+	+
Fusobacterium spp.	–	–	–	+	–	–	–	–
Haemophilus influenzae	–	+	+	–	+	+	–	–
Klebsiella pneumoniae	–	–	–	–	+	–	+	–
Lactobacillus spp.	–	–	+	+	–	–	+	+
Leptotrichia	–	–	–	+	–	–	–	+
Micrococcus spp.	+	–	–	+	–	–	+	–
Mycobacterium spp.	+	–	+	–	–	–	–	+
Mycoplasmas (PPLO)	–	–	–	+	+	+	+	+
Neisseria spp.	–	+	–	+	+	+	–	+
Proteus spp.	–	–	–	–	–	–	+	+
Pseudomonas aeruginosa	–	–	+	–	–	–	+	–
Staphylococci	+	+	+	+	+	+	+	+
S. aureus	+	–	+	+	+	–	–	–
S. epidermidis	+	+	+	+	+	–	–	–
Streptococci	+	+	+	+	+	+	+	+
S. mitis	+	+	–	+	+	–	–	–
S. pneumoniae	–	+	+	+	+	–	–	–
S. pyogenes	+	+	+	–	–	–	–	–
Veillonella spp.	–	–	–	+	–	–	+	–
Fungi								
Actinomyces spp.	–	–	–	+	–	–	–	–
Candida albicans	+	+	–	+	–	–	+	+
Cryptococcus spp.	+	–	–	–	–	–	–	–
Protozoa	–	–	–	+	–	–	+	+
Viruses	–	–	–	–	+	+	+	–

+, present; –, absent

near the mucosal openings of the body (the mouth, eyes, nose, anus, and genitalia) is inhabited by bacteria present in their secretions.

Frequent washing with soap and water removes most of the potentially harmful transient organisms harbored in sweat, oil, and other secretions from moist body parts. All persons involved in patient care must be particularly careful to keep their skin and clothing as free of transient microbes as possible, as an aid in preventing personal infections and to avoid transferring the pathogens to patients. Such persons should always remember that most infections following burns, wounds, and surgery result from the growth of resident or transient skin flora in these susceptible areas.

Flora of the Mouth

Nowhere in the body is there a more abundant and varied population of microorganisms than in the mouth and throat. These areas provide the moist, warm mucous membranes that furnish excellent conditions for microbial growth. Bacteria thrive especially well in particles of food and in the debris of dead epithelial cells around the teeth. The peculiar anatomy of the oral cavity and the throat affords shelter for numerous anaerobic and aerobic bacteria. Anaerobic organisms flourish in the gum margins, in crevices between the teeth, and in the deep folds (crypts) on the surface of the tonsils.

The list of microbes that have been isolated from normal human mouths reads like a manual of the main groups of microorganisms. It includes cocci, bacilli, and spirilla, as well as yeasts, moldlike organisms, protozoa, and viruses. The first such list was made by Leeuwenhoek as long ago as 1690.

Most organisms normally found in the mouth and throat are beneficial, or at least harmless; these include the diphtheroids, bacteroids, lactobacilli, and micrococci. Others, such as certain streptococci and staphylococci, are potentially pathogenic opportunists and are frequently associated with disease. Some people carry virulent pathogens in their throats but do not have the diseases associated with the pathogens, such as diphtheria, meningitis, pneumonia, and tuberculosis. These people are "healthy carriers" who can transmit the pathogens to susceptible persons.

Food remaining on and between the teeth provides a rich nutrient medium for the growth of many oral bacteria. Carelessness in dental hygiene allows growth of these bacteria, with development of dental caries (tooth decay) and gingivitis (gum disease). These bacteria include species of *Actinomyces, Lactobacillus, Streptococcus, Neisseria,* and *Veillonella.*

Many α-hemolytic streptococci are normal inhabitants of the mouth and oropharynx. When β-hemolytic streptococci are present, however, the person should be treated with an antibiotic to destroy these pathogens that may cause "strep" sore throat and its complications.

Flora of the Ear and Eye

The middle ear and inner ear are normally sterile, whereas the outer ear and the auditory canal contain the same types of microorganisms as are found on moist skin areas, such as the mouth and the nose. When a person coughs, sneezes, or blows his nose, these microbes are carried along the eustachian tube and into the middle ear where they can cause infection. Infection can also develop when the eustachian tube does not open and close properly to maintain correct air pressure within the ear.

Many microorganisms are found in the external opening of the eye, the conjunctiva which lines the eyelids, and the tears. But these microbes are not a frequent cause of disease because the intact membranes serve as a barrier. These mucous membranes are constantly flushed by the tears, which are provided with an enzyme called lysozyme that destroys bacteria. The normal flora in the eye area includes species of *Staphylococcus, Streptococcus,* and *Corynebacterium,* as well as *Branhamella (Neisseria) catarrhalis.*

Flora of the Respiratory Tract

The respiratory tract consists of the nose, pharynx (throat), larynx (voice box), trachea, bronchi, bronchioles, and alveoli. The lower respiratory tract, below the larynx, is normally free of microbes because the mucous membranes and lungs have defense mechanisms that efficiently remove the invaders. Thus, staphylococci, streptococci, *Pseudomonas* species, or yeasts found in sputum specimens would indicate either an infectious disease of the lungs or specimen contamination by the normal flora of the upper respiratory tract.

The membranes of the upper part of the tract, which includes the nasopharynx and the oropharynx, provide a suitable environment for the growth of many species of *Streptococcus, Staphylococcus, Neisseria, Corynebacterium,* and other microorganisms and yeasts. In susceptible persons, many of these opportunists can quickly cause disease.

Flora of the Urogenital Area

The normal kidney, ureters, and bladder are sterile. However, the external opening of the urethra houses many normal flora such as nonpathogenic *Neisseria* species, staphylococci, enterococci, diphtheroids, mycobacteria, mycoplasms, enteric (intestinal) gram-negative rods, yeasts, and viruses. As a rule, these organisms do not invade the bladder because it is constantly flushed by the acidic urine; however, persistent, recurring urinary infections can develop with obstruction or narrowing of the urethra and with infrequent urination, which allows the invasive organisms to multiply, thus causing urinary tract infections. Chlamydias and mycoplasmas are frequent causes of nongonococcal urethritis (NGU). All of these organisms are easily introduced into the urethra by sexual intercourse.

The reproductive systems of both men and women are normally sterile, with the exception of the vagina; here the flora varies with the stage of sexual development. During puberty and following menopause, the vaginal secretions are alkaline, supporting the growth of various diphtheroids, streptococci, staphylococci, and coliforms (enteric gram-negative rods); through the childbearing years, the vaginal secretions are acidic, encouraging the growth mainly of lactobacilli, along with a few α-hemolytic streptococci, staphylococci, diphtheroids, and yeasts.

The *Neisseria* species, particularly *Neisseria gonorrhoeae* (also called the gonococcus), can survive the acid environment of the vagina and the penis; hence, they may be harbored by infected persons who show no symptoms of gonorrhea. This disease, which is readily transmitted through sexual contact, is asymptomatic (causes no symptoms) in 80% of infected women and 20% of infected men.

Flora of the Gastrointestinal Tract

The acidic environment of the stomach prevents the growth of normal flora. However, a few microbes, protected by foods, manage to pass through the stomach during periods of low acid concentration. Also, when the amount of acid is reduced in the course of diseases such as stomach cancer, certain bacteria may be found in this site.

In the small intestine the upper portion, or duodenum, has little normal flora because bile inhibits the growth of most microbes, but many are found in the lower part of the small intestine. The most abundant organisms include many species of *Staphylococcus, Lactobacillus, Streptobacillus, Veillonella,* and *Clostridium perfringens.*

The colon, or large intestine, contains large numbers of microorganisms growing on the food wastes collected there. Obligate anaerobic bacteria make up most of the colon population including gram-positive *Clostridium* species and gram-negative *Bacteroides* and *Fusobacterium* species. Normally, less than 10% of the large intestine normal flora are facultative anaerobes that are easily grown in the laboratory, including *Escherichia coli, Enterobacter aerogenes,* and species of *Proteus, Pseudomonas, Streptococcus, Lactobacillus,* and *Mycoplasma.* Also, many fungi, protoza, and viruses are found in the intestine. Usually these normal flora are opportunists, often causing disease only when they lodge in the other areas or when the balance among the organisms is upset.

Beneficial Roles of Normal Flora

Many benefits are derived by humans from the symbiotic relationship established with their normal microbial population. Some nutrients, particularly vitamins K, B_{12}, pantothenic acid, pyridoxine, and biotin are obtained from an excess secreted by the coliform bacteria.

Evidence also indicates that these indigenous microbes provide a constant source of irritants and antigens to stimulate the immune system. Thus, the immune complex responds more readily by producing antibodies to other foreign invaders and substances, enhancing protection against disease-producing agents. It appears that by merely occupying a place and using the nutrients present, these normal flora prevent other organisms that may be pathogenic from establishing a site of infection. This protection is maintained by competition for food, controlled pH and oxygen levels, and antibiotic production by certain of the resident microbes.

When the delicate balance of the various species in the population of normal flora is upset by antibiotic or other chemotherapy, many complications may result. Certain organisms may flourish out of control, such as the yeast that is the cause of candidiasis. Also, diarrhea and intestinal upsets may occur. Frequently, cultures of *Lactobacillus* added to yogurt or present in medication are prescribed to reestablish and stabilize the microbial balance.

Symbiotic Relationships

The relationship between normal flora and the human host is an excellent example of *symbiosis*. This term is the name given to a general relationship between organisms living in close proximity. The symbionts (the organisms that live together) are two or more organisms of unlike species. The relationship may be beneficial, harmless, or harmful to one, several, or all of the symbionts. The types of relationships outlined in the following sections demonstrate that the pathogenicity of a microbe can be represented as a balance between the virulence of the pathogen and the resistance of the host. These factors are further discussed in later chapters.

Mutualism   In the symbiotic relationship called mutualism, both organisms benefit. An example is the intestinal bacterium *E. coli*, which obtains nutrients from food materials ingested by the host and produces vitamin K to be used by the host. Vitamin K is a blood-clotting factor that is essential in humans. Also, some protozoa live symbiotically in the intestine of the termite and enable the termite to digest the wood it eats by breaking down the wood cellulose into nutrients to be absorbed and used. In turn, the termite provides food and a place for the protozoa to live. Without these protozoa the termite would die of starvation. A stable marriage could also be a mutualistic relationship.

In some mutualistic relationships, two organisms work together to produce a result that neither could accomplish alone. This is called *synergism*, or a synergistic relationship. The fusiform bacillus and the spirochete, which together cause the disease trench mouth, represent such a relationship. Also, the nitrogen-fixing bacteria and the roots of legumes where they exist have a true synergistic relationship, for each depends on the other for nutrients.

Commensalism   A relationship in which one member is benefited but the host organism is neither benefited nor harmed is called commensalism. Most of the normal flora of humans are considered to be commensals, in that the microbes are provided nutrients and housing with no effect on the welfare of the host.

Neutralism   Indifference, or neutralism, exists when organisms occupy the same niche but do not affect each other, as with many bacteria that live in the human mouth and intestines. However, sometimes waste products of one microorganism will destroy certain neighboring bacteria. This situation is called *antagonism* or *antibiosis*. Penicillium mold growing on a culture plate of certain strains of staphylococci inhibits the growth of the staphylococci by producing penicillin.

Parasitism   The relationship in which an organism benefits at the expense of the host organism is called parasitism. Depending on the parasite and the circumstances, the damage may be slight or it may be fatal. However, the "wise" parasite does not kill its host but rather takes only the nutrients it needs to exist. Intestinal worms, such as pinworms and tapeworms, and external parasites, such as mites, lice, and ticks, usually cause only minor damage in humans. The presence of these multicellular parasites in or on a host is referred to as an *infestation*, whereas invasion and multiplication of the unicellular parasites (microorganisms) that cause cellular damage is called an *infection* by pathogens.

Pathogenic Relationships   When parasitic microorganisms cause damage to the host during the infection process, a pathogenic relationship exists. The pathogen may be only a displaced commensal; for example, the staphylococci that normally inhabit the skin can cause infection when the skin is wounded or burned. It may be a highly virulent airborne pathogen such as the common cold virus, or it may be carried in food and water such as the dysentery pathogen. An *opportunist* is a pathogen that causes disease only in a host who is physically impaired or debilitated, because his normal defenses against disease are weakened. Pneumonia developing in a bedridden patient is another example of a pathogenic relationship. Thus, in the normal course of events, the opportunist microbe is harmless; it moves in to cause damage when an abnormal situation develops, such as a wound or a burn, or destruction of the normal flora by antibiotic therapy.

Nonpathogenic Microbes   Microbes that never cause disease or do so only in rare circumstances in an extremely susceptible host are nonpathogenic.

Microbial Ecology

Ecology is the systematic study of the interrelationships of various organisms to other organisms and to their shared environment. The interreactions of microorganisms with animals, plants, and other microbes have far-reaching effects on our lives. We are all aware of diseases caused by microbial infections; this is just one example of the effects of one type of organism on another. Most of these relationships in nature are beneficial rather than harmful.

Bacteria are exceptionally adaptable and versatile and are found on the land, in all waters, in every animal and plant, and even in other microorganisms. Some bacteria and fungi serve a valuable function by recycling nutrients from dead, decaying animals and plants back into the soil, as discussed in Chapter 4. The free-living fungi and bacteria that decompose dead organic matter into inorganic materials are called saprophytes. These inorganic nutrients that are returned to the soil are used by autotrophic bacteria and plants for synthesis of cellular biochemicals necessary to their growth; the plants are eaten by animals, which eventually die and are recycled again with the aid of the saprophytes.

Good examples of the cycling of nutrients in nature are the nitrogen, carbon, oxygen, sulfur, and phosphorus cycles, in which the microorganisms play very important roles in the following manner. In the nitrogen cycle, the free atmospheric nitrogen (N_2) is converted by nitrogen-fixing bacteria and cyanobacteria into ammonia (NH_3), nitrite (NO_2^-), and nitrate (NO_3^-) compounds in the soil (Fig. 5-1). The plants

Fig. 5-1. The nitrogen cycle. Nitrogen of the air is converted by nitrogen-fixing bacteria and algae into ammonia, nitrites, and nitrates. These inorganic nitrogen compounds are also derived from the breakdown of fecal material, and from decaying plant and animal material. The nitrates are used as food nutrients by plants, which are eaten by animals. The cycle is completed by the denitrifying bacteria, which produce free nitrogen from the inorganic nitrogen compounds.

then use the nitrate to build plant proteins, which are eaten by animals, which then use these proteins to build animal proteins. The excreted waste products (such as urea in urine) are converted by certain bacteria to ammonia. Also, the dead plant and animal debris and fecal material are transformed by the saprophytic fungi and bacteria into ammonia, nitrites, and nitrates for recycling by plants. To replenish the free nitrogen in the air, a group of bacteria called denitrifying bacteria convert nitrites and ammonia to atmospheric nitrogen (N_2). Thus, the cycle continues.

The nitrogen-fixing bacteria are of two types, free-living and symbiotic ("living together"). The symbiotic bacteria live in and near the root nodules of plants called legumes—alfalfa, clover, peas, soy beans, and peanuts (Fig. 5-2). These plants are often used in crop-rotation techniques by farmers to return nitrogen compounds to the soil and thus avoid the loss of nutrients.

The type and number of microorganisms living in the soil depend upon many factors: amount of decaying organic material, available nutrients, moisture present, oxygen available, acidity, temperature, and the waste products of other microbes present. Likewise, the types and number of harmless microbes that live on and within the human body depend on the pH (acidity), moisture, nutrients, antibacterial factors, and the presence of other microorganisms.

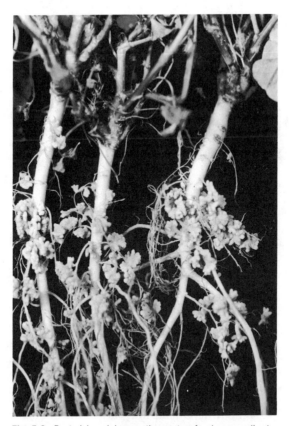

Fig. 5-2. Bacterial nodules on the roots of a legume. (Lech-avalier HA, Pramer D: The Microbes. Philadelphia, JB Lippincott, 1970)

Problems and Questions

1. What relationship exists between man and his normal flora?
2. Where would you find symbiotic relationships in your environment?
3. What are the differences between mutualism, commensalism, neutralism, antagonism, and parasitism?
4. Why are the microbial decomposers so necessary for life on earth?
5. What factors control the number of microorganisms in the soil and on the human body?

Chapter 6

Control of Microbial Growth

Objectives

After studying this chapter, you should be able to
1. List three reasons why microbial growth must be controlled
2. Define sterilization, disinfection, bactericidal agents, and bacteriostatic agents
3. Differentiate between sterilization, pasteurization, and lyophilization
4. Describe aseptic, antiseptic, and sterile techniques
5. List the factors that influence the growth of microbial life
6. Describe the following types of microorganisms: psychrophilic, mesophilic, thermophilic, halophilic, haloduric, alkaliphilic, acidophilic, and barophilic
7. List several factors that influence the effectiveness of antimicrobial methods
8. List the common *physical* antimicrobial methods
9. List the common *chemical* antimicrobial compounds
10. Describe the mode of action of sulfonamide drugs on bacteria
11. Describe the action of penicillin on bacteria
12. List four reasons why antibiotics should be used with caution

New Words to Pronounce and Understand

Antibiotic (an-tie-buy-ot'-tick). Substance produced by microorganisms that inhibits or destroys pathogens during the disease process

Antiseptic (an-ti-sep'-tick). A chemical disinfectant that is safe to use on living tissues

Asepsis (a-sep'-sis). Absence of infectious microorganisms on living tissue

Bactericide (back-tear'-i-side). An agent that kills bacteria

Chemotherapy (key-mow-ther′-uh-pee). The treatment of diseases and infection using chemicals

Disinfectant (dis-in-feck′-tant). A chemical agent used to destroy pathogens on or within nonliving materials

Facultative anaerobes (fack′-ul-tay-tive an′-air-robes). Microorganisms that prefer to live in the absence of free oxygen but that survive in an oxygen environment

Fungicide (fun′-juh-side). A substance that kills fungi

Germicide (germ′-uh-side). A substance that kills microorganisms

Haloduric (hey-low-dur′-ick). Surviving in a salty environment

Hypertonic (hi-per-tahn′-ick). Having a greater osmotic pressure outside the cell membrane than inside the cell

Hypotonic (hi-po-tahn′-ick). Having less osmotic pressure outside the cell membrane than inside the cell

Isotonic (i-so-tahn′-ick). Having the same osmotic pressure inside and outside a cell membrane

Lyophilization (lie-off-i-liz-za′-shun). Preservation by freeze-drying

Mesophilic (mess-oh-fill′-ick). Thriving at 30° to 45°C (86° to 113°F)

Microbial (my-crow′-bee-al). Pertaining to microbes

Microbistasis (my-crow-bi-stay′-sis). The inhibition of growth and reproduction of microorganisms

Microbicide (my-crow′-bi-side). An agent that kills microbes

Osmotic pressure (oz-mah′-tick). The pressure exerted on the cell membrane by the solution inside the cell

Pasteurization (pass-tur-uh-zay′-shun). A process by which heat is used to kill pathogens in foods

Plasmolysis (plaz-moll′-uh-sis). The shrinking of the cell membrane and cytoplasm from the cell wall, causing the cell to shrink

Plasmoptysis (plaz-mop′-ti-sis). Process in which water enters a cell through the cell walls, increasing the osmotic pressure

Psychroduric (sigh-crow-dur′-ick). Ability to endure − 20° to 5°C (−5° to 40°F)

Sporicidal (spor-uh-sigh′-dull). Killing spores

Thermoduric (ther-mow-dur′-ick). Ability to survive boiling

Thermophilic (ther-mow-fill′-ick). Ability to thrive at temperatures above 45°C (113°F)

Tuberculocidal (too-bur-cue-low-sigh′-doll). Killing the bacteria that cause tuberculosis (*Mycobacterium tuberculosis*)

Virucide (vi′-ruh-side). A substance that kills viruses

The factors or agents that influence the growth of microorganisms are under constant study. On the basis of these studies researchers learn how the beneficial microbes can be encouraged to grow while the pathogenic ones can be controlled, inhibited, or destroyed. The control of certain microorganisms is important (1) for the prevention and control of infectious diseases in man, animals, and plants; (2) for the preservation of food; (3) to prevent contaminating microbes from interfering with certain industrial processes; and (4) to prevent contamination of pure culture research. Preventing the spread of infectious diseases and controlling infections require many different procedures. The source of infection can be controlled by (1) destroying or inhibiting disease-causing microbes; (2) checking the sources, routes, and vectors of transmission of disease agents; and (3) protecting the infected person from the consequences of disease by building up resistance and administering appropriate chemotherapeutic drugs.

An *infectious disease* is any disease caused by the invasion and multiplication of pathogenic microorganisms in the body. Thus, an infection indicates the presence of pathogens in living tissues. *Contamination* means that pathogenic microorganisms are present on or in nonliving materials such as bed linens, discharges from human or animal sources, or food and water.

Long before people were aware of the existence of microorganisms, they tried to prevent the spoilage of food and wines, the transmission of diseases, and the infection of wounds. They developed many primitive procedures and "cures" that were often more harmful to the recipient than helpful. Today we know that the avoidance, inhibition, and destruction of potentially pathogenic microorganisms is imperative to control diseases. It is essential that those who work in the health fields appreciate the importance of controlling microbes in patient rooms, operating rooms, treatment rooms, and emergency rooms. They must be aware of proper aseptic procedures to be followed for dressing wounds, giving injections and respiratory treatments, and assisting physicians, dentists, and all other personnel who have the responsibility for patient care. Health workers must be able to properly handle contaminated linen and wound dressings, bedside equipment, and laboratory specimens to avoid infecting themselves, the patients for whom they are providing care, or other patients.

Definition of Terms

Before we can discuss the methods used to destroy or inhibit microbes, the following terms should be understood as they apply to microbiology:

Sterilization   The complete destruction of all living organisms is called sterilization. Sterilization of objects can be accomplished by heat, autoclaving (heat and steam or ethylene oxide under pressure), various chemicals (such as formaldehyde), and certain levels of radiation with ultraviolet or gamma rays. These procedures are discussed later in this chapter.

Disinfection   The destruction or removal of infectious or harmful microorganisms from nonliving objects by physical or chemical methods is disinfection. The heating process developed by Pasteur to disinfect beer and wines is called pasteurization. It is still used to eliminate pathogenic microorganisms from milk and beer. It should be remembered that pasteurization is not a sterilization procedure, since not all the microbes are destroyed. Chemical agents are also used to eliminate pathogenic agents. The chemicals used to disinfect inanimate objects, such as bedside equipment and operating rooms, are called *disinfectants.* An *antiseptic* is a solution used to disinfect the skin or other living tissues. Disinfectants are strong chemical substances and are more destructive to living tissues than antiseptics.

Microbicidal Agents   The suffix *-cide* or *-cidal* refers to killing. Thus, a microbicidal agent is one that kills microbes. A *bactericidal agent* (bactericide), kills bacteria. A disinfectant that kills fungi is a *fungicide* and, similarly, an agent that destroys viruses is a *virucide.* The general term *germicide* refers to any agent that destroys germs or harmful microorganisms.

Microbistatic Agents   The suffix *-stasis* or *-static* means the inhibition or cessation of growth and reproduction of microorganisms. A *bacteriostatic agent* is one that inhibits the metabolism and reproduction of bacteria so that they degenerate and die or are destroyed. Important microbistatic agents and processes include desiccation (drying), freezing temperatures, concentrated sugar and salt solutions, and some chemotherapeutic drugs (including the antibiotics).

Asepsis   Because sepsis refers to the growth of infectious microbes on living tissues, *asepsis* means the absence of infectious microorganisms on living tissues. Thus, *aseptic technique* is a procedure designed to eliminate and exclude all infectious microbes by sterilization of equipment, disinfection of environment, and cleansing of the body tissues with antiseptics. The *antiseptic technique* was developed by Lister in 1867. He used dilute carbolic acid to cleanse surgical wounds and equipment and a carbolic acid aerosol to prevent harmful microorganisms from entering the surgical field or contaminating the patient.

Sterile Technique   When it is necessary to prevent *all* microorganisms from gaining entrance into a laboratory or onto a surgical field, sterile technique is followed.

Factors Influencing Microbial Growth

There are many environmental factors that enhance or inhibit the growth of microorganisms, including temperature, moisture, osmotic pressure, pH, barometric pressure, gases, radiations, chemicals, and the presence of neighboring microbes. Many concepts involving these factors may be applied to our everyday lives as well as to laboratory and hospital situations.

Temperature

There is an optimum temperature at which an organism grows best, a minimum temperature at which it ceases to grow, and a maximum temperature at which it is destroyed. These temperature ranges differ greatly among organisms. Their rate of growth and metabolism is generally slower at low temperatures and faster at higher temperatures, with the effect of temperature changes varying according to the species of organism. Microbes that thrive at 20° to 40°C (68°–104°F) are called *mesophiles*, a group that includes most of the species that grow on plants and animals and in soil and water. *Psychrophiles* are capable of growth at temperatures near the freezing point; they thrive in oceans, soil, and refrigerated foods at temperatures between 0° and 20°C (30°–68°F). Microorganisms that grow at temperatures above 45°C (113°F) are called *thermophiles*. These heat-loving microbes may be found in hot springs, compost pits, and silage; because they thrive at high temperatures, boiling is not an effective means of killing them. Refer to Table 6-1 for the minimum and maximum temperature ranges of psychrophilic, mesophilic, and thermophilic bacteria.

Most pathogens and normal flora are mesophilic because they grow best at normal body temperature, 37°C (98.6°F). Thus, most pathogens are easily destroyed by boiling. The exceptions are the spores from spore-forming bacteria, the mycobacteria with resistant cell walls, and those microbes that are encased in a protective coating of organic material such as mucus, vomitus, pus, or feces.

Microorganisms that can survive or endure very cold temperatures and can be preserved in the frozen state are known as *psychroduric* organisms. The fecal material left by early arctic explorers contained psychroduric *E. coli* that survived the arctic temperatures. Also, many microbes and endospores can survive boiling and are, therefore, called *thermoduric* organisms. These microbes cause much of the color observed in hot springs.

Moisture

Living organisms require water to continue their normal metabolic processes. However, some microorganisms can survive the complete drying process called *desiccation*. Such organisms are in a dormant or resting state after they have been dried; then, as soon as they are placed in a moist environment, they grow and reproduce normally.

Table 6-1 Bacteria Named on the Basis of Temperature Tolerance

Group	Temperature Range (°C)		
	Minimum	*Optimum*	*Maximum*
Psychrophiles	−20 to 5	0 to 20	19 to 35
Mesophiles	10 to 15	20 to 40	35 to 47
Thermophiles	40 to 45	55 to 75	60 to 90

Another method of inhibiting growth of microbes is by dehydration of frozen organisms, a process often called *lyophilization*. The lyophilized materials are frozen in a vacuum, which is then sealed to maintain the inactive state. This freeze-drying method is widely used in industry to preserve foods, antibiotics, antisera, microorganisms, and other biological materials. It should be remembered that lyophilization cannot be used as a method to sterilize or kill microorganisms, but rather, it is used to prevent them from reproducing.

Osmotic Pressure

The osmotic pressure is that pressure on the cell membrane exerted by the solution inside the cell (Fig. 6-1). When cells are suspended in a solution, the normal osmotic pressure inside the cell should equal that outside the cell so the cell will neither shrink nor swell; the solution outside the cell is then said to be an *isotonic solution*. Red blood cells in serum and bacterial cells in a nutrient broth remain normal in size because these solutions are isotonic—the osmotic pressure is equalized. When red blood cells are suspended in a *hypotonic* (more dilute than normal) solution, they increase in size because the water moves across the cell membrane into the concentrated cytoplasm of the cell. Often the cell membrane ruptures; this is called *hemolysis*. However, when bacterial cells are placed in water (a hypotonic solution), more water enters the cell than leaves the cell, greatly increasing the osmotic pressure inside the bacterial cell, because the rigid cell wall prevents an increase in size. This condition is referred to as *plasmoptysis*, and is found in plants and bacteria, which have rigid cell walls. If red blood cells are suspended in a *hypertonic* (more concentrated than normal) salt or sugar solution, water will be drawn from the cytoplasm of the cell to the surrounding solution, and the result will be shrinking or *crenation* of the cell. If a bacterial cell is placed in a hypertonic solution, the cell membrane and cytoplasm will shrink away from the cell wall; this condition is called *plasmolysis*, and it inhibits

Fig. 6-1. Changes in osmotic pressure. No change in pressure occurs inside the cell in an isotonic solution; pressure is increased in a hypotonic solution; pressure is decreased in a hypertonic solution. Arrows indicate direction of water flow.

bacterial cell growth and metabolism. Refer to Figure 6-1 for a comparison of the differences of various solution concentrations on bacteria and human body cells.

Sugar solutions for jellies, and pickling brines (salt solutions) for meats, preserve these foods by inhibiting the growth of microorganisms. However, many types of molds and some types of bacteria can survive and even grow in a salty environment. Such organisms are known as *haloduric,* while those that thrive in concentrated salt water, such as the Great Salt Lake, are called *halophilic.*

pH

The term *p*H refers to the acidity or alkalinity of a solution (refer to Chap. 3). Most microorganisms prefer a neutral growth medium (about *p*H 7), but the *acidophilic* microbes, which can live in the stomach and in pickled foods, prefer a *p*H of 2 to 5. *Alkaliphiles* prefer an alkaline environment such as is found inside the intestine, about *p*H 9.

Barometric Pressure

Most bacteria are not affected by minor changes in pressure. They thrive at normal atmospheric pressure, and some thrive deep in the ocean and in oil wells, where the atmospheric pressure is very high.

Autoclaves and home pressure cookers kill microbes by a combination of high pressure and high temperature. The increase in pressure raises the temperature above the temperature of boiling water. (At a pressure of 15 pounds per square inch, the temperature of boiling water is 121°C.) However, home canning done without the use of a pressure cooker does not destroy the spores of certain bacteria, notably *Clostridium botulinum.* Occasionally, the local newspapers carry an account of cases of food poisoning resulting from the release of *C. botulinum* spores in improperly canned vegetables and meats.

Gases

The types of gases present and their concentrations determine which species of microbes will be able to live in a particular environment. Most microbes are *aerobic;* that is, they grow best in an atmosphere containing oxygen. *Anaerobes* prefer to live without oxygen, usually in 5% carbon dioxide in an atmosphere from which the oxygen has been removed or deep within the body tissues. *Facultative anaerobes* can survive in oxygen, whereas *obligate anaerobes* die when exposed to oxygen. For this reason oxygen is sometimes forced into wound infections caused by anaerobes. For instance, wounds that may contain tetanus bacteria are lanced (opened) to expose them to the air. Another example is gas gangrene, a deep wound infection, which is often treated by placing the patient in a hyperbaric (greatly increased pressure) oxygen chamber or in a room with high oxygen pressure, because the causative bacteria, *Clostridium perfringens,* cannot live in the presence of oxygen.

Antimicrobial Methods

The methods used to destroy or inhibit microbial life are either physical or chemical, and sometimes both types are used. The effectiveness of any antimicrobial procedure depends on (1) the length of time it is applied, (2) temperature, (3) concentration, (4) nature and number of microbes and spores present (bioburden), and (5) presence of protective materials such as the proteins in feces, blood, vomitus, and pus (Fig. 6-2).

Physical Methods

The physical methods commonly used in hospitals, clinics, and laboratories to destroy or control pathogens are heat, pressure, drying, radiation, sonic disruption, and filtration.

Heat   Heat is the most practical, efficient, and inexpensive method of disinfection and sterilization of objects that can withstand high temperatures. Because of these advantages, it is the means most frequently employed.

Two factors, *temperature* and *length of time*, determine the effectiveness of heat for sterilization. There is considerable variation from organism to organism in susceptibility to heat; pathogens usually are more susceptible than nonpathogens. Also, the higher the temperature, the shorter the time required to kill the organisms. The *thermal death point* of any specific species of microorganism is the lowest temperature that will kill all the organisms in a standardized pure culture within a specified period of time. The *thermal death time* is the length of time necessary to sterilize a pure culture at a specified temperature.

In practical applications of heat for sterilization, one must consider the material in which a mixture of organisms and their spores may be found. Pus, feces, vomitus,

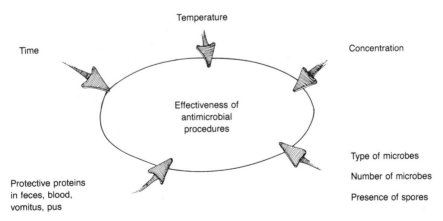

Fig. 6-2. The factors that determine the effectiveness of any antimicrobial procedure: time, temperature, concentration, presence of other microbes or spores, and presence of protein materials.

mucus, and blood contain proteins that serve as a protective coating to insulate the pathogens; when these discharges are present on bedding, bandages, surgical instruments, and syringes, very high heat is required to destroy the microorganisms and spores. In practice, the most effective procedure is to wash away the protein debris with strong soap, hot water, and a disinfectant, then sterilize the equipment with heat.

Heat applied in the presence of moisture, such as by boiling or steaming, is more effective than dry heat because moist heat causes the proteins to coagulate. Because cellular enzymes are proteins, they are also inactivated. This is exactly what happens when an egg is hard-boiled: the combination of heat and moisture causes the proteins to coagulate. Moist heat sterilization is faster than dry heat, and can be done at a lower temperature; thus, it is less destructive to many materials that otherwise would be damaged by higher temperatures.

The vegetative forms of most pathogens are quite easily destroyed by boiling; however, bacterial spores are particularly resistant to heat and drying. The autoclave, which combines heat and pressure, offers the most effective yet inexpensive means of destroying the spores. Two examples of sporeformers are *Clostridium tetani*, the causative agent of tetanus, and *Clostridium botulinum*, which causes a food poisoning; they are usually found in contaminating dirt and dust. Botulism food poisoning is preventable by properly washing and pressure cooking (autoclaving) the food.

Certain viruses are remarkably resistent to heat. A case in point is the hepatitis virus, which is frequently transferred from one person to another by the reuse of contaminated syringes and needles that have not been adequatly sterilized. It is recommended that all equipment used in the transfer of blood be autoclaved at 121°C (250°F) for 20 minutes, boiled for 30 minutes, or baked at 180°C (356°F) for 1 hour.

Dry heat. Dry heat baking in a thermostatically controlled oven provides effective sterilization for metals, glassware, some powders, oils, and waxes. These items must be baked at 160° to 165°C (320°–329°F) for 2 hours or at 170° to 180°C (338°–356°F) for 1 hour. An ordinary oven of the type found in most homes may be used if the temperature remains constant. The effectiveness of dry heat sterilization depends on how deeply the heat penetrates throughout the material, and the items to be baked must be placed so that the hot air circulates freely among them.

Incineration, or burning, is an effective means of destroying contaminated disposable materials. An incinerator must never be overloaded with moist or protein-laden materials such as feces, vomitus, or pus; within these moist substances the contaminating microorganisms may not be destroyed if the heat does not readily penetrate and burn them. Flaming the surface of heat-resistant material is an effective way to kill microorganisms on forceps and bacteriological loops and is a common laboratory procedure. Flaming is accomplished by holding the end of the loop or forceps in the yellow portion of a gas flame (Fig. 6-3).

Moist heat. As was stated, moist heat causes the cellular proteins (enzymes) in the microorganism to become inactivated, and the cell dies. Boiling water and steam are favored in disinfection because no expensive equipment is necessary and the

Fig. 6-3. The technique for flaming the bacteriological loop.

required time is short. Most pathogens die after 10 minutes of steaming at 70°C (158°F), and boiling for 10 to 30 minutes at 90° to 100°C (194°–212°F), depending on the altitude, destroys most viable bacteria, fungi, and viruses. Clean articles made of metal and glass, such as syringes, needles, and simple instruments, may be disinfected by boiling for 30 minutes. However, this technique is not always effective because heat-resistant bacterial spores, mycobacteria, and viruses may be present. As mentioned in Chapter 2, the spores of the bacteria that cause anthrax, tetanus, gas gangrene, and botulism, as well as the hepatitis viruses, are notably heat resistant and often survive normal disinfection procedures.

An effective way to disinfect clothing, bedding, and dishes is to use hot water, above 60°C (140°F) with a detergent or soap and to agitate the solution around the items. This combination of heat, mechanical action, and chemical inhibition is deadly to most pathogens.

Pressurized steam. An autoclave is a large pressure cooker that uses steam under pressure to completely destroy all microbial life. Pressure raises the temperature of the steam and shortens the time necessary to sterilize materials that can tolerate the high temperature and moisture. Autoclaving at 15 pounds per square inch of pressure at a temperature of 121.5°C (250°F) for 20 minutes will kill viable microorganisms, viruses, and exposed bacterial spores, if they are not hidden in pus, feces, vomitus, blood, or other protein substances. Some types of equipment and certain materials, such as rubber, which may be damaged by high temperatures, can be autoclaved at lower temperatures for longer periods. The timing must be carefully determined based

Fig. 6-4. Pressure-sensitive autoclave tape shows dark stripes after sterilization. (Volk WA, Wheeler MF: Basic Microbiology, 5th ed. Philadelphia, JB Lippincott, 1984)

on the contents and compactness of the load. All articles must be properly packaged and arranged within the autoclave to allow steam penetration of each package (Fig. 6-4). Cans should be open, bottles covered loosely with foil or cotton, and instruments wrapped in cloths. Sealed containers should not be autoclaved.

Cold Microorganisms are not killed by cold temperatures and freezing; their metabolic activities are slowed so that their growth is greatly inhibited. Thus, freezing is a microbistatic method of preservation in which the microorganisms are in a state similar to suspended animation. When the temperature is raised above the freezing point, the metabolic reactions speed up and the organisms slowly begin to reproduce again. Refrigeration merely slows the growth of microorganisms; it does not altogether inhibit them. Many foods, biologic specimens, and bacterial cultures are preserved by rapid freezing to very low temperatures. It should be noted that slow freezing will cause ice crystals to form within the cells and may rupture the cell walls of a few bacteria; hence, if it is important to preserve a pure culture of bacteria, such slow freezing should be avoided and rapid freezing should be performed.

Persons who are involved in the preparation and preservation of foods must be aware that thawing to room temperature allows bacterial spores to germinate and microorganisms to resume growth. This is why the public is reminded time and again that refreezing of thawed foods is an unsafe practice because it preserves the millions of microbes, and the food will deteriorate quickly when it is rethawed. Also, if bacterial endospores of *C. botulinum* or *C. perfringens* were present, the viable bacteria would begin to produce toxins that would cause food poisoning.

Drying For many centuries, foods have been preserved by drying. When moisture and nutrients are lacking, many dried microorganisms remain viable, although they cannot reproduce. Foods, serums, toxins, antitoxins, antibiotics, and pure cultures of microorganisms are often preserved by the combination of freezing and drying. This process, in which the frozen material is dried in a vacuum, is called *lyophilization.*

In the hospital or clinic environment, health care workers should keep in mind that dried viable pathogens may be lurking in dried blood, pus, fecal material, and dust as found on floors, in bedding, on clothing, and in wound dressings. Should these dried materials be disturbed, such as by dry dusting, the microbes would be easily transmitted through the air or by contact. They would then grow rapidly should they settle in a suitable moist, warm nutrient environment such as a wound or a burn. Therefore, important precautions must be observed: wet mop and damp dust floors and furniture, roll the bed linens and towels carefully, and properly dispose of wound dressings.

Radiation The sun is not a particularly reliable disinfecting agent because it kills only those microorganisms that are exposed to direct sunlight. The rays of the sun include the long infrared (heat) rays, the visible light rays, and the shorter ultraviolet (UV) rays. The UV rays do not penetrate glass and building materials but are effective only in the air and on the surface of equipment. They do, however, penetrate cells and thus can cause damage to the DNA molecule. When this occurs, the genes may be so severely damaged that the cell will die (especially unicellular microorganisms) or be drastically changed.

In practice, the UV lamp is useful for reducing the number of microorganisms in the air. The UV lamp often is called a germicidal lamp. Its main component is a low-pressure mercury vapor tube. Such lamps are found in newborn nurseries, operating rooms, elevators, entryways, cafeterias, and classrooms, where they are incorporated into louvered ceiling fixtures designed to radiate across the top of the room without striking persons in the room. The sterility of an area may also be maintained by having a UV lamp placed in a hood or cabinet containing instruments, paper and cloth equipment, liquid, and other inanimate articles. Many biologic materials such as serums, antiserums, toxins, and vaccines are sterilized with UV rays.

Those whose work involves the use of UV lamps must be particularly careful not to expose their eyes or skin to the rays, because the rays can cause serious burns and therefore cellular damage. Because UV rays do not penetrate cloth, metals, and glass, these materials may be used to protect persons working in a UV environment. It has been shown that skin cancer can be caused by excessive exposure to the UV rays of the sun; thus, extensive suntanning is not always beneficial.

X-rays and gamma and beta rays of certain wavelengths from radioactive materials may be lethal or cause mutations in microorganisms and tissue cells because they damage the large molecules or macromolecules (DNA and proteins) within those cells. Work done in radiation research laboratories has demonstrated that these radiations can be used for the prevention of food spoilage, for preparation of organs for transplantation, for the sterilization of heat-sensitive surgical equipment, for the preparation of vaccines, and for the treatment of some chronic diseases such as cancer, all of which are very practical applications for laboratory research. When these radiations are used in the treatment of disease, care must be taken to focus the rays precisely on the specific area being treated to minimize damage to normal cells.

Ultrasonic Waves   In hospitals and clinics, ultrasonic waves are a frequently used means of cleaning and sterilizing delicate equipment. Ultrasonic cleaners consist of tanks filled with liquid solvent (usually water); the short sound waves are then passed through the liquid. The sound waves mechanically dislodge organic debris on instruments and glassware.

Glassware and other articles that have been cleansed in ultrasonic equipment must be washed to remove the dislodged particles and solvent, then be sterilized by another method before they are used.

Filtration   Filters of various pore sizes are used to filter or separate cells, larger viruses, bacteria, and certain other microorganisms from the liquids or gases in which they are suspended. The filtered solution or filtrate is not necessarily sterile, because the small viruses may not be filtered out. The variety of filters is large and includes sintered glass (in which uniform particles of glass are fused), plastic films, unglazed porcelain, asbestos, diatomaceous earth, and cellulose membrane filters. Small quantities of liquid can be filtered through a syringe; large quantities require larger apparatuses.

A cotton plug in a test tube, flask, or pipette is a good filter for preventing the entry of microorganisms. Dry gauze and paper masks prevent the outward passage of microbes from the mouth and nose, at the same time protecting the wearer from inhaling airborne pathogens and foreign particles that could damage the lungs.

Chemical Methods

Chemical disinfection means the use of chemical agents to inhibit the growth of microorganisms, either temporarily or permanently. How effective a chemical disinfectant will be depends on many factors: the concentration of the chemical; the time allowed for the chemical to work; the pH or acidity of the solution; the temperature; and the presence of proteins, blood, pus, feces, mucous secretions, and vomitus. Directions for the preparation and dilution of the disinfectant must be carefully followed and the proper concentration, pH, and temperature must be maintained for the specified period to ensure the best results. The items to be disinfected must first be washed to remove any material in which pathogens may be hidden. Although the washed article may then be clean, it is not safe to use until it has been properly disinfected. Health personnel need to understand an important limitation of chemical disinfection: namely that many disinfectants that are effective against pathogens in the controlled conditions of the laboratory become ineffective in the actual hospital or clinic environment. Furthermore, the stronger and more effective antimicrobial chemical agents have limited use because of their destructiveness to human tissues and to certain other substances.

Almost all bacteria in the vegetative growing state as well as fungi, protozoa, and most viruses are susceptible to many disinfectants, although the mycobacteria of tuberculosis and leprosy, the endospores of bacteria, fungal spores, and the hepatitis viruses are notably resistant. Therefore, chemical disinfection should never be attempted when it is possible to use proper physical sterilization techniques.

The disinfectant most effective for each situation must be carefully chosen. Chemical agents used to disinfect respiratory therapy equipment and thermometers must destroy all pathogenic bacteria, fungi, and viruses that may be found in sputum and saliva. One must be particularly aware of the oral and respiratory pathogens, including the tubercle bacillus, *Pseudomonas,* staphylococci, and the fungi that cause candidiasis, blastomycosis, coccidioidomycosis, and histoplasmosis, as well as all the respiratory viruses.

Because most disinfection methods do not destroy all bacterial spores that are present, any instrument or dressing that was used in the treatment of an infected wound or of a disease caused by spore-formers must be autoclaved or burned. Gas gangrene, tetanus, and anthrax are examples of diseases caused by spore-formers that require the health worker to take such precautions. Formaldehyde and ethylene oxide, when properly used, are highly destructive to spores, mycobacteria, and viruses. Certain articles are heat sensitive and cannot be autoclaved or safely washed before disinfection; such articles are soaked for 24 hours in a strong detergent and disinfectant solution, washed, and then sterilized in the ethylene oxide gas autoclave. The use of disposable equipment whenever possible in these situations will help protect the patient as well as the health care team members.

How effective a chemical agent will be depends to some extent on the physical characteristics of the article on which it is used. A smooth, hard surface is readily disinfected, whereas a rough, porous, or grooved surface is not. For similar reasons, thought must be given to selection of the most suitable germicide for cleaning patient rooms and all other areas where patients are treated.

The most effective antiseptic or disinfectant should be chosen for each specific purpose, each environment, and each pathogen likely to be present. The characteristics of a good chemical antimicrobial agent are as follows:

1. It must kill pathogens within a reasonable period and at specified concentrations.
2. It must be nontoxic to human tissues and noncorrosive and nondestructive to materials on which it will be used.
3. It must be soluble in water and easy to apply. If a tincture (alcohol–water solution) is used, the concentration should be checked. Evaporation of the alcohol solvent can cause a 1% solution to increase to a 10% solution, and at this concentration it may cause tissue damage.
4. It should be inexpensive and easy to prepare for use with simple, specific directions.
5. It must be stable in the dissolved or solid form so that is can be shipped and stored for a reasonable period.
6. It should be stable to *p*H and temperature changes within reasonable limits.

Antisepsis   Most antimicrobial chemical agents are too irritating and destructive to be applied to the mucous membranes and the skin. Those that may be safely used on human tissues are called *antiseptics*. An antiseptic merely reduces the number of organisms on a surface but does not penetrate the pores and hair follicles to destroy microorganisms residing there. To remove organisms lodged in pores and folds of the skin, health personnel use an antiseptic soap and scrub with a brush. The surgeon wears sterile gloves on freshly scrubbed hands, and a mask and hood to cover face and hair, to prevent resident normal flora from contaminating the surgical field. Also, an antiseptic is applied at the site of the surgical incision to destroy local micro-organisms.

How Antimicrobial Chemicals Work   *Injury of cell membranes.* Soap and detergents are referred to as surfactants; this means that they are surface-active agents that help to disperse the bacteria so they are more readily rinsed away. These agents concentrate on the surface and thus reduce the surface tension; this characteristic makes them good wetting and dispersing agents. Some agents, such as Dial and Safeguard soaps, contain disinfectants, which also aid in killing bacteria. Certain concentrations of weak acids such as acetic acid and benzoic acids may be used.

Inactivation of enzymes. Alcohols, such as ethyl and isopropyl, are good skin antiseptics at 70% solution. They have a low toxicity for humans, hence they are frequently used to disinfect clinical thermometers and other instruments. Alcohols are tuberculocidal (destructive of tuberculosis-causing organisms) but not sporicidal (destructive of spores).

Carbolic acid, cresol soaps, and such commercial preparations as Lysol are germicidal but are too irritating and toxic to be used on the skin. They also are not sporicidal.

Salts of heavy metals such as mercury chloride (Merthiolate, Mercurochrome, Metaphen) and silver nitrate (Argyrol, Protargol) are bacteriostatic antiseptics, but they are not sporicidal and are ineffective against many pathogens. Silver nitrate in low concentrations is used in the eyes of newborns to kill the gonococcus organism; this prevents gonorrheal infections, which could cause blindness.

Chemical oxidizing agents are useful disinfectants. Two of these are hydrogen peroxide and sodium perborate, which destroy bacteria and tissue debris and prevent anaerobic growth in damaged tissues. A third, potassium permanganate, is employed in weak solutions to treat urethral infections and fungal infections of the skin. Another agent in this group is ethylene oxide (Carboxide, Cryoxide, Oxygume), which is used as a sterilant in gas autoclaves to sterilize heat-sensitive materials. It is a good micro-bicide and sporicide but must be used with great care because it is inflammable and is toxic to humans.

The elements and many compounds of chlorine, iodine, bromine, and fluorine are also useful disinfectants. For example, chlorine compounds (Clorox, Halozone, hypochlorites, Warexin) are used to disinfect water and sewage and for sanitation of dishes, floors, and plumbing fixtures. It has been found that the HIV (AIDS virus) can be destroyed on syringes and needles by soaking them in Chlorox. The iodine compounds, such as Wescodyne, Betadine, Isodine, and tincture of iodine, are effective skin antiseptics and disinfectants. These compounds can be dangerous, however; if an alcohol solution of iodine is left open to the air, allowing the alcohol to evaporate, the solution may become too concentrated, and an iodine burn may result if it is used on the skin. Most compounds of bromine and fluorine are too toxic at the effective concentrations to be used as antiseptics. All of these compounds are viricidal, bactericidal, and tuberculocidal, but not sporicidal.

Damage to the genetic material. The DNA of cells is inactivated by caustic compounds such as formalin. Formalin is a 37% aqueous solution of gaseous formaldehyde that inactivates proteins and nucleic acids. It is one of the few antimicrobial agents that also are sporicidal; however, it is so irritating to the skin and mucous membranes that it cannot be used on living tissues. Frequently it is used to preserve tissue specimens.

Basic aniline dyes also inactivate the nucleic acids. In this group are included gentian violet and crystal violet, which are useful in treatment of fungal skin infections (ringworm) and vaginal infections caused by yeasts (*Candida*) and gram-positive bacteria, as well as intestinal infestations of roundworms. Pyridium is a dye classified in the same group. It is prescribed for urinary infections caused by gram-negative enteric organisms.

Chemotherapy

For thousands of years, people have been finding and using herbs and chemicals to cure diseases. The native witch doctors in Central and South America long ago discovered that ipecac, an herb, aided in the treatment of dysentery and that an extract of quinine bark was effective in treating malaria. During the 16th and 17th centuries, the alchemists of Europe searched for a way to cure smallpox, syphilis, and the many other diseases that were rampant during that period of history. Many mercury and arsenic chemicals used frequently caused more damage to the patient than to the pathogen.

The true beginning of modern chemotherapy was in the late 1800s when Paul Ehrlich began his search for chemicals that would destroy bacteria yet would not affect normal body cells. By 1909 he had tested and discarded more than 600 chemicals. Finally, in that year, he discovered an arsenic compound that proved effective against syphilis. Because this was the 606th compound Ehrlich had tried, he called it "compound 606." The technical name for it was arsphenamine and the trade name was Salvorsan. Until the purification of penicillin in 1938, Salvorsan was used to treat syphilis.

In 1928 Alexander Fleming noted that the waste products of a mold, *Penicillium notatum*, inhibited the growth of staphylococci on an agar plate. He also found that broth cultures of the mold not only were not toxic to his laboratory animals, but that they destroyed staphylococci and other bacteria. During World War II, two biochemists, Howard Florey and Ernst Boris Chain, purified penicillin and demonstrated its effectiveness in treatment of various bacterial infections. By 1942, the American drug industry was able to produce sufficient penicillin for human use, and the search for other antibiotics began.

In 1935, a chemist named Gerhard Domagk discovered the dye Prontosil, which was effective against streptococcal infections in mice. Further research demonstrated that Prontosil was degraded or broken down in the body into sulfanilamide, and that the sulfanilamide was the effective agent. For their outstanding contributions to scientific progress, these investigators received the Nobel Prize at various times.

A *chemotherapeutic agent* or *antimicrobial drug* is any chemical used to treat infectious disease by inhibiting or killing pathogens *in vivo* (in the living animal). A chemotherapeutic substance that is derived from a living organism and that in small amounts kills or inhibits the growth of microorganisms is labeled an *antibiotic;* these substances are produced by molds, bacteria, and some plants. The term antibiotic was intended to distinguish between chemical therapeutic agents, such as sulfonamide drugs, and those that are extracted from the waste products of living organisms, such as penicillin, streptomycin, and erythromycin; however, many of these drugs are now synthesized or manufactured in the laboratory.

The ideal chemotherapeutic agent should (1) kill or inhibit the growth of pathogens, (2) cause no damage to the host, (3) cause no allergic reaction in the host, (4) be stable so that it can be stored in the solid or liquid form, (5) be retained in specific tissues in the body long enough to be effective, and (6) kill the pathogens before they mutate and become resistant to it. However, almost all chemotherapeutic agents either have some side-effects or produce allergic reactions or enable resistant mutant pathogens to develop.

How Chemotherapeutic Drugs Work

To be effective an antimicrobial drug must inhibit or destroy the pathogen without damaging the host. The agent does this by disrupting the pathogen's metabolism in an area that is slightly different from normal human metabolism. Some examples will illustrate how, through scientific research, we have learned to "trick" pathogens in such a way as to improve the lot of humanity.

The sulfonamide drugs inhibit production of folic acid in those bacteria that require para-aminobenzoic acid (usually abbreviated PABA) to synthesize folic acid. The folic acid (a vitamin) is essential to the bacteria. Because the sulfonamide molecule is similar in shape to the PABA molecule, the bacteria attempt to metabolize the sulfonamide to produce folic acid (Fig. 6-5). However, the enzymes that convert the PABA to folic acid do not function on the sulfonamide molecule. Without the folic acid, the bacteria cannot produce some essential proteins and finally die. The sulfa drugs therefore are called *competitive inhibitors,* that is, by competing with an enzyme that metabolizes an essential nutrient, they inhibit the growth of the microorganisms. In other words, they are bacteriostatic. The cells of humans and animals do not synthesize folic acid from PABA (they get it from the food they eat) and consequently they are unaffected by the sulfa drugs.

Fig. 6-5. The effect of sulfonamide drugs.

In most of the gram-positive bacteria, including the streptococci and staphylococci, penicillin interferes with the synthesis of peptidoglycan required in the bacterial cell wall. Thus, by inhibiting cell wall synthesis, the penicillin destroys the bacteria. Why does penicillin not also destroy human cells? Human cells are eucaryotic cells and do not have a cell wall.

There are other chemotherapeutic drugs that have similar action: they inhibit a specific step that is essential to the microorganism's metabolism and thereby cause its destruction. Antibiotics are employed in this way against bacteria, and they are highly effective. Some destroy the gram-positive bacteria; some destroy the gram-negative bacteria; those that are destructive to many gram-negative and gram-positive bacteria are called *broad-spectrum antibiotics*. Examples of broad-spectrum antibiotics are tetracycline, streptomycin, and ampicillin. Table 6-2 lists some of the antimicrobial drugs most frequently used against many common pathogens.

Antimicrobial drugs work well against bacterial pathogens because the bacteria (being procaryotic) have different cellular structures and metabolic pathways that can be disrupted by drugs that would not damage the host (eucaryotic) cells. These antibacterial agents work in one of several ways.

1. To inhibit peptidoglycan cell wall synthesis, *e.g.*, penicillins, vancomycin, and cephalosporins
2. To act as competitive enzyme inhibitors to block the formation of essential metabolites; these "antimetabolites" include the sulfa drugs, trimethoprim, and ethambutol
3. To inhibit protein synthesis by acting on 70S ribosomes, *e.g.*, tetracyclines, erythromycin, streptomycin, neomycin, and chloroamphenicol
4. To damage plasma membranes, such as polymyxin B

(Text continues on p. 136)

Table 6-2 Some Chemotherapeutic Agents Employed Against Important Pathogens

Pathogen	Disease	Chemotherapy or Treatment
Bacteria		
Bacillus anthracis	Anthrax	Penicillin, tetracyclines, erythromycin
Bordetella pertussis	Whooping cough	Tetracyclines, penicillin, ampicillin
Brucella abortus and B. melitensis	Brucellosis, undulant fever	Tetracyclines, streptomycin
Chlamydia trachomatis	Lymphogranuloma venereum	Sulfonamides, tetracyclines
Clostridium botulinum	Botulism (food poisoning)	(Antitoxin), penicillin, kanamycin
Clostridium perfringens	Gas gangrene, wound infections	(Antitoxin), penicillin, kanamycin
Clostridium tetani	Tetanus (lockjaw)	(Antitoxin), penicillin, kanamycin
Corynebacterium diphtheriae	Diphtheria	(Antitoxin), penicillin, erythromycin
Escherichia coli	Urinary infections	Sulfonamides, gentamicin, cefazolin, nalidixic acid, norfloxacin
Francisella tularensis	Tularemia	Streptomycin, tetracyclines
Haemophilus ducreyi	Chancroid	Streptomycin, tetracyclines
Haemophilus influenzae	Meningitis, pneumonia	Ampicillin, streptomycin, tetracyclines, cefamandole
Klebsiella pneumoniae	Pneumonia	Colistin, cefazolin, gentamicin
Legionella pneumophila	Legionnaires' disease	Erythromycin
Mycobacterium leprae	Leprosy	Dapsone, tetracyclines, rifamide
Mycobacterium tuberculosis	Tuberculosis	Isoniazid, streptomycin, PAS, rifamide, ethambutol
Mycoplasma pneumoniae	Atypical pneumonia	Tetracyclines, erythromycin
Neisseria gonorrhoeae	Gonorrhea	Pencillin, tetracyclines, spectinomycin
Neisseria meningitidis	Nasopharangitis, meningitis	Penicillin, sulfonamides, ampicillin, tetracyclines, rifamide
Proteus vulgaris and P. morgani	Gastroenteritis, urinary infections	Kanamycin, streptomycin, nalidixic acid
Pseudomonas aeruginosa	Respiratory and urogenital infections	Gentamicin, sulfonamides, mezlocillin, amikacin
Rickettsia rickettsii	Rocky Mountain spotted fever	Tetracyclines, chloramphenicol
Salmonella typhi	Typhoid fever	Chloramphenicol, ampicillin, tetracyclines

Table 6-2 Some Chemotherapeutic Agents Employed Against Important Pathogens *(continued)*

Pathogen	Disease	Chemotherapy or Treatment
Salmonella spp.	Gastroenteritis	Chloramphenicol, ampicillin, tetracyclines, co-trimoxazole
Shigella spp.	Shigellosis (bacillary dysentery)	Ampicillin, tetracyclines, sulfonamides, nalidixic acid
Staphylococcus aureus	Boils, carbuncles, pneumonia, septicemia	Bacitracin, erythromycin, gentamicin, vancomycin, cephalosporins
Streptococcus pyogenes	Strep throat, scarlet fever, rheumatic fever, septicemia	Penicillin, lincomycin, erythromycin
Streptococcus pneumoniae	Pneumonia	Penicillin, lincomycin, erythromycin
Treponema pallidum	Syphilis	Penicillin, erythromycin, tetracyclines
Vibrio cholerae	Cholera	Streptomycin, chloramphenicol
Yersinia pestis	Plague	Streptomycin, tetracyclines
Fungi		
Dermatophytes	Tineas	Nystatin, amphotericin B, griseofulvin
Candida	Mucosal candidiasis	Clotrimazole, micanazole, nystatin
Blastomyces	⎫	5-Flucytosine, amphotericin B
Histoplasma	⎪	5-Flucytosine, amphotericin B
Cryptococcus	⎬ Systemic mycosis	5-Flucytosine, amphotericin B
Coccidioides	⎪	5-Flucytosine, amphotericin B
Candida	⎭	Amphotericin B
Protozoa		
Trichomonas	Trichomoniasis	Metronidazole, griseofulvin
Giardia lamblia	Giardiasis	Metronidazole, quinacrine
Entamoeba histolytica	Amebiasis	Emetine, metronidazole
Toxoplasma	Toxoplasmosis	Clindamycin
Plasmodium spp.	Malaria	Clindamycin, chloroquine, pyrimethamine, sulfadiazine
Pneumocystis carinii	Pneumonia	Pentamidine, co-trimoxazole
Viruses		
Herpes spp.	Eye and lip	Idoxuridine, acyclovir
	Genital	Acyclovir
	Encephalitis	Vidarabine, acyclovir
Influenza A	Influenza	Amantidine, rimantadine
Human immunodeficiency virus (HIV)	AIDS	Azidothymidine (AZT), dideoxycytidine, ribavirin, suramin

5. To inhibit nucleic acid synthesis, *e.g.*, rifamycin, nalidixic acid, and norfloxacin

It often happens that a single chemotherapeutic agent is not sufficient to destroy all the pathogens that develop during the course of a disease, so two or more drugs may be used simultaneously to prevent resistant mutant pathogens from emerging. In tuberculosis, for example, three drugs are routinely prescribed, and as many as twelve drugs may be required in resistant cases. Many urinary, respiratory, and gastrointestinal infections respond particularly well to a combination of trimethoprim and sulfamethoxazole; this combination is called co-trimoxazole.

It is much more difficult to use antimicrobial drugs against fungal and protozoan pathogens because they are eucaryotic cells, thus the drugs are much more toxic to the host. Antifungal agents work by (1) binding with plasma membrane sterols, *e.g.*, nystatin and amphotericin B; (2) by interfering with sterol synthesis, *e.g.*, clotrimazole and micanazole; (3) by blocking mitosis or nucleic acid synthesis, *e.g.*, griseofulvin and 5-flucytosine. Antiprotozoan drugs are usually quite toxic and work (1) by interfering with DNA and RNA synthesis, *e.g.*, chloroquine, pentamidine, and quinacrine; or (2) by interfering with protozoan metabolism, *e.g.*, metronidazole.

Antiviral chemotherapeutic agents are particularly difficult to find and use because the viruses are being produced within the host's cells. A few have been found to be effective in certain conditions, and these work by interfering with the action of certain enzymes necessary for viral replication. These include amantadine and rimantadine (for influenza), acyclovir (for herpes), and azidothymidine (AZT, for AIDS). Some may interfere with DNA replication and RNA transcription; the action of others is unknown.

In cancer, in which the malignant cells are dividing more rapidly than the normal cells, the chemical agents that inhibit DNA and RNA synthesis can be used, provided the dosage and total period of administration are carefully controlled. Cancer drugs interfere with normal DNA function in rapidly dividing cells, whether the cells are normal or malignant. Thus, the normal cells that are rapidly dividing, including skin cells, the erythroblasts that later become blood cells, and the sperm cells, are damaged along with the malignant cells. This is why blood cell counts are done frequently in cancer patients: the physician must be able to determine at what point the chemotherapy must be discontinued to avoid critical damage to the patient's normal cells.

There are many reasons why chemotherapeutic drugs should not be used indiscriminately:

1. The microorganisms may mutate and become resistant to the antibiotic. Their metabolism may change, and they may produce an enzyme that can destroy the antibiotic, or one that uses the antibiotic as a nutrient; or they may become impermeable to the antibiotic. To prevent these developments, several drugs, each of which has a different mode of action, often are administered simultaneously.

2. The patient may become allergic to the antibiotic. For example, penicillin G in low doses often sensitizes those who are prone to allergies; when these persons receive a second dose of penicillin at some later date, they may have a severe reaction known as anaphylactic shock, or they may break out in hives. This reaction is described in more detail in Chapter 11.

3. Many chemotherapeutic drugs are toxic to humans, and some are so toxic they are administered only for serious diseases for which there are no other antibiotics available. One such drug is chloramphenicol (Chloromycetin) which, if given in high doses for a long period, may cause a very severe type of anemia called aplastic anemia. Another is streptomycin, which can damage the auditory nerve and cause deafness.

4. With prolonged use, the broad-spectrum antibiotics may destroy the normal flora of the mouth, intestine, or vagina. The person no longer has the protection of the normal flora and, thus, becomes much more susceptible to infections caused by opportunists or secondary invaders. The result is a superinfection. An example of such an infection is diarrhea, which can result from prolonged antibiotic therapy owing to the loss of the normal protective microbes. This topic is discussed more fully in Chapter 5.

Therefore, chemotherapeutic drugs, including antibiotics, should be taken only when prescribed and only under a physician's supervision. Also, the proper dosage must be administered for the recommended period to prevent resistant organisms gaining a foothold.

In recent years, science research has developed new antibiotics at such a rapid pace that many thoughful people, including some of the researchers, are beginning to fear that pathogens are becoming so resistant to antibiotics that the human race may be destroyed. Some problems already have arisen; a case in point is pneumonia. In the developed countries of the world, the types of pneumonia occurring at present are different from those that were seen 30 years ago, and sometimes they are highly resistant to treatment. Our hope is that antibiotics will be used with greater care and that effective vaccines may become available. We now have *H. influenzae* and a *Streptococcus pneumoniae* vaccine on the market to protect against some types of pneumonia, but not all. Also, resistant strains of gonococci, *Neisseria gonorrhoeae*, have developed, and we hope to soon see a vaccine against gonorrhea, syphilis, and AIDS. The difficulty then will be to convince the American public to take the vaccines to protect themselves against these pathogens.

Problems and Questions

1. Discuss why it is necessary to control microbial growth.
2. Give the definitions for sterilization, disinfection, pasteurization, and lyophilization.
3. What are the differences between sterile, aseptic, and antiseptic techniques? In what circumstances might each be used?

4. What are the characteristics of bacteria indicated by the following terms: psychrophilic, mesophilic, thermophilic, halophilic, haloduric, alkaliphilic, acidophilic?

5. What are the characteristics of a good antimicrobial agent?

6. List some effective physical and chemical means of controlling microbial growth.

7. How do chemotherapeutic agents destroy microbes without also killing the patient?

8. Discuss why antibiotics should be used discriminately.

Chapter 7

Microbes versus Humans

Objectives

After studying this chapter, you should be able to
1. Differentiate between infectious, communicable, and contagious disease
2. List six reasons why an infection may not occur when a pathogen is present
3. Discuss the disease process
4. Define acute and chronic disease
5. State the difference between primary and secondary diseases
6. State the difference between local and generalized infections
7. List three factors associated with the virulence of a pathogen
8. List and discuss eight factors that affect the pathogenicity of bacteria

New Words to Pronounce and Understand

Botulism (bot'-you-lis-um). A disease caused by a bacterial exotoxin in food

Coagulase (co-ag'-you-laze). An enzyme that clots plasma around bacteria

Collagenase (col-lodge'-in-aze). An enzyme that breaks down collagen in connective tissue

Encephalitis (en-seff-uh-lie'-tis). A disease involving inflammation of the brain

Fibrinolysin (fy-brin-oh'-li-sin). An enzyme that breaks down fibrin clots

Hemolysin (he-moll'-uh-sin). An enzyme that breaks down red blood cells

Hyaluronic acid (high'-ah-lu-ron'-ick). A chemical in connective tissue

Hyaluronidase (high'-ah-lu-ron'-uh-days). An enzyme that
breaks down connective tissue

Leukocidin (lew-co-side'-in). An enzyme that destroys white
blood cells

Pathogenicity (path-oh-gin-iss'-city). The ability of an organism
to cause disease

Streptokinase (strep-tow-kine'-aze). An enzyme that aids
streptococci to invade the body by dissolving blood clots

Toxigenicity (tox-uh-gin-iss'-city). The ability of a pathogen to
produce a toxin, causing damage to the host

Toxin (tox'-in). A toxic or damaging substance

Virulence (veer'-you-lence). The properties of an organism that
make it pathogenic

There are many diseases that are not caused by pathogens. Included among
them are those caused by malfunction of an organ, such as diabetes and hyper-
thyroidism; those caused by a vitamin deficiency, such as scurvy and rickets; those
caused by an allergic response, such as asthma and hay fever; and those caused by
uncontrolled cell growth, such as tumors and cancer. However, the object of our
interest in this chapter is the many infectious diseases caused by the growth of
pathogens on and in living tissues.

The ability of a pathogen to invade and infect the host, cause damage, and
produce disease is termed its *virulence*. Those microbes that can cause disease with
relative ease are referred to as *virulent* pathogens; microorganisms incapable of causing disease, except in rare circumstances, are described as *avirulent*. Within a single
genus and species, some strains may be virulent and others avirulent, as determined
by the genetic characteristics of the microorganism. Thus, when a person is exposed
to a pathogen, disease may or may not result depending on many factors, including
the host's resistance and the virulence of the microorganism.

The potential for infections always exists when organisms live in a parasitic
relationship. When a pathogen finds the appropriate places and conditions in which
it can grow and cause damage, it produces an infectious disease.

An *infection* occurs when a pathogenic microbe is able to multiply in the tissues
where it lodges. Thus, an *infectious* disease results from the growth of a pathogenic
microorganism. A *communicable* disease can be transmitted from one person to another, as with measles, gonorrhea, and diphtheria. A *contagious* disease is a communicable disease that is easily transmitted from person to person via droplets in the air,
such as occurs with the common cold and influenza.

The severity of an infectious disease and the amount of damage inflicted is
determined by the host's ability to resist invasion and to neutralize the damaging
enzymes and toxins from the pathogen.

$$\text{Severity of infection} = \frac{\text{microbial virulence}}{\text{host defenses}}$$

Why Infection Does Not Always Occur

Many persons who are exposed to pathogenic microbes do not get sick. There are several reasons for this.

1. The microbe may alight in the wrong place and be unable to multiply. For example, when a respiratory pathogen falls on the skin, it may be unable to grow because the skin lacks the necessary warmth, moisture, and nutrients required for the growth of the particular microbe.
2. Many pathogens must be able to attach to specific host receptor sites before they can multiply and cause damage.
3. There may be antibacterial factors present that destroy or inhibit growth, such as lysozyme in the tears, saliva, and perspiration.
4. The normal flora present may inhibit the growth of the foreign microorganism in regions such as the mouth, vagina, and intestine, by occupying the space and using the available nutrients.
5. The microbes already growing in the region may produce antibacterial factors (called bacteriocidins) that have a local antibiotic effect, as when streptococci inhibit the diphtheria pathogen.
6. Antibodies may be present because the person had previously had the infection or had been immunized against it. These antibodies will attack and destroy the pathogen before it can multiply.
7. Phagocytes present in the mucous membranes will attempt to engulf and destroy the invader.

The Development of Infection

Infection occurs when the pathogens are able to enter the host, attach, adhere, multiply, and cause damage to the tissues of the host.

The body responds to the infection via the inflammatory process (Fig. 7-1). The symptoms of inflammation are swelling (edema), redness, heat (fever), and pain. The swelling is due to the escape of large quantities of fluid from the highly permeable capillaries. The area becomes reddened because more blood is brought to it. The heat is caused by increased metabolic activity in the cells. Pain usually results from pressure on the nerve endings. Phagocytes rush in to help destroy the invaders and rid the area of dead tissue. Pus is often found at the site of inflammation; it consists of lymph, serum, tissue cells, dead leukocytes, and sometimes bacteria.

The production of antibodies begins slowly; the body attempts to isolate the infection by forming a connective tissue wall that will inhibit deeper penetration by the pathogens around the site of infection. If the pathogen is pyogenic (pus-forming), such as a staphylococcus or a streptococcus, the inflamed area will contain much more pus than is normally present during the inflammatory process. Inflammation and antibody production are further discussed in Chapters 10 and 11, which are devoted to mechanisms of defense against disease.

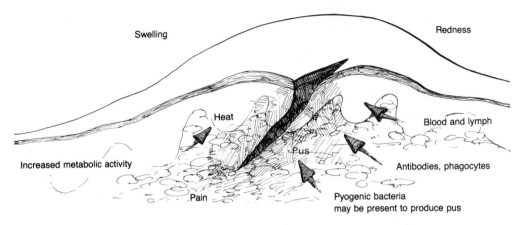

Fig. 7-1. The development of infection and the inflammatory process. The symptoms of inflammation include swelling, redness, heat, and pain. Pus may also be present whether or not pyogenic bacteria are present.

The Disease Process

If the body wins the battle against the invading pathogens at the site of inflammation, the local infection is stopped. The person then has some antibodies to protect him against a later similar infection, but he may become a "carrier" if all of the pathogens have not been destroyed. A person may recover from a sore throat without complications, yet he may harbor the pathogen (become a carrier) and transmit it to others.

Clinical disease occurs when the body's primary defenses lose the war with the pathogen. The disease may be a *local* infection in which the pathogen is confined to a single area; this is the situation in diphtheria, "staph" boils or carbuncles, "strep" sore throat, tuberculosis, primary syphilis, and gonorrhea. But if the pathogen is not stopped at the local level, it may deeply invade the tissues or be carried by the bloodstream as a *generalized* or *systemic* infection; this occurs in systemic streptococcal infection, staphylococcal septicemia, and meningitis.

A disease may be acute, chronic, or both, beginning as an acute response that becomes a chronic illness. An *acute* disease has a rapid onset followed by a rapid recovery, as with measles, mumps, and influenza. A *chronic* disease is one of long duration and slow onset, such as tuberculosis, leprosy (Hansen's disease), and syphilis. Some diseases, such as gonorrhea, often have an acute inflammatory phase, then become chronic, causing slow deterioration of the infected tissues.

A disease may also reach a stage in which there are no symptoms (asymptomatic disease); it is then known as a *latent infection* or *latent stage*; tuberculosis, syphilis, gonorrhea, and herpes cold sores are examples. In tuberculosis, when the tubercles of *Mycobacterium tuberculosis* are successfully walled off in the lungs, the symptoms disappear temporarily; the infection then is said to be latent. Syphilis progresses through primary, secondary, latent, and tertiary stages (Fig. 7-2). The lesion, or chancre, of the primary stage appears at the site of entry of the spirochete

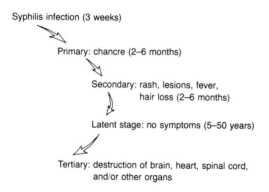

Syphilis infection (3 weeks)

Primary: chancre (2–6 months)

Secondary: rash, lesions, fever,
hair loss (2–6 months)

Latent stage: no symptoms (5–50 years)

Tertiary: destruction of brain, heart, spinal cord,
and/or other organs

Fig. 7-2. Stages of syphilis.

Treponema pallidum. A few weeks after the spirochete has invaded the bloodstream, the chancre disappears, and the symptoms of the secondary stage arise, including rash, fever, and lesions of the mucous membranes. This is the most contagious stage of syphilis. These symptoms also disappear after a few weeks when the disease enters the latent stage, which may last from 1 to 50 years and may cause few or no symptoms. In tertiary syphilis the organism causes destruction of the organ where it had been hiding: the brain, the heart, or bone tissue.

Gonorrhea, caused by *Neisseria gonorrhoeae,* is often an *asymptomatic disease* in the early phase when the organism lives in the mucous membranes of the urogenital tract, rectum, or mouth. After many months, during which the organism causes damage, scarring, and constriction of the fallopian tubes or vas deferens, localized pain is experienced. Gonorrhea is very contagious by direct mucous membrane-to-mucous membrane transfer, usually sexual. It is particularly difficult to detect because it has been shown to be asymptomatic in most infected women and in many infected men.

Cold sores, or fever blisters, and venereal herpes are caused by latent herpes virus infections. The viruses remain dormant inside the cell and do not destroy it until some type of stress acts as a trigger. These stresses may be fever caused by illness; heat and ultraviolet rays from the sun (sunburn); a bruise; extreme cold; or an emotional upset.

An infection that is the first or original illness is called the *primary* disease, such as a cold or influenza. A *secondary* disease or infection is caused by a pathogen that can invade only a weakened person with lowered resistance. Examples of secondary diseases or infections are pneumonia and ear or sinus infections following a primary case of influenza.

Once exposure to the pathogen has occurred, the course of infectious disease has three periods: (1) the incubation period when there are no symptoms, (2) the period of illness with progression of symptoms, and (3) the convalescent period, disability, or death (fortunately the final stage is usually the convalescent period; Fig. 7-3). The communicable diseases are most contagious during the second period. For

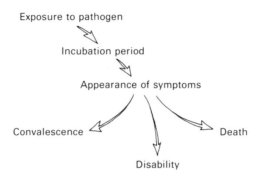

Fig. 7-3. The course of infectious disease.

instance in measles the incubation period lasts 10 to 12 days after the initial exposure to the virus. The early symptoms are much like those of a cold, with an eye infection and low-grade fever, and Koplik's spots (red with white centers) can be seen inside the cheeks. During this early stage the virus is easily transmitted in secretions from the eyes, nose, and mouth. As the illness progresses a skin rash appears; it disappears during the convalescent stage. Usually, measles is considered contagious only from the time the fever begins until the second day of the rash. Complications are frequent because body defenses are lowered by the initial virus infection; thus, the virus and possibly opportunistic bacteria can invade deeper to cause pneumonia, ear and sinus infections, or encephalitis.

Although the patient may recover from the illness itself, there may be permanent damage caused by the disease; brain damage may follow encephalitis or meningitis; paralysis may follow poliomyelitis; deafness may follow ear infections. This type of damage is caused by destruction of tissues in the affected area.

Mechanisms of Disease Causation

The capacity of pathogens to cause disease (virulence) is related to their ability to (1) infect the host or protect themselves against the body defenses, (2) invade and multiply in tissues, and (3) cause damage or destruction to tissue. In other words,

virulence = infectivity + invasiveness + toxigenicity.

Each species of pathogenic microbes has specific characteristics, including its unique metabolism, that determine its pathogenicity and virulence. It would be impossible to list every individual pathogen and its disease-causing mechanism in this text; in fact, the mechanism frequently is not completely understood. With these limitations in mind, we will discuss some of the factors associated with virulence and pathogenicity.

The ability of a pathogen to settle upon a susceptible tissue and to survive the shock of landing is largely a matter of chance, but once it finds itself in a moist, warm environment, it must be able to resist the body's bacteriolytic enzymes, antibodies, and phagocytes if it is to multiply successfully.

Bacterial Morphology Associated with Infectivity

Some structural aspects of pathogens actually enable them to attach to tissues in certain areas of the host and survive to multiply and cause an infection. These structures include capsules, flagella, and pili.

Capsules Capsules are often regarded as a portion of the cell envelope (including cell membrane, cell wall, and outer slime layer). Capsular constituents vary among the different species of procaryons. Many bacteria have slimy capsule layers consisting of polysaccharides only; others have proteins within the polysaccharide capsule. Both serve to enable the bacteria to attach to tissues and to resist phagocytic digestion (Fig. 7-4). Most bacteria infecting the body have some type of capsule, but it is frequently not seen when they are grown on an artificial medium.

Some colonies of bacteria secrete polysaccharide fibers (glycocalyx) to increase adherence to teeth and mucous membranes. This additional polysaccharide layer also protects the colony from antibodies, phagocytes, and other antimicrobial agents.

The cell envelope of group A *Streptococcus pyogenes* contains a certain antigenic protein (protein M) that appears to be antiphagocytic, and other substances that aid the organism in adhering to pharyngeal cells.

Flagella Although flagella serve useful functions by making certain bacteria motile, they also can aid bacteria in invading the aqueous areas of the body. In spite of the flushing action and continuous peristaltic movement of the ureters, some flagellated pathogens are able to reach the kidney where they cause serious infections and complications.

Pili Frequently, the piliated pathogens are able to adhere to cells within mucous membranes to establish an infection when other pathogens cannot; for example, *N.*

Fig. 7-4. Electron micrograph of *Streptococcus pneumoniae*, type 1. The capsule has been reacted to accentuate its visibility. (Mudd S, et al: J Exp Med 78:327, 1943. By copyright permission, Rockefeller University Press)

gonorrhoeae with pili attach to urethral cells and multiply while other pathogens are flushed away by urination. Enterotoxigenic *E. coli* also appear to be piliated and are able to attach to cells in the intestine where they multiply and secrete the exotoxins that cause gastroenteritis (see Fig. 2-9 for an example of a piliated *E. coli*).

Enzymes Associated with Invasiveness

Pathogens excrete some enzymes that step up their ability to invade body tissues. These substances include (1) coagulase, (2) streptokinase, (3) hyaluronidase, and (4) collagenase. Note that the *-ase* ending always indicates that the material is an enzyme, that is, it catalyzes (speeds up) a particular reaction.

Coagulase Pathogenic staphylococci are noted for the production of the extracellular (outside the cell) enzyme coagulase. This enzyme enables the staph organisms to clot plasma and thereby to form a sticky coat of fibrin around themselves for protection. In the laboratory the coagulase-positive staphylococci cause citrated blood plasma to clot.

Streptokinase Sometimes referred to as fibrinolysin, streptokinase has the opposite effect of coagulase. Streptokinase lyses, or dissolves, a fibrin clot, thus enabling the streptococci to invade and spread throughout the body. A similar enzyme produced by staphylococci is called *staphylokinase*.

Hyaluronidase The spreading factor, as hyaluronidase is sometimes called, enables pathogens to spread through connective tissue by breaking down the tissue's hyaluronic acid. It is secreted by several pathogenic species.

Collagenase The enzyme collagenase breaks down collagen, the supportive protein found in tendons, cartilage, and bones. *Clostridium perfringens,* which causes gas gangrene, spreads deeply within the body by secreting collagenase and hyaluronidase.

Toxins and Enzymes Associated with Toxigenicity

The ability to damage host tissues may depend upon the excretion of hemolysin, leukocidin, and exotoxins. Endotoxins (*endo* = within), which are an integral part of the pathogen's cell wall, may also be toxic to the host.

Hemolysin Hemolysin (*hemo* = blood; *lysis* = breakdown or dissolution) causes damage to the host's red blood cells, the erythrocytes. This hemolysis of red blood cells in blood agar is useful as a diagnostic tool for identifying α-hemolytic and β-hemolytic streptococci, as described in Chapter 5. The pathogenicity and invasiveness of the streptococci may not depend on the amount of hemolysin produced, although it is certainly related to the amount of damage the organisms can cause to the host.

Leukocidin This enzymelike exotoxin (*exo* = outside) secreted by some staphylococci and streptococci causes destruction of the white blood cells, the leukocytes. The effect of leukocidin has been shown by observation of lysis on a laboratory slide of leukocytes in the presence of streptococci.

Lecithinase The alpha (α) toxin of *Clostridium perfringens* is called lecithinase. It is destructive to the cell membranes of red blood cells and other tissues.

Exotoxins Bacterial exotoxins are usually proteins secreted by living (vegetative) pathogens. Exotoxins are often described by the target organs they affect. The most toxic exotoxins are *neurotoxins;* they are the cause of nerve destruction in botulism and diphtheria and of spasmodic muscle contractions (tetany) in tetanus. *Enterotoxins,* those toxins that affect the vomiting centers of the brain and cause gastroenteritis, are secreted by *Staphylococcus aureus, Vibrio cholerae, Shigella dysenteriae,* and a few other enteric pathogens. Some new strains of *E. coli* are known to produce an enterotoxin causing a form of dysentery. Toxic shock syndrome (TSS) symptoms are caused by exotoxins (C and F) secreted by the staphylococci. The *exfoliatins* of TSS cause the epidermal layers of the skin to slough away, and *erythrotoxins* cause rash and redness in the skin. Pathogens of diphtheria secrete toxins that affect the heart muscle (cardiotoxins), nerves (neurotoxins), and kidneys (nephrotoxins).

Endotoxins The cell walls of certain gram-negative bacteria contain endotoxins that cause disease when the bacteria are present in large numbers. With the destruction and death of the bacteria in the digestive tract, the lipopolysaccharide and protein molecules in the cell wall cause fever, vomiting, and diarrhea. Diseases associated with endotoxins include dysentery, meningitis, typhoid fever, gonorrhea, and cholera.

Endotoxins appear to destroy phagocytes, to upset the water and salt balance in the intestine, and to weaken the infected host by dehydration (because of water loss in diarrhea); as a result, the person is a prime target for secondary infections.

Pathogenicity and Virulence

In summary, all of the terms presented in this chapter concerning the pathogenicity and virulence of pathogens are useful in discussing general concepts of disease causation. Pathogenicity and virulence are sometimes used synonymously, but this is not entirely accurate; virulence refers to the degree of pathogenicity.

Pathogenicity refers to the ability of a species or genus of microorganisms to produce disease. This implies that there may be some avirulent strains or species within those groups. For instance, we know there are some avirulent strains of *N. gonorrhoeae, Corynebacterium diphtheriae,* and *M. tuberculosis.*

Because virulence depends on infectivity, invasiveness, and toxigenicity, one might observe that pathogens that occur in large numbers or that are highly infective but low in invasiveness might produce a large carrier rate. This large group of pathogens would include the opportunists found among the normal flora. Likewise, if the infectivity of a pathogen were low but its invasiveness and toxigenicity were high, there would be sporadic outbreaks of the disease.

The production of toxic products by pathogens is the most influential factor in their pathogenicity. Toxin-producing bacteria differ greatly in the amount of exotoxin they produce, depending on growth conditions. For example, virulent strains of some pathogens will become avirulent when grown in the laboratory under artificial conditions; some virulent encapsulated pathogens will lose their ability to produce capsules when grown on artificial media in the laboratory, as has been shown to occur in gonococci. Also, some toxin producers cease producing exotoxins on artificial media.

These changes can be regarded as the pathogen's response to different environments. On a completely artificial medium in the incubator where a constant temperature is maintained, life is easy for the microorganisms. There are plenty of nutrients, the temperature is ideal, there is no overcrowding by other microbes, and there are no phagocytes or antibodies, so pathogens have no need to arm themselves with capsules and toxins, as they do when attempting to grow in human tissues.

It should also be noted that virulence usually increases in pathogens that are transmitted from animal to animal and human to human, which explains why the virulence may increase during an epidemic. This factor may also account for the relatively high virulence of pathogens in a hospital environment, where there is a constantly changing population of susceptible persons. The rampaging hospital staphylococcal infections are caused by virulent staphylococci that continue to mutate and to become resistant to the antibiotics that are used in ever greater varieties and numbers to fight infections.

Problems and Questions

1. Define *infectious, communicable,* and *contagious disease.* Why are some diseases more contagious than others?
2. List several ways that the human body resists infection by foreign invaders.
3. Define and illustrate the following terms used to describe infectious diseases: (a) acute, (b) chronic, (c) latent, (d) primary, (e) secondary, (f) local, (g) systemic.
4. Name three phases in the course of infectious diseases.
5. On what general properties does virulence and pathogenicity depend?
6. Compare exotoxins with endotoxins. List some diseases produced by each.
7. Name some general types of exotoxins.

Chapter 8

Epidemiology and Transmission of Diseases

Objectives

After studying this chapter, you should be able to
1. Write the meaning of these terms: epidemiology, epidemic, endemic, and pandemic
2. Describe the difference between sporadic and nonendemic diseases
3. List three factors that contribute to an epidemic
4. List six reservoirs of infection
5. List five modes of disease transmission
6. Discuss the procedure for stopping an epidemic

New Words to Pronounce and Understand

Amebiasis (ah-me-buy'-uh-sis). A disease caused by a protozoan, *Entamoeba histolytica*

Arthropod (ar'-throw-pod). A phylum classification of animals including insects, mites, lice, ticks, and fleas

Diphtheria (diff-ther'-ee-uh). A disease caused by the bacterium *Corynebacterium diphtheriae*

Endemic (en-dem'-ick). A disease present in normal numbers in a community

Epidemic (ep-i-dem'-ick). More than the normal number of cases of a disease in a community at a particular time

Epidemiology (ep-i-deem-ee-ol'-oh-gee). The systematic study of epidemics

Fecal (fee'-kull). Referring to feces or bowel movement

Fomite (foe'-mite), pl. *fomites* (fo'-mi-teez). An object such as a book or an item of clothing that is not in itself harmful but that is able to harbor pathogenic organisms and thus serve as an agent for transmission of an infection

Gonorrhea (gon-or-ee′-uh). A venereal disease caused by the bacterium *Neisseria gonorrhoeae*

Hepatitis (hep-uh-tie′-tus). A disease of the liver, usually caused by a virus

Herpes (her′-peas). A viral disease (cold sores) caused by *herpes simplex*

Pandemic (pan-dem′-ick). A worldwide epidemic

Parenteral injection (pear-ren′-ter-al). Intramuscular or intravenous

Poliomyelitis (pole-ee-oh-my-uh-lie′-tus). A viral disease

Salmonella (sal-moe-nell′-uh). A genus of bacteria that causes diarrhea and typhoid fever

Shigella (shig-el′-uh). A genus of bacteria that usually causes dysentery or diarrhea

Syphilis (sif′-fill-us). A venereal disease caused by the spirochete *Treponema pallidum*

Trichinella (trick-i-nell′-uh). A worm that infects pork muscle, causing the disease trichinosis

Tuberculosis (tu-ber-cue-low′-sis). A disease caused by the bacterium *Mycobacterium tuberculosis*

Vector (veck′-tore). A carrier (especially an arthropod) of pathogenic organisms from one host to another

Epidemiology is the science that deals with the frequency and distribution of diseases and the factors that contribute to the spread of disease. These contributing factors include the virulence of the pathogen; susceptibility of the population because of overcrowding, lack of immunization, or inadequate sanitation procedures; and the mode of transmission of the pathogen.

Definition of Terms

Several terms are used to describe the prevalence of disease in an area at a particular time:

Endemic Diseases

Endemic diseases are those that are constantly present in a community, usually involving only a few people. The number of cases increases and decreases at various times, but the disease never dies out completely. The endemic infections that occur regularly in the United States include tuberculosis, staphylococcal and streptococcal infections, and virus diseases such as the common cold, influenza, chickenpox, and mumps. Tuberculosis remains endemic in the world as well as in the United States particularly among the poor, who live in crowded conditions; however, the number of deaths has been greatly reduced by drug therapy. In some parts of this country, plague is endemic among rats, prairie dogs, and other rodents; as a result, endemic plague in humans is occasionally observed. The actual incidence of an endemic disease at any particular time depends on a balance among several factors: environment, the genetic susceptibility of the population, behavioral factors, the number of people who are immune, the virulence of the pathogen, and the reservoir or source of infection.

Epidemic Diseases

Infections that are usually endemic may become epidemic. An *epidemic* is defined as more than the normal number of cases of a disease in an area within a particular period.

A current example of an historically important epidemic of a new disease is the acquired immune deficiency syndrome (AIDS) epidemic of the 1980s (Fig. 8-1). Evidently, a mutant virus was picked up from monkeys by African natives. It was transmitted among the Africans through the mucous membranes, semen, and blood, usually by sexual contact or blood transfer. From Africa, it spread to Haiti, where gay males carried the virus to New York and Miami. After spreading into other areas of homosexual men in the United States, it spread into the IV drug-using communities, and through blood banks to hemophiliacs. Finally it moved into the heterosexual society throughout the world. The virus was quickly isolated and identified as an HTLV-III (human T-cell lymphotrophic virus, type 3), LAV (lymphadenopathy-associated virus), and later named the HIV (human immunodeficiency virus) by international agreement. In 1986, over a million people in the United States were believed to be infected, and at least 20% were expected to develop AIDS in the next few years. This sexually transmitted or blood-borne virus has a long incubation period during which it destroys the T4 helper lymphocytes, crippling the immune system so that most victims succumb to secondary infections (see Chaps. 11 and 13). One significant outcome of this epidemic is the reduction of other sexually transmitted diseases (gonorrhea, syphilis, herpes) because of the increased awareness of these infections in people with many sex partners.

Another example of a disease becoming epidemic is the 1976 epidemic of a respiratory illness following an American Legion convention in Philadelphia, Pennsylvania (Legionnaires' disease, or legionellosis). The organism was finally isolated, identified, and named *Legionella pneumophila* (Fig. 8-2). Other such epidemics have been identified through constant surveillance and accumulation of data by the U.S. Centers for Disease Control (CDC). Epidemics usually follow a specific pattern in which the number of cases of a disease increases to a maximum and then decreases rapidly, because the number of susceptible and exposed individuals is limited.

Epidemics may occur in communities that have not been previously exposed to a particular pathogen. People from populated areas who travel into isolated communities frequently introduce a new virulent pathogen to susceptible natives of that community; then the disease spreads like wildfire. There have been many such examples described in history. The syphilis epidemic in Europe in the early 1500s was caused by a highly virulent spirochete carried back from the West Indies by Columbus's men

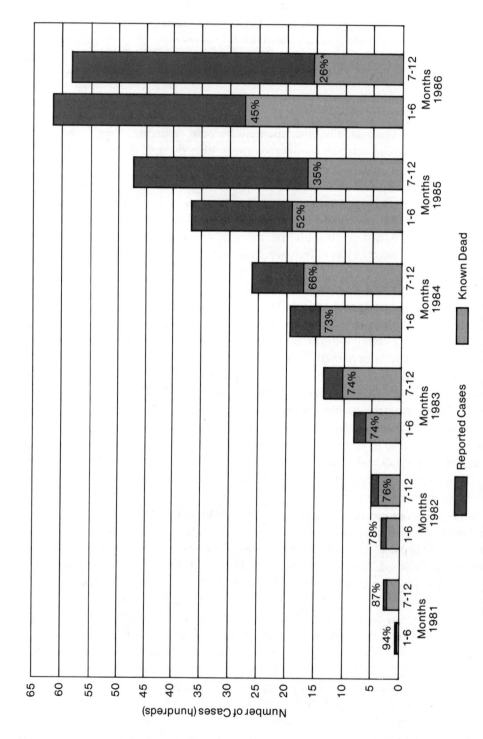

Fig. 8-1. Relationship of AIDS cases diagnosed and the number of deaths to date within each 6-month interval. *Number may not be accurate because all end-of-year reports may not be in. (Prepared from data provided by U.S. Public Health Service, Centers for Disease Control, Atlanta, Georgia)

Fig. 8-2. *Legionella pneumophila* cultured in human embryonic lung fibroblasts. (Courtesy of Mae C. Wong, Centers for Disease Control, Atlanta, Georgia)

in 1492. Also, measles and tuberculosis introduced to American Indians by early explorers and settlers almost destroyed many tribes. Recently, we have observed devastating outbreaks of measles and other contagious diseases in Australia, Africa, Greenland, and other relatively isolated areas.

In communities in which normal sanitation practices are relaxed, allowing fecal contamination of water supplies and food, epidemics of typhoid, cholera, giardiasis, and dysentery frequently occur. Visitors to these communities are particularly aware of this situation because they are more susceptible to the diseases, never having developed a natural immunity by being exposed to them in childhood.

In the 1970s gonorrhea reached epidemic proportions in the United States and most of the world because no immunity remains after the disease is cured (Fig. 8-3). This disease runs rampant in a promiscuous, mobile society where the use of birth control pills makes women more susceptible to the disease by changing the environment of the vagina. Also, the careless use of penicillin allowed the gonococcus to mutate into penicillin-resistant strains, making control by antibiotics more difficult. An effective vaccine might produce antibodies to prevent the pathogen from adhering to mucous membranes. An additional complicating factor is that this disease is asymptomatic in 80% of infected women and 20% of infected men; that is, the gonococcus lives and multiplies in the urogenital areas yet produces no symptoms. As noted in Figure 8-3, a significant reduction in the number of cases has occurred during the herpes and AIDS epidemics since 1980.

During certain times of the year diseases, such as the various types of influenza,

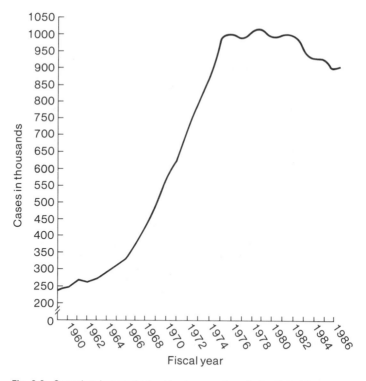

Fig. 8-3. Gonorrhea has reached epidemic proportions in the United States; the graph shows the number of reported cases. (Prepared from data provided by U.S. Public Health Service, Centers for Disease Control, Atlanta, Georgia)

occur in many areas and involve most of the population because the immunity developed to influenza usually is temporary. Thus, the disease recurs each year among those who are not revaccinated or naturally resistant to the infection.

Pandemic Diseases

A *pandemic* is a worldwide epidemic of a specific disease. Pandemics of influenza ("flu") have been recorded in 1898, 1917–1918, 1955, 1968, 1972, 1975, and 1978. Recent influenza pandemics have been named for the point of origin or first recognition, such as the Taiwan flu, Hong Kong flu, London flu, Port Chalmers flu, and Russian flu.

Sporadic and Nonendemic Diseases

Certain diseases follow neither the endemic nor the epidemic pattern but occur only sporadically; these are *sporadic* diseases such as tetanus, gas gangrene, and botulism. Diseases that are controlled as a result of immunization and sanitation procedures are termed *nonendemic;* these include smallpox, poliomyelitis, and diphtheria (in most parts of the world). Occasionally, outbreaks of these controlled diseases occur where vaccination programs have been neglected for one reason or another.

The entire concept of communicability of pathogens is built on the survival of infectious agents during their transfer from one host to another. Thus, health professionals should be thoroughly familiar with pathways of transfer and sources of potential pathogens. For instance, a hospital staphylococcal epidemic begins when aseptic conditions are relaxed and a carrier of a staphylococcal infection introduces the organism to the many susceptible patients (babies, surgical patients, and debilitated persons). Such an epidemic may quickly spread from one person throughout the entire hospital population.

Reservoirs of Infectious Agents

The sources of microorganisms that cause infectious diseases are many and varied. They are known as *reservoirs of infection*. A reservoir of infection is any site where the pathogen can multiply or merely survive until it is transferred to its host. Reservoirs of infection may be living hosts or inanimate objects or materials.

Living animal reservoirs include humans, horses, cattle, pigs, cats, dogs, wildlife, insects, ticks, mites, and many others. Humans may acquire pathogens from other humans and animals, which may or may not be diseased; through direct contact and bites; by eating meat or other products from diseased animals; or through the bites of mosquitoes, flies, fleas, mites, ticks, and other arthropod vectors. The most important reservoir of human infections is man himself, because many human pathogens are species-specific, which means they can cause disease in only one species of animal; thus, human pathogens usually cause disease only in humans.

Some people who do not have the disease may harbor the pathogen and transmit it to susceptible people who then develop the disease symptoms. Those who "carry" the pathogen without manifesting symptoms are called *carriers*. Human carriers are infected with the pathogen, but they are asymptomatic. *Active carriers* have recovered from the disease but continue to harbor the pathogen for a long time. *Passive carriers* carry the pathogen without having the disease. *Convalescent carriers* harbor the pathogen during their recovery from the disease. Usually, the respiratory secretions and the intestinal or urinary excretions are the vehicles by which the disease agent is transferred to food and water, and thus to many other persons. Human carriers are very important in the spread of staphylococcal and streptococcal infections as well as hepatitis, diphtheria, dysentery, meningitis, and the sexually transmitted diseases.

The inanimate reservoirs of infection include air, soil, food, milk,, water, and fomites. Air is contaminated by dust, smoke, and respiratory secretions of humans expelled into the air by breathing, blowing, sneezing, and coughing. The most highly contagious diseases are those such as colds and influenza, in which the respiratory viruses can be transmitted through the air on droplets of water or by the hands to another person. Dust particles also can carry spores of certain bacteria and dried bits of human and animal excretions that contain pathogens. Bacteria cannot multiply in the air but can be easily transported to a warm, nutrient site for growth via airborne particles. All personnel in hospitals and other facilities where housekeeping is done for large numbers of people must be especially aware of air currents that carry dust and pathogens throughout the facility. The fomites are articles of clothing, bedding, eating and drinking utensils, and hospital equipment, such as bedpans, and urinals, that are easily contaminated by pathogens from the respiratory tract, intestinal tract, and the skin of patients. Great care must be taken by the nursing and hospital staff to prevent transmission of pathogens to patients, causing a nosocomial (hospital-acquired) infection.

Modes of Disease Transmission

There are five principal modes of transfer of pathogens from an infected person to a susceptible person (Fig. 8-4 and Table 8-1).

Direct person-to-person contact with the skin of a diseased person or carrier
Direct mucus-to-mucus contact by kissing or sexual intercourse

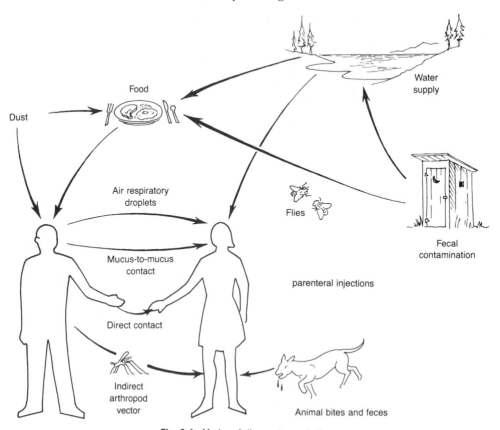

Fig. 8-4. Modes of disease transmission.

Table 8-1 Modes of Disease Transmission

Mode	Common Diseases
Direct skin contact	Staphylococcal and streptococcal infections, eczema, boils, acne, smallpox, measles, chickenpox, colds, influenza, pneumonia, tuberculosis, poliomyelitis, diphtheria
Mucus-to-mucus contact	Syphilis, gonorrhea, chancroid, herpes cold sores, AIDS, staphylococcal and streptococcal infections
Air, droplets, dust	Colds, influenza, measles, mumps, chickenpox, smallpox, pneumonia
Food, water, soil	Cholera, typhoid, dysentery, botulism, staphylococcal food poisoning, poliomyelitis, hepatitis, amebiasis, trichinosis, giardiasis
Blood contamination	Malaria, Rocky Mountain spotted fever, typhus, plague, Q fever, tularemia, trench fever, relapsing fever, African sleeping sickness, encephalitis, yellow fever, AIDS

Indirectly through the air on droplets or dust

Indirect contamination of food and water by fecal material, dead or live animals, soil, and other sources

Blood contamination indirectly by arthropod and other animal vectors and directly by parenteral injection by nonsterile syringes and needles, as well as by IV transfusions and kidney dialysis

Most diseases transferred by direct contact are those in which the causative organism can be carried on the skin; usually the pathogen is transferred by the hands and face. Many viruses and opportunistic bacteria are thus transferred and cause colds, influenza, staphylococcal and streptococcal infections, pneumonia, tuberculosis, polio, and diphtheria. In hospitals, this mode of transfer is particularly prevalent. Even the dysentery organisms, *Salmonella* and *Shigella,* can be transferred by the fecal material on the hands of one person to the hands, mouth, and food of another.

The mucus-to-mucus mode of transfer by kissing or sexual intercourse has been called the venereal route because the sexually transmitted diseases (STD), such as syphilis and gonorrhea, can be transmitted only in this manner. However, many other pathogens, including the herpes and AIDS viruses, may be conferred upon another in this manner.

Most of the contagious airborne diseases are due to respiratory pathogens carried in droplets of moisture to susceptible people. Some respiratory pathogens may dry as they settle in dust particles and be carried long distances through the air and into a building's ventilation system (as observed in the Legionnaires' disease epidemic). Improperly cleaned inhalation therapy equipment can easily transfer these pathogens from one patient to another. Diseases that may be transmitted in this manner include colds, influenza, measles, mumps, chickenpox, smallpox, and pneumonia. A respiratory infection that may be acquired from infected birds is psittacosis, or parrot fever. Also, some fungal respiratory diseases (*e.g.*, histoplasmosis) are frequently transferred via dried bird feces.

Indirect transfer of organisms to a susceptible person frequently occurs through contamination of foods and water. Human and animal fecal material from outhouses, cesspools, and feed lots often is carried into water supplies. Improper disposal of sewage and inadequate treatment of drinking water contribute to the spread of fecal and soil pathogens. Food and milk may be contaminated by careless handling so that pathogens enter from dust particles, dirty hands, hair, and respiratory secretions. If these pathogens and bacterial spores are not destroyed by proper processing and cooking, food poisoning can develop. Diseases frequently transmitted through foods and water are tuberculosis, botulism, staphylococcal and streptococcal infections, diarrhea caused by *Salmonella* and *Shigella* species, typhoid fever, amebiasis (caused by an ameba), giardiasis (diarrhea caused by *Giardia*) and trichinosis (caused by *Trichinella* worms in pork).

Normally the blood is sterile; thus, the discovery of organisms in the blood indicates the presence of a pathogen. A vector is necessary to carry pathogens from

Fig. 8-5. Medical instruments and apparatus are inanimate vectors of infection. (Rosdahl CB: Textbook of Basic Nursing, 4th ed. Philadelphia, JB Lippincott, 1985)

the blood of one person to another. Living vectors are animals, usually arthropods (ticks, fleas, lice). Included among the arthropod vectors are insects such as mosquitoes and flies, which bite an infected person or animal, then carry the pathogens to a healthy one.

To better understand this mode of transmission, let us take an example: the tick. (If you own a dog, you probably have a well-placed fear of ticks.) The pathogen in question goes by the name *Rickettsia rickettsii* which causes Rocky Mountain spotted fever (see Chap. 2). The organisms are widespread in the animal population and in ticks themselves. If an infected tick bites a person, the pathogen may be injected, causing an infection. Ticks may also carry the pathogens of Q fever, typhus, and tularemia. In similar fashion, body lice and head lice are the vectors of epidemic typhus, trench fever, relapsing fever, trachoma, impetigo, and even cholera. The blood-sucking fleas carry the pathogens of plague and endemic typhus. Deer flies transmit tularemia, and tsetse flies carry African sleeping sickness. Certain strains of mosquitoes transmit malaria, encephalitis, and yellow fever.

Many pets and other animals are important reservoirs of *zoonoses* (infections of animals transmissible to humans). Dogs, cats, bats, skunks, and other animals are known vectors of rabies, transmitting the rabies virus to man via the saliva injected when they bite. Salmonellosis and shigellosis are frequently acquired from the feces of turtles, dogs, and poultry. Cat and dog bites easily transfer *Pasteurella, Staphylococcus,* and *Streptococcus* species into the tissues where severe infections may result. Toxoplasmosis, a protozoan disease carried by cats and other animals, may cause severe brain damage to the fetus when contracted by a woman during the first 3 months of pregnancy. The infective agent can be contracted from cat feces in cat boxes as well as from infected raw meats.

Common inanimate vectors of blood and internal infections are the instruments and apparatus handled by medical personnel, most often nonsterile syringes, needles, and solutions, and blood-processing equipment such as kidney dialyzers and blood-transfusing apparatus (Fig. 8-5). One reason disposable sterile tubes, syringes, and various other types of hospital equipment have become very popular is that they are effective in preventing blood infections. Any blood disease can be transferred by improperly sterilized instruments and equipment. Hepatitis, syphilis, malaria, AIDS, and systemic staphylococcal infections are the diseases most often seen. Individuals using illegal IV drugs easily transmit these diseases to each other by sharing needles and syringes.

Control of Epidemic Diseases

The World Health Organization and the U.S. Public Health Service constantly strive to prevent epidemics and to identify and eliminate those that do occur. One way in which health personnel and community workers participate in this massive program is by reporting cases of communicable diseases to the proper agencies. They also can help to educate the public by describing the transmission of diseases, by explaining proper sanitation procedures, by identifying and attempting to eliminate reservoirs of infection, by carrying out measures to isolate diseased persons, by participating in immunization programs, and by helping to treat sick persons. Through measures like these, diphtheria, poliomyelitis, and smallpox have been practically eliminated in most parts of the world. Everyone in our society should contribute in whatever way possible to eliminating infectious diseases from the human environment.

Problems and Questions

1. Define and give examples of epidemic, endemic, pandemic, sporadic, and nonendemic diseases.
2. In what way do infected persons, who carry pathogens but have no symptoms, influence epidemics?
3. Discuss how the reservoirs of infection could be reduced or destroyed.
4. How could each of the five modes of transmission be interrupted to prevent diseases transmitted in that way?
5. If you were called to a distant island to stop an epidemic, what measures would you take?

Chapter 9

Preventing the Spread of Communicable Diseases

Objectives

After studying this chapter, you should be able to
1. List the six factors that have contributed to an increase in hospital-acquired infections
2. Write the names of three microorganisms that commonly cause hospital infections
3. List areas in the hospital where infections are most probable
4. List several types of patients who are extremely vulnerable to infectious diseases
5. Write a brief description of reverse isolation and source isolation
6. Briefly describe three important procedures to follow in isolation techniques
7. List the sources of water contamination
8. Describe how water and sewage are treated
9. Discuss how epidemics are controlled and prevented

New Words to Pronounce and Understand

Asepsis (a-sep'-sis). Without the growth of pathogens

Clostridium botulinum (clos-strid'-ee-um bot-you-lin'-um). The species of anaerobic bacteria that causes botulism, a toxic food poisoning

Clostridium perfringens (clos-trid'-ee-um per-frin'-genz). The species of anaerobic bacteria that causes gas gangrene

Nosocomial (nos-o-ko'-me-al). Of hospital origin

Proteus (pro'-tea-us). A genus of intestinal pathogens

Staphylococcus aureus (staff-fill-oh-cock'-us or'-ee-us). A species of bacteria that causes boils, wound infections, and hospital "staph" infections

Streptococcus pneumoniae (strep-toe-cock'-us new-moan'-ee-aye).
A species of bacteria that causes pneumonia

Prevention of Hospital Infections

How Hospital Infections Develop

The importance of microbiology to those who work in the health-related occupations can never be overemphasized. Whether employed in a hospital, an institution, or a clinic, or as health workers caring for sick persons in their homes, all must follow the same procedures to prevent the spread of communicable diseases.

Thoughtless or careless actions when giving patient care can cause preventable infections. A preventable nosocomial infection often adds several weeks to the patient's stay in the hospital, and may give rise to serious complications or may even result in the patient's death. Cross-infections because of hospital personnel, including physicians, are not infrequent; this is particularly true when hospitals and clinics are overcrowded and the staff is overworked. However, these infections *can* be avoided through proper care and the disciplined use of aseptic techniques.

Nurses and physicians play the major roles in preventing nosocomial infections; nevertheless, respiratory therapists, physical therapists, laboratory technicians, occupational therapists, radiologic technologists, and all others who deal with patients must be equally knowledgeable about methods of preventing the spread of pathogens. Members of the hospital housekeeping staff and central supply department, and those who prepare, dispense, and dispose of food, as well as administrative personnel, can help to prevent cross-contamination among patients or, through their carelessness, can contribute to its spread. Of course, sick and debilitated hospitalized patients are much more susceptible to even minor opportunistic pathogens than are the healthy people caring for them. In all situations, health workers must protect themselves from infectious agents as well.

There has been a definite increase in the number of nosocomial or hospital-acquired infections during the past 25 years, despite the availability of new disinfectants and antibiotics. There are many reasons for this situation: (1) the indiscriminate use of broad-range antibiotics, which may allow opportunistic pathogens to mutate and become resistant to them; (2) a false sense of security about the effectiveness of antibiotics, with a corresponding neglect of aseptic techniques; (3) current lengthy, more complicated types of surgery; (4) overcrowding of hospitals and shortage of staff; (5) increase in both numbers and types of health workers who often are not aware of the importance of aseptic and sterile techniques; (6) increased use of anti-inflammatory and immunosuppressant agents such as radiation, steroids, anti-cancer chemotherapy, and antilymphocytic serum. The presence of even one of these factors is sufficient to enable opportunistic pathogens to rush in and cause problems; taken together, they are the cause of approximately 60% of hospital-acquired infections. The most prevalent of these opportunistic bacteria are *Staphylococcus aureus,*

Escherichia coli, Streptococcus pneumoniae, and *Pseudomonas* and *Proteus* species, which cause most wound, burn, respiratory, and surgical infections.

The operating room, the delivery room, the nursery, and the central supply area are the most critical areas from the standpoint of disease transmission. In the operating theater and delivery areas, particular care must be taken because portals of entry into the body are readily accessible to the pathogens. The nursery is critical because newborns have very little resistance to disease. The central supply department must take great care not to distribute contaminated materials or supplies, since these might expose patients to a myriad of pathogens.

In a hospital, the most vulnerable patients are (1) newborn and premature babies, (2) women in labor and during delivery, (3) surgical and burn patients, (4) diabetic and cancer patients, (5) those receiving treatment with steroids, anticancer drugs, antilymphocyte serum, and radiation, (6) those with a deficient immune response, and (7) patients who are paralyzed or who are undergoing renal dialysis or catheterization.

General Control Measures

Using general principles of sanitation, disinfection, and sterilization, a general state of cleanliness must be maintained throughout the hospital or institution. Each area, from the trash disposal area to the operating rooms, must be thoroughly cleaned to remove organic wastes and carefully dusted to prevent the growth and spread of microorganisms. Dry dusting and sweeping should not be practiced because they aid dispersal of microorganisms on dust particles in the air.

Medical Asepsis

Once basic cleanliness is achieved, it is not difficult to maintain asepsis. The goal of medical asepsis is to exclude all pathogenic microorganisms from the immediate environment. Medical asepsis includes all the precautionary measures necessary to prevent direct transfer of pathogens from person to person and indirect transfer of pathogens through the air or on instruments, bedding, equipment, and other inanimate objects (fomites).

Hospitals vary greatly in their specific requirements for the maintenance of medical asepsis, but there is general agreement about sanitary methods for handling food and dishes, proper cooking and storage of food, proper disposal of waste products and contaminated materials, proper hand-washing and personal hygiene of hospital personnel, proper use of gown and mask in isolation rooms, proper washing and sterilization of hospital equipment, proper use of disposable equipment, and proper disinfection of a room after the patient has been discharged.

Handling Food and Dishes   Contaminated food provides an excellent environment for the growth of pathogens. Most often, human carelessness is responsible for this contamination: failure to take precautions with fecal material, hand-washing, flies and insects, dust, dirt, and domestic animals and pets. The microbes most frequently carried in food are *Staphylococcus* species (from skin and dust); *Clostridium botulinum* (from dust and dirt); *Clostridium perfringens* (from dust, dirt, and hands); *Salmonella* species (from feces, hands, flies, and pets); *Shigella* species (from feces, hands, flies, and pets); *Proteus* species (from feces, hands, flies, and pets); and *Pseudomonas* species (from dirt, hands, and contaminated equipment).

Regulations for safe handling of food and dishes are not difficult to follow. They include

- The use of high quality fresh food
- Proper refrigeration and storage of food
- Proper washing, preparation and cooking of food
- Proper disposal of uneaten food
- Thorough washing of hands and fingernails before handling food and after visiting a restroom
- Proper disposal of nasal and oral secretions in tissues
- Covering hair and wearing clean clothes and aprons
- Providing periodic health examinations for kitchen workers
- Prohibiting anyone with an infection or intestinal upset from handling food or dishes
- Keeping all kitchen equipment and all other equipment scrupulously clean
- Rinsing and then washing dishes in a dishwasher in which the water temperature is above 80°C (176°F).

Hand-washing   Hands should be kept clean at all times and should be washed before and after each patient contact to preclude carrying pathogens from one patient to another. A disinfectant soap containing hexachlorophene is often used to control staphylococci. Common-sense rules that one should always follow include

- Using gloves or tongs to handle contaminated materials
- Washing hands with disinfectant soap before and after contact with a patient
- Rinsing hands under running water
- Drying hands and applying antiseptic lotion to prevent chapping

Handling of Fomites   As previously described, fomites are any articles or substances other than food that may harbor and transmit microbes. Examples of fomites are dishes, bedpans, urinals, thermometers, washbasins, bed linen, and clothing and other personal patient items. Transmission of pathogens by these items may be prevented by observing the following rules:

Use disposable equipment and supplies wherever possible.
Disinfect or sterilize equipment as soon as possible after use.

Use individual equipment for each patient.

Use an individual thermometer for each patient and store each thermometer in a disinfectant solution.

Empty bedpans and urinals, wash them in hot water, and store them in a clean cabinet between uses.

Place bed linen and soiled clothing in bags to be sent to the laundry.

Prevention of Airborne Contamination   Respiratory infections are most often transmitted through the air. Observe the following measures to decrease the number of pathogens transmitted by this means:

Cover the mouth and nose when coughing or sneezing.

Limit the number of persons in a room.

Remove the dirt and dust from floor and furniture by damp dusting.

Open the room to fresh air and sunlight whenever possible.

Roll linens together carefully to prevent dispersal of microbes in the air.

Remove bacteria from the air by a filtered air-conditioning system.

Isolation of Patients

Patients are placed in isolation for one of two reasons: (1) to prevent the spread of pathogens to other susceptible people, or (2) to protect a very susceptible patient from exposure to pathogens.

Reverse Isolation   Certain patients are especially vulnerable to infection; among them are patients with severe burns, those who have leukemia, patients who have received a transplant, immunodeficient persons, and those receiving radiation treatments. Premature babies are also highly susceptible. All such patients are protected through isolation procedures. This type of isolation is referred to as reverse isolation. The room must be thoroughly cleaned and disinfected before the patient is admitted. Those entering the room must wear sterile gowns and masks to prevent carrying microorganisms into the room on their clothes and from their respiratory tract. Proper hand-washing procedures must also be followed before entering the room.

Source Isolation   Whenever possible, patients with contagious diseases should be isolated in private air-conditioned rooms with a private bath. In this manner infectious agents are isolated within a definite area, and thereby spread of the pathogens to other patients is prevented. Isolation procedures should be determined by

The mode of transmission of the disease from one person to another

The location of the pathogen causing the infection, its portal of exit (intestinal, respiratory, or wound drainage), and its portal of entry

The virulence of the pathogen and its susceptibility to antibiotics

Isolation Techniques   Isolation techniques are designed to immediately destroy the pathogenic organisms in the infectious discharges of the patient. Nondisposable items are disinfected, with a minimum of handling, then cleaned thoroughly and resterilized. If the patient's infection involves spore-forming bacteria such as those found in gas gangrene and tetanus, then contaminated equipment must be autoclaved to destroy the spores before the item can be reused. Disposable equipment must be incinerated or thoroughly autoclaved before disposal.

Hand-washing   Doctors, nurses, and other hospital personnel entering the room must be particularly careful to wash their hands before and after caring for a patient. Hand contact with door knobs, telephones, elevator buttons, and furniture easily transmits pathogens to and from the patient. Fingernails should be kept short and clean, and jewelry should not be worn in an isolation room.

Gowns   In every isolation room, gowns should be used. A clean fresh gown should be available for each person who enters the isolation room on each occasion and discarded after each use. To be protective, gowns should be large enough to be fastened securely. They must be kept dry—remember that a moist environment is required for growth of pathogens, so if an area is moist, the pathogens may gain access to clothing worn under the gown.

Masks   Masks generally are not worn outside the operating room. However, if a patient is isolated because of a respiratory infection, he should be masked whenever it is necessary to take him out of his room for treatment in other parts of the hospital. Personnel working closely with an isolated respiratory patient may wish to wear masks for self-protection. Remember that wet masks are not effective. Used masks should be promptly discarded, or laundered and autoclaved. Hands should be washed again after touching a used mask.

Surgical Asepsis

The goal of surgical asepsis is to exclude *all* microorganisms from the immediate environment. Surgical aseptic techniques include those practices that make and keep all objects and the area itself sterile. These practices are necessary during all surgical procedures, as well as any other procedure that involves exposure of the deep body tissues, to prevent the entry of any microorganisms into those tissues.

The surgical area of the patient's skin must be shaved and thoroughly cleansed and scrubbed with soap and antiseptic. If the surgery is to be extensive, the surrounding area is covered with a plastic film or sterile cloth drapes so that a sterile surgical field is established. The surgeon and all surgical assistants must scrub for 10 minutes with a disinfectant soap and then cover their clothes, mouth, and hair because these might shed microorganisms onto the operative site. These coverings include sterile gloves, gowns, caps, and masks. All instruments, sutures, and dressings must be sterilized; as soon as they are contaminated they must be discarded and replaced with sterile ones. Any instruments or equipment that cannot be autoclaved must be disinfected properly or destroyed.

The floors, walls, and all equipment in the operating room must be cleaned and disinfected before each use. Proper ventilation must be maintained so that fresh, filtered air is circulated through the room at all times.

Surgical aseptic techniques should be followed in treating postoperative wounds for the first few days after surgery until the tissues heal sufficiently to provide some natural protection. Surgical asepsis must also be applied in the delivery room and the nursery to prevent infections in these very susceptible patients.

Maintenance of Aseptic Conditions

Even though every department of the hospital or institution endeavors to maintain aseptic conditions, the total environment is constantly bombarded with microbes from the outside. These must be destroyed for the protection of patients (Fig. 9-1).

Hospital personnel (infection control committee or nurse) entrusted with this aspect of health care work diligently and constantly to maintain the proper environment. The microbiology laboratory cooperates to keep constant watch over asepsis within the hospital and consults, as necessary, with various personnel to ensure the maintenance of aseptic conditions throughout the hospital. Laboratory tests can demonstrate the presence and location of contaminating microbes as well as the effectiveness of the disinfection processes. The laboratory should also be able to trace the sources of infections and make recommendations to prevent recurrence. In case of an epidemic, the laboratory or infection control committee notifies city, county, and state health authorities so they can concentrate their efforts toward bringing the epidemic to an end.

Environmental Disease Control Measures

Public Health

Massive networks involving the World Health Organization (WHO), public health agencies at all levels, and community groups work together to coordinate preventive health programs and to maintain constant surveillance for sources and causes of epidemics. WHO also develops international regulations for disease control and standardization of drugs, and plays an active part in the distribution of technical information. When an epidemic strikes, teams of epidemiologists are sent to the scene to investigate the situation and assist in bringing the outbreak under control. Because of this assistance, many countries have been successful in their fight to control smallpox, diphtheria, malaria, trachoma, and numerous other diseases. In fact, it appears that smallpox has been completely eradicated from the face of the earth; hence, vaccination of a population or of international travelers may no longer be required.

In the United States, the Department of Health and Human Services administers the U.S. Public Health Service and the Centers for Disease Control, which assist

Strict Isolation

Visitors—Report to Nurses' Station
Before Entering Room

1. Private Room—*necessary;* door must be kept closed.

2. Gowns—must be worn by all persons entering room.

3. Masks—must be worn by all persons entering room.

4. Hands—must be washed on entering and leaving room.

5. Gloves—must be worn by all persons entering room.

6. Articles—must be discarded, or wrapped before being sent to Central Supply for disinfection or sterilization.

Enteric Precautions

Visitors—Report to Nurses' Station
Before Entering Room

1. Private Room—necessary for children only.
2. Gowns—must be worn by all persons having direct contact with patient.
3. Masks—not necessary.
4. Hands—must be washed on entering and leaving room.
5. Gloves—must be worn by all persons having direct contact with patient or with articles contaminated with fecal material.
6. Articles—special precautions necessary for articles contaminated with urine and feces. Articles must be disinfected or discarded.

Protective Isolation

Visitors—Report to Nurses' Station
Before Entering Room

1. Private Room—*necessary;* door must be kept closed.
2. Gowns—must be worn by all persons entering room.
3. Masks—must be worn by all persons entering room.
4. Hands—must be washed on entering and leaving room.
5. Gloves—must be worn by all persons having direct contact with patient.

Wound & Skin Precautions

Visitors—Report to Nurses' Station
Before Entering Room

1. Private Room—desirable.
2. Gowns—must be worn by all persons having direct contact with patient.
3. Masks—not necessary except during dressing changes.
4. Hands—must be washed on entering and leaving room.
5. Gloves—must be worn by all persons having direct contact with infected area.
6. Articles—special precautions necessary for instruments, dressings, and linen.

Respiratory Isolation

Visitors—Report to Nurses' Station
Before Entering Room

1. Private Room—*necessary;* door must be kept closed.
2. Gowns—not necessary.
3. Masks—must be worn by all persons entering room if susceptible to disease.
4. Hands—must be washed on entering and leaving room.
5. Gloves—not necessary.
6. Articles—those contaminated with secretions must be disinfected.
7. Caution—all persons susceptible to the specific disease should be excluded from patient area; if contact is necessary, susceptibles must wear masks.

Fig. 9-1. Hospital precaution signs used for the protection of patients, staff, and visitors. (Volk WA, Wheeler MF: Basic Microbiology, 5th ed. Philadelphia, Harper & Row, 1984) state and local health departments in the application of all aspects of epidemiology. Through the valiant efforts of these agencies working with local physicians, nurses and other health workers, educators, and community leaders, many diseases are no longer endemic in the United State. A list of the diseases that no longer pose a threat to the community would include diphtheria, smallpox, typhoid fever, and cholera.

The prevention and control of epidemics is a never-ending community quest. To be effective, it must include measures to

Increase host resistance through development and administration of vaccines that induce active immunity and maintain it in susceptible persons.

Ensure that persons who have been exposed to a pathogen are protected against the disease; for instance, injections of gamma globulin or antiserums are effective against outbreaks of diphtheria.

Segregate, isolate, and treat those who have contracted a contagious infection to prevent the spread of pathogens to others.

Identify and control the potential reservoirs and vectors of infectious diseases. This may be accomplished by prohibiting "healthy carriers" from working in restaurants, hospitals, and other institutions where they may carry pathogens to susceptible people, and by instituting effective sanitation measures to control diseases transmitted through water supplies, sewage, and food, including milk.

Water Supplies and Sewage Disposal

Water is the single most essential resource necessary for the survival of humanity. The main sources of community water supplies are surface water from rivers, natural lakes, and reservoirs, and groundwater from wells. However, two types of water pollution are present in our society that are making it increasingly difficult to provide safe water supplies; these come from chemical and biological sources. *Chemical pollution* of waters occurs when industrial installations dump waste products into local waters without proper pretreatment and when pesticides are used indiscriminately and thoughtlessly. The main source of *biological pollution* is the waste products of humans—fecal material and garbage—which swarm with pathogens. The pathogens of cholera, typhoid fever, bacterial and amebic dysentery, giardiasis, infectious hepatitis, and poliomyelitis can all be spread through contaminated water. Water-borne epidemics today are the result of failure to make use of the available existing knowledge and technology. In those countries that have established safe sanitary procedures for water purification and sewage disposal, outbreaks of typhoid fever, cholera, and dysentery only rarely occur.

Source of Water Contamination   Rainwater falling over a large area collects in lakes and rivers and thus is subject to contamination by soil microbes and raw fecal material. For example, an animal feed lot located near a community water supply source harbors

Fig. 9-2. Sources of water contamination.

innumerable pathogens, which are washed into lakes and rivers. A city that draws its water from a local river, processes it, and uses it, but then dumps inadequately treated sewage into the river at the other side of town may be responsible for a serious health problem in another city downstream on the same river. The city downstream must then find some way to rid its water supply of the pathogens. In many communities untreated raw sewage and industrial wastes are dumped directly into local waters; then, a storm or a flood may result in the local drinking water being contaminated with sewage (Fig. 9-2).

Groundwater from wells also can become contaminated. To prevent such contamination, the well must be dug deep, so that the surface water is filtered before it reaches the level of the well. Outhouses, septic tanks, and cesspools must be situated in such a way that the surface water passing through these areas does not carry the fecal microbes directly into the well water. With the growing popularity of trailer homes in recent years, a new problem has arisen because of trailer sewage disposal tanks being located too near the water supply.

In some very old cities where the water pipes are old and the sewage pipes leak, the sewage has easy access to the water pipes wherever there is a break in the pipe at a point just before it enters the dwelling. This is often the case in the old cities of Europe and Asia.

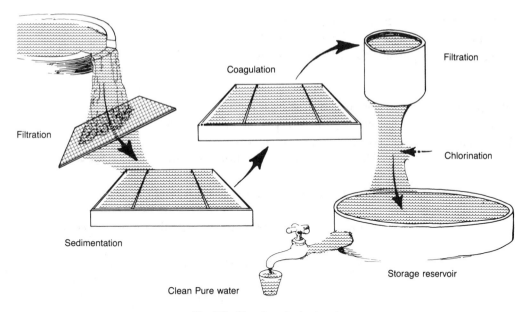

Fig. 9-3. Steps in water treatment.

Water and Sewage Treatment   Water must be properly treated to make it safe for human consumption. It is interesting to trace the many steps involved in such treatment (Fig. 9-3). The water first is filtered to remove large pieces of debris such as twigs and leaves. Next, it is held in sedimentation ponds where alum is added to coagulate bacteria and organic materials so they settle more rapidly. The water is then filtered through sand filters to remove the remaining bacteria and other small particles. Finally, chlorine gas or sodium hypochlorite is added to a final concentration of 0.2 to 1 part per million (ppm); this kills any remaining bacteria.

In the laboratory, water can be tested for fecal contamination by checking for the presence of the coliform bacteria (*E. coli*). These bacteria normally live in the human intestine, so their presence in drinking water is a sure sign that the water was subjected to fecal contamination.

If one is unsure about the purity of drinking water, boiling for 20 minutes will destroy any pathogens present. It can then be cooled and used.

When sewage is adequately treated in a disposal plant, the water in it can be returned to lakes and rivers to be recycled. Raw sewage consists mainly of water, fecal material including intestinal pathogens, and garbage from the drains of human habitations. In the sewage disposal plant, large debris first is filtered out; then the bacteria break down some of the organic material. Next, the "activated sludge," which includes the solid matter and bacteria, is settled out in a settling tank. In some communities, the sludge is heated to kill the bacteria, then dried and used as fertilizer. The remaining liquid is filtered and chlorinated so that the effluent water can be returned to the rivers or oceans. In some desert cities where water is at a premium, the effluent water from the sewage disposal plant is distilled so it can be returned directly to the drinking water system. In some other cities the effluent water is used to irrigate lawns; however, it is expensive to install a separate water system for this purpose.

Problems and Questions

1. What is meant by the phrase *hospital infections?*
2. What groups of people are responsible for the development of nosocomial infections?
3. How can hospital infections be eliminated or reduced in number?
4. Which patients are most susceptible to nosocomial infections?
5. Which pathogens are most frequently found in nosocomial infections?
6. Why are gowns and masks used in various areas of the hospital? Name the places where they would be used.
7. If the hands are clean, why must sterile gloves be worn in surgery?
8. What are the differences between surgical and medical asepsis?
9. Who must be notified to help control an epidemic?
10. How is water treated to make it safe for human consumption?
11. If a laboratory test showed that *Escherichia coli* were present in a sample of drinking water, what would this indicate?

Chapter 10

Nonspecific Mechanisms of Defense Against Disease

Objectives

After studying this chapter, you should be able to

1. List and describe the nonspecific defenses of the human body systems, or the first line of defense
2. Define phagocytosis, the body's second line of defense
3. List the cellular types of phagocytes
4. Describe the process of inflammation

New Words to Pronounce and Understand

Antibody (an'-tea-body). A glycoprotein produced by the body in response to antigens

Antigen (an'-ti-gin). A foreign substance that stimulates the production of antibodies.

Bactericidal (back-teer-i-sigh'-dull). Bacteria-killing action

Bacteriolytic (back-teer-ee-oh-li'-tick). A substance that lyses or breaks apart bacteria

Chemotaxis (keem-oh-tacks'-sis). Movement of cells in response to a chemical substance (the attraction of phagocytes to an area of injury is due to release of complement fragments.)

Cilia (sill'-ee-uh). Short, hairlike structures that provide for movement (characteristic of protozoa, Class Ciliata)

Complement (com'-ple-ment). A blood serum protein group involved in inflammation, chemotaxis, and lysis of bacteria

Encapsulate (en-cap'-sue-late). To surround by a capsule

Exudate (x'-you-date). A substance expelled or given off

Histamine (hiss'-tuh-mean). Potent chemical released from cells during some immune reactions, causing swelling and inflammation

Innate (in-ate'). Present in a person at birth

Interferon (in-ter-fear'-on). Antiviral, soluble protein substances produced by cells infected with an animal virus; also regulates immune function (Interferon is cell-specific and species-specific, but not virus-specific.)

Peristalsis (pear-i-stall'-sis). Waves of contraction passing along tubular organs, particularly the intestine, mixing contents and moving them along

Phagocyte (fag'-oh-site). White blood cells capable of ingesting foreign particles including microorganisms

Properdin (pro-pair'-din). A blood serum protein involved in destruction of certain bacteria and viruses in the presence of complement; an alternate complement pathway

Pyogenic (pie-oh-jen'-ick). Pus producing

Virulent (veer'-you-lent). Able to produce disease

Humans and the lower animals have survived on earth for millions of years because they have many built-in mechanisms of defense against harmful microorganisms and the infectious diseases caused by them. The ability of any animal to resist these invaders and recover from disease is due to many complex interacting functions within the body.

Humans have three lines of defense against bacteria, viruses, fungi, and other parasitic organisms. The first two lines of defense are nonspecific, that is the body attempts to destroy all types of substances that are foreign to it. However, the third line of defense, the immune response, is very specific: antibodies are formed in response to the presence of particular foreign substances. These foreign substances are called antigens because they cause the production of specific antibodies. The immune response is discussed in Chapter 11.

Nonspecific defense mechanisms are general in nature and serve to protect the body against most harmful substances. One of the nonspecific defenses is innate, or inborn, resistance observed in some species of animals, some races of humans, and some persons who have a natural resistance to some diseases. These innate or inherited characteristics make these people and animals more resistant to some diseases than to others. Cholera is an example of species resistance. Human beings can contract human cholera but not chicken cholera. The exact factors that produce this innate resistance are not well understood but are probably due to chemical, physiological, and temperature differences between the species, as well as the general state of physical and emotional health of the person and the environmental factors that affect certain races and not others.

Although we are usually unaware of it, our bodies are, more or less, constantly in the process of defending against microbial invaders. Nonspecific defense mechanisms include such things as mechanical and physical barriers to invasion, chemical factors, microbial antagonism by our normal body flora, phagocytic host cells, fever, and the inflammatory response.

First Line of Defense

The body protects itself against invasion by foreign microorganisms and other substances by defending the body openings to the respiratory, digestive, urinary, and reproductive systems with mucous membranes that entrap the invaders. Also, the skin provides an unbroken and complete external covering for all other parts of the body.

The unbroken skin acts as a physical or mechanical barrier to pathogenic microorganisms; only when it is cut, abraded (scratched), or burned can they gain entrance. There are several factors that account for the skin's ability to resist pathogens. One is the skin's normal secretions, which destroy the bacteria or inhibit their growth on its surface. These bactericidal secretions include the acidic perspiration of the sweat glands and the fatty acids of the oil glands. In addition, the pathogens may not be able to establish themselves and multiply because there are many normal flora (microorganisms) already living in the pores and in the moist parts of the head, underarms, hands, feet, and perianal and urethral regions.

The respiratory system would be particularly accessible to invaders that could ride on dust or other particles inhaled with each breath, were it not for the hair, mucous membranes, and the irregular chambers of the nose that serve to trap much of the inhaled debris. The cilia (mucociliary covering) of the epithelial (surface) cells of the posterior nasal membranes, nasal sinuses, bronchi, and trachea sweep the trapped dust and microbes toward the throat, where they are swallowed or expelled in sneezing and coughing. Phagocytes in the mucous membranes may also be involved in this mucociliary clearance mechanism. Lysozymes and other enzymes that lyse or destroy bacteria, are present in nasal secretions, saliva, and tears. The normal flora residing in the nose and mouth may also serve a protective function.

The digestive system is protected, to a large degree, by the process of digestion, the digestive enzymes, the acid condition of the stomach, and the alkalinity of the intestine. Bile, which is secreted from the liver into the intestine, lowers the surface tension and causes chemical changes in the bacterial cell wall and membrane that make the bacteria more digestible. Many invading microorganisms are trapped in the mucous lining of the digestive tract where they may be destroyed by bactericidal enzymes and phagocytes, a type of white blood cell. The normal flora that use available nutrients and occupy the space in the intestines include *Escherichia coli*, *Enterobacter aerogenes*, *Streptococcus faecalis*, and many other enteric (intestinal) bacteria. Peristalsis and the expulsion of feces serve to flush the bacteria from the intestine, as well.

The urinary tract is normally sterile in healthy persons; therefore, urine drawn in an aseptic manner (catheterization) should have no microorganisms present. Also, the reproductive system of the male and most of the reproductive organs in the female lack normal flora. However, the normal flora and pathogens from the anus and surrounding skin may grow in the vagina and vaginal opening, and may attempt to invade the urethral opening to the bladder. These two areas continually flush out the invading normal flora (which act as opportunists in this circumstance) by frequent urination and the expulsion of mucous secretions. Many bladder infections occur simply as a result of infrequent urination, especially following intercourse. Normally the acid urine and vaginal secretions also inhibit microbial growth. Many women who are taking certain oral contraceptives are particularly susceptible to some infections because those chemicals reduce the acidity of the vagina.

The prevention of colonization of potential microbial pathogens by the normal flora of a given anatomical site is called *microbial antagonism;* this is another example of a nonspecific defense mechanism. The inhibitory capability of the normal flora has been attributed to a competition for nutrients and the production of certain inhibitory substances. Examples of such inhibitory substances are the *colicins* produced by certain strains of *Escherichia coli.* Similar substances are produced by some strains of *Pseudomonas* and *Bacillus* species, as well as by other bacteria. Collectively these antibacterial substances (proteins), produced by other bacteria, are known as *bacteriocins.* The effectiveness of microbial antagonism is frequently decreased following prolonged administration of broad-spectrum antibiotics. The antibiotics reduce or eliminate certain members of the normal flora (*e.g.,* the vaginal and gastrointestinal flora) and permit overgrowth by bacteria and/or fungi that are resistant to the antibiotic being administered. This overgrowth of organisms, *e.g., Candida albicans,* is called a superinfection.

Second Line of Defense

The nonspecific cellular and chemical responses to microbial invasion are considered the second line of defense. Virulent pathogens that penetrate the first line of defense usually are destroyed by this series of defense mechanisms, known as the *inflammatory response.* Inflammation is a complex sequence of events involving the cellular secretions (interferon, prostaglandins, histamine), activation of serum proteins (complement, properdin), chemotaxis, phagocytosis, neutralization of toxins, clean-up and repair of damaged areas. We will consider this process step by step.

Interferon

When certain body cells (leukocytes, fibroblasts, and T lymphocytes) are infected by some viruses, the cells respond by producing interferon, a group of small proteins. The interferons are absorbed by surrounding cells and inhibit the synthesis of viruses within those cells. Thus, the spread of the viral infection is inhibited, allowing the other body defenses to fight the disease more effectively. In this way many viral diseases (*e.g.,* colds, influenza, and measles) are self-limiting in duration. Similarly, the acute phase of herpes simplex cold sores is of limited duration, but then the virus enters a latent phase and hides in nerve cells where it is protected until the person's defenses are down and the cycle of disease is repeated.

The interferons are species-specific, that is, they are effective only in the animals that produce them; only human interferon is effective for humans. Now human interferons are industrially produced by bacteria with recombinant DNA (interferon genes inserted) and are used in clinical trials for viral infections, cancer and tumors, and in some immunodeficiency diseases. *Interleukins* are types of interferons that aid in stimulating the immune (antibody) response.

Serum Proteins

Complement   A series of 11 proteins (C1–C9) found in normal blood serum constitute the complement system, so called because it "complements" the action of antibodies in immune and allergic reactions. Complement is a nonspecific defense mechanism because it will bind to many antigen–antibody complexes. Once bound it becomes activated (1) to enhance the inflammatory response, (2) to aid in the destruction (lysis) of cells and microorganisms, (3) to attract phagocytes into the region (chemotaxis), and (4) to aid in neutralizing the toxins of certain microorganisms.

Properdin   The defense serum protein properdin works in tandem with complement C3 and C5 protein in the absence of an antigen–antibody complex. It also enhances phagocytosis, inflammation, and the destruction of bacteria and certain viruses.

Prostaglandins

The prostaglandins are membrane-associated lipids, acting much like local hormones. They are biologically reactive in controlling platelet aggregation, immune response, inflammation, increased capillary permeability, pain production, diarrhea, and many other conditions in health and disease.

Phagocytosis

The process by which phagocytes surround and engulf (swallow) foreign material is called phagocytosis. These foreign materials not needed by the body include dead cells, unused secretions (such as milk), dust, debris, and microorganisms. These phagocytes serve as the "clean-up crew" to rid the body of these unwanted and often harmful substances.

The white blood cells (leukocytes) that act as phagocytes are microphages and macrophages. Microphages are phagocytic granulocytes, including neutrophils, eosinophils, and basophils. The most efficient and abundant phagocytes are the neutrophils. Eosinophils become more plentiful and play a phagocytic role in allergic responses, whereas basophils become the mast cells in tissues involved in inflammatory reactions. Macrophages develop from monocytes during the inflammatory response to infections. These cells leave the blood and migrate to the infected area as *wandering macrophages* and are very efficient phagocytes. *Fixed macrophages*, or histocytes, are those macrophages that remain in tissues and organs and serve to trap foreign debris. They may be found in tissues of the organs of the reticuloendothelial system (RES); this defensive system includes the liver (Kupffer cells), spleen, lymph nodes, and bone marrow as well as the lungs (dust cells) and brain (microglia). Thus, it appears that the macrophages are more efficient scavenger cells than the neutrophilic microphages, but both are able to destroy most of the microorganisms they ingest.

The principal function of the entire RES is the engulfment and removal of foreign and useless particles, living or dead, such as excess cellular secretions, dead and dying leukocytes, erythrocytes, and tissue cells, as well as foreign debris and microorganisms that gain entrance to the body.

Phagocytosis begins when a phagocyte moves to within 100 μm of a foreign object such as a bacterium. The phenomenon that causes the phagocyte to be attracted to the bacterium is called chemotaxis. This chemical attraction is not well understood but is believed to be the result of lymphokines produced by T lymphocytes in many circumstances (as discussed in Chap. 11).

When the phagocyte touches a pathogen, the phagocyte's membrane indents (invaginates), and the phagocyte moves around the microbe until it surrounds the latter completely (Fig. 10-1). The membrane-bound vesicle (pouch) that surrounds the pathogen, which is now inside the phagocyte, is called the phagosome, or phagocytic vacuole. The phagosome fuses with nearby lysosomes to form a digestive vacuole, and killing and digestion of the microbe begins. Within 10 to 30 minutes after ingestion the microorganism is killed by lactic acid and hydrogen peroxide from the lysosome. Then lysosomal digestive enzymes, including lysozyme and β-lysin, digest and degrade the carbohydrates, lipids, proteins, and nucleic acids. The products of this digestion, which may be used by cells as nutrients, are then absorbed into the cytoplasm. Undigested materials are retained within the membrane, thus the digestive vacuole becomes the residual body until the undigested wastes are expelled from the phagocyte.

It should be noted that not all bacteria engulfed by phagocytes are destroyed by the digestive enzymes. Usually the encapsulated bacteria are resistant to digestion; thus, they may be carried to another part of the body before the phagocyte expels them. Also, some pathogens secrete an enzyme, leukocidin (discussed in Chap. 7), that destroys leukocytes, including the phagocytes that ingest them. Other pathogens, such as *Mycobacterium* species, are able to multiply within the phagosome and destroy the phagocyte. The causative agents of brucellosis and tularemia may remain dormant within the phagocyte for months or years before they escape to cause disease. These types of virulent pathogens usually win the battle with phagocytes. Unless antibodies are present to activate the complement to aid in the destruction of these pathogens, the infection may progress unchecked (Fig. 10-2).

Inflammation

The body normally responds to any local injury, irritation, microbial invasion, or bacterial toxins by a complex series of events called inflammation. The purposes of the inflammatory response are to localize an infection, to prevent the spread of microbial invaders, to neutralize toxins, and to aid in the repair of damaged tissue (Fig. 10-3). In this process, all the nonspecific defenses come into play. These interrelated physiological reactions result in the signs and symptoms of *edema* (swelling of

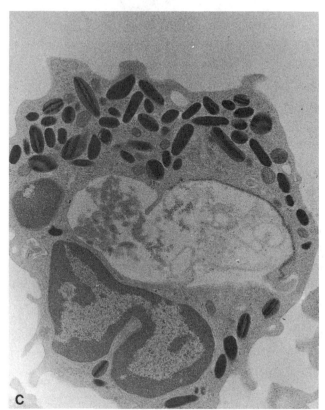

Fig. 10-1. Phagocytosis of a Giardia trophozoite. (*A*) Attachment. (*B*) Ingestion. (*C*) Digestion. Note the cross sections of cilia in *A* and *B*, and the lysosomes in *C*. (From S. Koester and P. Engelkirk)

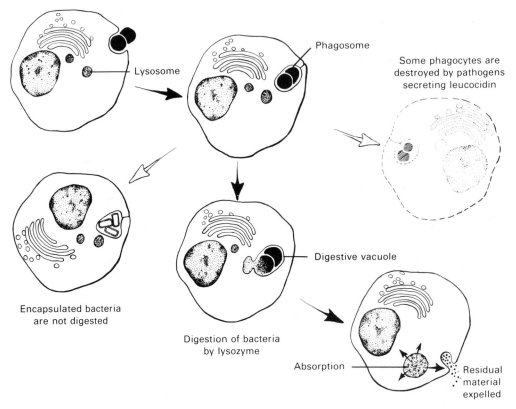

Fig. 10-2. Not all pathogens are destroyed by the phagocytes. Encapsulated bacteria and bacteria that secrete leukocidin are the two types that are not destroyed if antibodies are lacking.

the area), *redness, heat* (fever), *pain,* and often pus formation and occasional loss of function of the damaged area.

A complex series of physiological events occurs immediately following the initial damage to the tissue. Some of the injured cells (mast cells, basophils, and platelets) release certain chemicals (histamine, bradykinin, other kinins, and heparin) that increase the permeability of the capillaries and venules, and prevent immediate clotting of the blood. Vasodilation and increased capillary permeability allow more blood (plasma, clotting agents, and cells) to enter the area, including more leukocytes for phagocytosis and antibody production. Macrophages are also attracted to the region by the chemotaxis of the secretions from the damaged cells.

The surrounding tissue becomes engorged with fluids, and edema results. Red blood cells collecting in the irritated area cause redness. Heat is generated and fever produced by increased cellular activity in the destruction and detoxification of foreign materials, microbes, dead cells (tissue and phagocytic), and toxic chemicals, including waste products released by invading microorganisms.

Pain or tenderness usually accompanies inflammation. It may result from actual

1. Skin puncture
2. Histamine released
3. Capillaries dilate
4. Increased capillary permeability
5. Increased plasma in tissues
6. Increased phagocytosis of microorganisms and injured tissue
7. Fibrocytes wall off and heal area

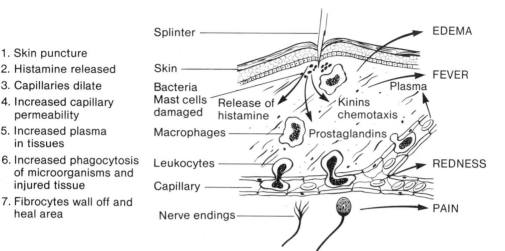

Fig. 10-3. The inflammatory response.

damage of the nerve fibers because of the injury, from irritation by microbial toxins or other cellular secretions (such as prostaglandins), or from the edema causing increased pressure on the nerve endings (Fig. 10-4).

The accumulation of fluid and cells within the inflamed site is referred to as the *inflammatory exudate.* If the exudate is thick and yellow with many dead leukocytes it is known as a purulent exudate or pus. However, it should be noted that in many inflammatory responses, such as arthritis or pancreatitis, there is no exudate and no invading microorganisms. When pyogenic (*pyo* = pus) microorganisms, such as some staphylococci and streptococci, are present, even more pus is produced as a result of the killing effect of the bacterial toxins on phagocytes and tissue cells. Most pus has a yellow color, but in infections caused by *Pseudomonas aeruginosa,* the exudate may be blue-greenish owing to the pigments produced by the bacteria.

When the inflammatory response is over and the body has won the battle, the

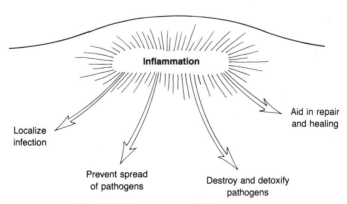

Fig. 10-4. The purposes of inflammation.

phagocytes continue to clean up the area and help to restore order. Then the cells and tissues can repair the damage and begin to function normally again in a homeostatic state, although some permanent damage and scarring may have occured.

The lymphatic system, including the lymph fluid, lymph vessels, lymph nodes, and lymph organs (tonsils, spleen, and thymus gland) plays an important role in defending the body against invaders. The primary functions of this system include draining and circulating intercellular fluids from the tissues and transporting digested fats from the digestive system to the blood. Also, the macrophages and the B- and T-cell lymphocytes in the lymph nodes serve to filter the lymph by removing foreign matter and microbes and by producing antibodies and other factors to aid in the destruction and detoxification of any microorganisms that are attempting to invade through this pathway.

The body continually wages war against damage, injury, malfunction, and microbial invasion. The outcome of each battle depends on the person's age, hormonal balance, genetic ability for resistance, and overall state of physical and mental health, as well as the virulence of the pathogens presented.

Problems and Questions

1. What factors contribute to natural resistance to disease?
2. List the nonspecific defenses of the skin, respiratory system, digestive system, and urogenital tract.
3. List some serum proteins that aid in the destruction of invading microorganisms.
4. Describe the process of phagocytosis.
5. What is the function of the lysosome? Of the residual body?
6. What are the four main symptoms of inflammation?
7. What are the causes of the symptoms of inflammation?
8. What are pyogenic bacteria? Give an example.
9. Describe inflammatory exudate.

Chapter 11

Immunology and Specific Mechanisms of Defense Against Disease

Objectives

After studying this chapter, you should be able to

1. Describe the immune response, or "third line of defense"
2. Define *antigen, antibody,* and *immunoglobulin*
3. Differentiate between active and passive immunity
4. Compare natural and artificial immunity
5. List three ways in which vaccines are prepared
6. Describe congenital naturally acquired passive immunity
7. Draw a graph representing the primary and secondary antibody responses to antigens
8. Differentiate between immediate and delayed hypersensitivity
9. Describe how anaphylactic shock and serum sickness occur
10. Define autoimmunity and give examples
11. List the serological tests used to determine the presence of a specific antibody in human serum
12. Describe and name *in vivo* toxin neutralization tests

New Words to Pronounce and Understand

Agglutination (uh-glue-ten-ay'-shun). The clumping of cells following reaction with antibodies

Allergen (al'-ur-jen). An antigen that causes an allergic reaction

Allergy (al'-ur-gee). A disease resulting from exposure to an antigen

Anamnestic response (an-am-nest'-tick). Memory response following antigen exposure in sensitized individuals

Anaphylactic shock (an-na-fill-lack'-tick). A severe allergic reaction that may result in death

Antibody (an-tea-body). A glycoprotein produced by lymphocytes in response to antigens

Antigen (an'-ti-gin). A foreign substance that stimulates the production of antibodies

Antitoxin (an-tea-tock'-sin). An antibody that neutralizes a toxin

Arthus reaction (ar'-thus). An immune complex skin reaction at the site of repeated injections

Attenuated (uh-ten'-you-ay-ted). A weakened, less pathogenic organism

Autoimmune disease (au-to-im-mune'). A disease in which the body produces antibodies to its own tissues

Cytotoxic (sigh-toe-tock'-sick). A substance harmful to cells

Exotoxin (x'-oh-tock-sin). A toxic substance secreted by a living organism

Hapten (hap-ten'). A nonantigenic small molecule that becomes antigenic when combined with a large molecule

Hypersensitivity (hi-purr-sens-uh-tiv'-it-tea). A cell-mediated immunological reaction that causes tissue destruction or inflammation

Immunity (im-mew'-ni-tea). Resistance to disease by means of antibodies

Immunoglobulin (im'-mew-no-glob'-you-lin). An antibody

In vitro (in vee'-tro). In the laboratory, in an artificial environment

In vivo (in vee'-vo). In the living organism

Lymphokines (lim'-fo-kines). T-cell secretions following antigenic stimulation

Lysis (lie'-sis). Cellular destruction

Monoclonal antibodies (mon-o-clone'-al). Antibodies for a single antigenic determinant produced by hybridoma cells (lymphocytes fused with tumor cells), *in vitro*

Mutation (mew-tay'-shun). A permanent change in the genetic constitution of an organism

Opsonization (op-son-i-zay'-shun). The engulfment of cells or bacteria by phagocytes, caused by the presence of specific antibodies

Precipitin (pre-sip'-i-tin). The precipitation of soluble antigenic material by the specific antibody

Serological tests (sero-o-lodge'-eh-cal). Antigen–antibody tests used for diagnostic purposes

Toxoid (tox'-oid. An inactivated toxin that can stimulate antitoxin production but not cause disease

Vaccine (vack-scene'). An inactivated agent used to cause the production of antibodies to protect against disease

As discussed in the preceding chapter, there are three lines of defense against infectious disease agents. The first is the mechanical barrier presented by the skin, mucous membranes, and hair covering, with their related antimicrobial secretions. The second consists of the nonspecific biochemicals and cellular reactions of phagocytosis and inflammation that are directed against damaged tissues and any organisms that invade the body. The *immune response* is the third line of defense against pathogens. Usually, in this protective type of immunity, antibodies are produced by lymphocytes to bind with, inactivate, and destroy specific microorganisms. These humoral circulating antibodies are normally found in serum, lymph, and other body secretions where they readily protect against those specific pathogens that stimulated their formation. Thus, a person has an immunity to a disease because of the presence of specific protective antibodies to the causative agent of that disease. In addition, there are protective cell-mediated immune responses that do not involve the presence of antibodies (see Fig. 11-4).

Although the immune system protects against disease and aids in fighting cancer, it may also cause damage to its host, as you will learn from the discussions on cell-mediated hypersensitivity and autoimmunity.

Immunity

Immunity is the resistance to disease afforded by the presence of antibodies to the causative pathogens (etiologic agents) of that disease. The innate, or native, resistance to disease found in certain individuals, races, and species of animals is not a type of immunity conferred by antibodies but, rather, is a resistance resulting from natural nonspecific factors. A person who is susceptible to a disease usually has inadequate levels of protective antibodies or insufficient nonspecific defenses, which may simply reflect a very poor state of health or the presence of an immunodeficiency disease.

Acquired Immunity

Immunity that results from the production of or transfer of antibodies to protect a person against infection is termed acquired immunity. If the antibodies are formed by the lymphocytes of the protected person, the immunity is called *active acquired immunity.* In *passive acquired immunity,* antibodies are transferred from one person (or from an animal) to another person to temporarily protect the latter against infection (Table 11-1).

Active Acquired Immunity When people have had a specific infection, they will have some resistance to reinfection by the causative pathogen because of the presence of antibodies and stimulated lymphocytes. This is called *naturally acquired active immunity.* Symptoms of the disease may or may not have been present for antibodies to be formed naturally. Such resistance to reinfection may be permanent (as with mumps,

Table 11-1 Types of Acquired Immunity

Active		Passive	
Natural	*Artificial*	*Natural*	*Artificial*
Clinical or subclinical disease	Vaccines: Dead or extract Attenuated Toxoids	Congential (across placenta) Colostrum	Antiserum Antitoxin Gamma globulin

measles, smallpox, diphtheria, whooping cough, poliomyelitis, plague, and typhoid fever), or it may be only temporary (as happens with pneumonia, influenza, gonorrhea, and streptococcal and staphylococcal infections). There is no immunity to reinfection following recovery from syphilis and tuberculosis.

Artificially acquired active immunity is the second type of actively acquired immunity. It occurs when a person receives a vaccination, which is the administration of a vaccine that causes specific antibodies to be produced. Sufficient antigens of a pathogen are contained in the vaccine for the person to form antibodies against that pathogen before exposure to the disease. A good vaccine is one that (1) contains enough antigens to protect against infection by the pathogen; (2) contains antigens from all of the strains of the pathogen that cause that disease (*e.g.*, three strains of virus cause "polio"); (3) is not too toxic; and (4) will not cause disease in the vaccinated person.

A successful vaccine for colds has not been developed because there are so many different viruses that causes colds. It is also difficult to maintain a successful vaccine for influenza because the viruses continually change.

Vaccines are made from living or dead pathogens or from certain toxins they excrete (Fig. 11-1). In general, vaccines made from living organisms are most effective, but they must be prepared from harmless organisms that are antigenically closely related to the pathogens or from weakened pathogens that have been genetically changed so they are no longer pathogenic. The process of weakening pathogens is called attenuation. The smallpox (variola) vaccine is derived from the cowpox virus (vaccinia), which causes a mild pox infection in cattle and humans. Most other live vaccines are avirulent (nonpathogenic) mutant strains of pathogens that have been derived from the virulent organisms; this is done by growing them for many generations under various conditions or by exposing them to mutagenic chemicals or radiations. In this way Pasteur developed the vaccine for rabies and Sabin developed the oral vaccine for poliomyelitis. Other attenuated living vaccines include those for measles (rubeola), mumps, German measles (rubella), yellow fever, and typhus.

Vaccines made from dead pathogens, which have been killed by heat or chemicals, can be produced faster and more easily, but they are less effective than live vaccines because the antigens on the dead cells are usually less effective and produce a shorter period of immunity. The dead vaccines are safer to use during the experimental phase of vaccine production because of the remote possibility that an avirulent

Vaccines

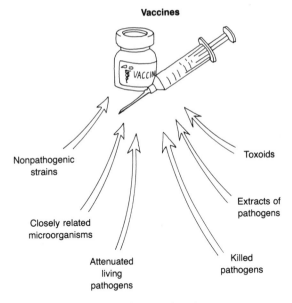

Nonpathogenic strains

Toxoids

Closely related microorganisms

Extracts of pathogens

Attenuated living pathogens

Killed pathogens

Fig. 11-1. Sources of vaccines.

strain of a living organism may revert to the virulent strain before the strain's stability has been proved. For example, the first poliomyelitis virus vaccine, which was developed by Jonas Salk, contained the killed organisms of three strains of polioviruses, which had to be injected to produce adequate immunity against the disease. A few years later, it was found that the live virus vaccine, developed by Sabin and others, was safe when taken by mouth. Killed pathogens or their extracts are used to vaccinate against whooping cough (pertussis), typhoid fever, paratyphoid fever, cholera, plague, Rocky Mountain spotted fever, and many respiratory diseases including influenza. The use of such vaccines shows us a very important and practical application of principles of microbiology.

Another type of vaccine used to prevent tetanus and diphtheria, called a *toxoid* vaccine, is prepared from exotoxins that have been inactivated or made nontoxic by heat or chemicals. These toxoids can be injected safely to cause the formation of antibodies that will neutralize the exotoxins of the pathogens, such as those that cause tetanus and diphtheria. Antiserum containing antibodies against toxoids prepared in this way is called *antitoxin*.

As microbiologists made further studies of the characteristics of vaccines, they found that it was practical to vaccinate against several diseases by combining the specific vaccines in a single injection. Thus, diphtheria–pertussis–tetanus (DPT) vaccine contains toxoids for diphtheria and tetanus and killed organisms for whooping cough (pertussis). Sometimes, the Salk poliovirus vaccine is added to form the "quad" vaccine (*quad* = four). A second example is the measles, mumps, rubella (MMR) vaccine that is recommended for all children.

An *autogenous vaccine* is one prepared from a localized infection, such as a staphylococcal boil. The pathogens are killed, then injected into the same person to induce production of more antibodies.

Passive Acquired Immunity   Passive immunity differs from active immunity in that antibodies formed in one person are transferred to another to protect the latter from an infection to which he has been exposed. Because the person receiving the antibodies did not produce them, the immunity thus derived is temporary, lasting about 3 to 6 weeks. The antibodies of passive immunity may be transferred naturally or artificially.

In *naturally acquired passive immunity*, the small antibodies (IgG) present in the mother's blood cross the placenta to reach the fetus while it is in the uterus. Also, the milk or colostrum secreted for a few days following delivery contains maternal antibodies to protect the infant during the early months of life.

Artificially acquired passive immunity is accomplished by transferring antibodies from an immune person to a susceptible person. When a patient has been exposed to a disease, the length of the incubation period usually does not allow sufficient time for vaccination to be an effective preventive measure. This is because a span of at least 2 weeks is needed before sufficient antibodies are formed to protect the exposed person.

To provide temporary protection in these situations, the patient is given "pooled" immune serum globulin (ISG), that is, antibodies taken from the blood of many immune people. Thus, the patient receives some antibodies to all of the diseases to which the donors are immune.

The ISG may be given to provide temporary protection against measles, mumps, polio, diphtheria, and hepatitis in people, especially infants, who are not immune and have been exposed to these diseases.

Hyperimmune serum globulin has been prepared from the serum of people with high antibody levels (titer) against certain diseases. For example, hepatitis B immune globulin (HBIG) is given to protect those who have been, or are apt to be, exposed to hepatitis; tetanus immune globulin (TIG) is used for nonimmunized patients with deep, dirty wounds; and rabies immune globulin (RIG) may be given following a bite by a rabid animal. In botulism food-poisoning cases, antitoxin antibodies are used to neutralize the toxic effects of the botulin toxin. Remember that passive immunity is always temporary because the antibodies are not produced by the lymphocytes of the protected person.

Immunology

Immunology is the scientific study of immune responses. In this book only the basic fundamentals of immunology can be presented. The topics briefly discussed in this chapter include active and passive immunity to infectious agents, processes involved in antibody production, cell-mediated immune responses, allergies and other types of hypersensitivities, autoimmunity, and serologic testing for antibodies and antigens.

An *antigen* can be any *foreign* organic substance that is large enough to stimulate the production of antibodies; in other words, it is *immunogenic*. Antigens may be proteins of more than 10,000 molecular weight, or polysaccharides larger than 60,000 molecular weight, large molecules of DNA or RNA, or any combination of biochemical molecules (*e.g.,* glycoproteins, lipoproteins, nucleoproteins) that make up cells of either microorganisms or macroorganisms. As antigen has one or more antigenic determinants (or sites) to which antibodies or lymphocytes can bind. The important point is that they must be *foreign* materials that the human body does not recognize as *self* antigens, and large enough to be acknowledged by a macrophage. Certainly, all microorganisms fall into this category. Some small molecules called *haptens* may act as an antigen if they are coupled with a large carrier molecule such as a protein. Then the antibodies formed against that antigenic determinant site will combine with the haptens when they are no longer coupled with the carrier protein. As an example, penicillin and other low-molecular-weight chemical molecules may act as haptens, causing people to become allergic to them.

Antibodies are glycoproteins produced by a lymphocyte (a white blood cell) in response to the presence of an antigen, and will bind specifically with that antigen. (Actually, the antibody-producing cells are a type of lymphocyte called B cells, which usually work in coordination with T-cell lymphocytes and macrophages, as described later.) A bacterial cell has many antigenic determinant sites on its cell membrane, cell wall, capsule, or flagella that will stimulate the production of many antibodies. However, those antibodies are considered to be "specific" for a particular group of identical bacterial cells. Occasionally, similar antigenic sites are found on other microorganisms or even on tissue cells, and those antibodies that will bind to these similar antigenic sites are referred to as cross-reacting antibodies.

All antibodies are also called *immunoglobulins* (Ig) because they are the globular glycoproteins in the serum that participate in the immune reaction. We usually refer to antibodies as those specific immunoglobulins with particular specificity for an antigen, whereas the term *immunoglobulin* represents all the antibodies a person possesses. Immunoglobulins are also found in lymph, tears, saliva, and colostrum (Fig. 11-2). Colostrum is the clear fluid secreted by the mother's mammary gland following the birth of an infant. This fluid contains a large number of antibodies and some lymphocytes from the mother that serve to protect the newborn during the first few months of life.

The number and type of antibodies produced by antigenic stimulation depends upon the nature of the antigen, the site of antigen stimulus, the amount of antigen, and the number of times the person is exposed to the antigen. Figure 11-3 shows that following the first exposure to the antigen (such as a vaccine), there is a delayed primary response in the production of antibodies. This delayed response is called the *lag phase.* During this time the antigen must be processed by macrophages and T lymphocytes which then stimulate the small B lymphocytes to develop into large B lymphocytes (plasma cells) that are able to produce antibodies by protein synthesis in the presence of helper T lymphocytes. This initial immune response is the *primary response.* When the antigen is used up, the number of antibodies in the serum declines

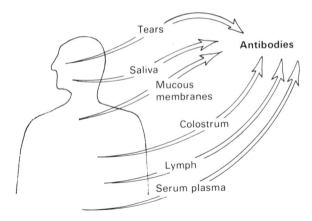

Fig. 11-2. Body structures and sites in which antibodies are produced.

as the plasma cells die off. Other antigen-stimulated B lymphocytes become "memory" cells, which are small lymphocytes that can be stimulated to produce antibodies quickly when later exposed to the same antigens. This increased production of antibodies following the second exposure to the antigen (a booster shot) is the *secondary response,* or the *anamnestic* or *memory response.* A second booster shot of antigen many months later will return the antibody concentration to the level of the secondary response. This is the reason for the immunization of infants and for booster shots given during their first year, before they attend school, and at specific intervals throughout life if the person is continually exposed to those pathogens, as with tetanus.

Some persons are born without the built-in protection given by antibodies. Because they are unable to produce antibodies, they have no gamma globulin in their blood. This abnormality is called *agammaglobulinemia.* These persons are very susceptible to infections by even the most harmless microorganisms in their environment. One treatment of agammaglobulinemia that is often successful consists of a bone

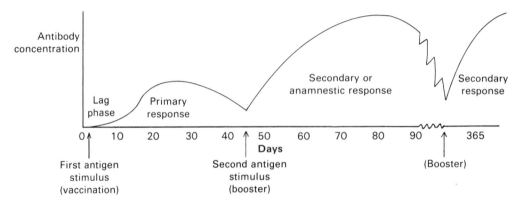

Fig. 11-3. Antibody production following exposure to antigen.

marrow transplant. This is the transfer of precursor white blood cells from a closely related person. Some of these cells become lymphocytes. These lymphocytes may be implanted in the lymph nodes and become immunocompetent, that is, they can be stimulated by antigens to produce antibodies.

Persons who produce an insufficient amount of antibodies are said to have *hypogammaglobulinemia.* Their resistance to infection is lower than normal, so they usually do not recover from infectious diseases as readily as most other persons.

Some patients are immunosuppressed (unable to make antibodies) following the administration of immunosuppressive drugs or agents such as antilymphocytic serum before organ transplant surgery. Others are infected with a virus (HIV virus, that causes AIDS) which destroys helper T_4 lymphocytes that induce plasma cells to make antibodies and are also involved in cell-mediated immune responses. These patients usually succumb to secondary infections for which they have little resistance.

The Immune System

The immune system encompasses the whole body, but the lymphoid system is the site and source of most immune activity. The cells involved in the immune responses originate in bone marrow (from which blood cells also develop; Fig. 11-4). At least two lines of lymphocytes, B cells and T cells and probably NK cells, derive from the lymphoid stem cells of bone marrow. About half of these stem cells migrate to the thymus gland where they differentiate into T cells (T for thymus) of the helper, suppressor, or cytotoxic type. This thymus processing of the T cells begins shortly before birth. T cells are small lymphocytes found in the blood, lymph, and lymphoid tissues. They do not produce humoral antibodies but aid in the control of antibody production and are involved in the cell-mediated immune responses (tissue transplant rejection; cellular immunity to *Mycobacteria,* fungi, and viruses; cytotoxicity of viral-infected cells and tumor cells).

Other lymphocytic stem cells differentiate into B cells (named for the bursa lymphoid area in birds). B cells migrate to the lymphoid tissues where they will produce antibodies to be circulated through lymph and blood to protect the individual (humoral immunity). Thousands of B cells exist in the body even though these cells live only about 1 to 2 weeks. Each B cell is capable of producing specific antibodies when stimulated by an antigen.

The Immune Response

Many chemicals, cells, and reactions are involved in the immune responses. Some chemicals and complexes are nonspecific and yet depend on the antigen–antibody complex for activation, as does complement. The specific humoral response always depends on the presence of specific antibodies for each antigen or antigenic determinant. However, some types of cell-mediated responses occur in the presence of antibodies, but others do not involve the antigen–antibody complex, as summarized in Figure 11-4.

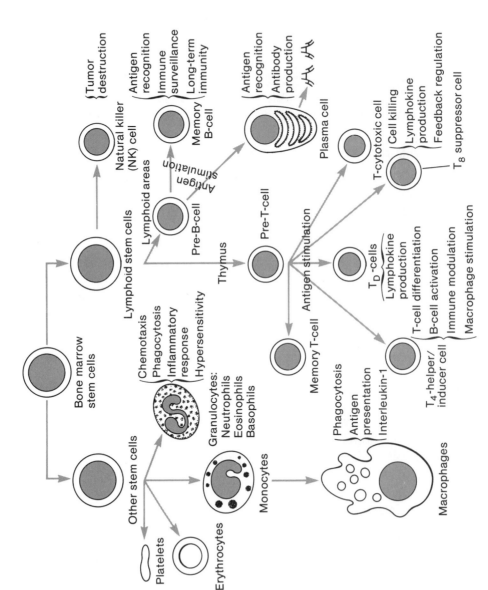

Fig. 11-4. Differentiation of blood and lymph cells from bone marrow cells; development of cell-mediated immunity and antibody production.

Antibody Production

For antibodies to be produced, a complex series of events must occur, some of which are not completely understood. It is known that macrophages, T cells, and B cells are involved in a cooperative effort.

When bacteria invade they are first processed by macrophages. It appears that macrophages prepare and present bacterial antigens to the T cells and B cells; apparently these antigens appear on the surface of the macrophage. T cells serve to control the production of antibody by the B cells, but do not manufacture antibodies themselves. T cells are sensitized or primed by the antigen on the macrophage. *Helper T cells* encourage the B plasma cells to synthesize more antibody, and *suppressor T cells* inhibit antibody production in B plasma cells. In this way, the level of antibodies is neither excessive nor insufficient if the control mechanism is working properly. When the antigen is presented to the B cells and T cells by the macrophages, some B cells are activated and stimulated to enlarge, differentiate, and divide into clones of antibody-producing *plasma cells* (large B lymphocytes). Antibodies are expelled in gunfire fashion for several days until the plasma cell dies. Each plasma cell clone makes only one type of antibody, the one that will bind with the antigen responsible for activating the B cell. This specificity is probably determined by the IgD-type antibodies on the surface of the B cell. Those activated B cells that did not become plasma cells, and some primed T cells, remain as memory cells, to respond more quickly when the antigen appears again at a later date.

When the antigen–antibody complex is formed, complement may be activated to destroy the bacterial cell, increase phagocytosis, and neutralize bacterial toxins. Thus, antibody-mediated immunity (AMI) almost entirely controls acute extracellular bacterial infections.

Cell-Mediated Immunity   Antibodies cannot enter cells containing intracellular pathogens; however, the macrophage–T cell-mediated immunity (CMI) serves the body by controlling chronic infections of intracellular parasites (bacteria, protozoa, fungi, viruses). For example, in cytolytic viral infections (*e.g.*, herpes), the virus moves in the body fluids from one lysed cell to another, during which time the virus can be neutralized and destroyed by the antibody–complement complex, and viral infections can be prevented in this manner. However, when the virus is established with the body cells, the cell-mediated immune response (macrophages, T-cytotoxic cells) can destroy many virus-infected cells and damaged tissues but cannot completely destroy the virus once it becomes latent in nerve ganglion cells.

Cell-mediated immunity results from several types of antigen-stimulated T lymphocytes. The helper T cells (T_4) cooperate with B cells to initiate the antibody-mediated response; suppressor T cells (T_8) reduce the intensity of antibody-mediated response and moderate the activities of cytotoxic T killer cells so that the immune response is effective but not destructive.

Another T cell (T_D) is involved in the delayed hypersensitivity reaction. Its action is delayed because it is formed following antigen sensitization and reacts to produce lymphokines after a subsequent antigen stimulation. This response will be discussed later in this chapter.

Nonspecific NK Cells   Some specialized lymphocytes (neither T nor B cells) become nonspecific *natural killer cells* (NK cells). These cells leave the lymphoid area and migrate to the inflammatory site of microbial invasion or area of tumor growth. There they attach to invading pathogens or tumor cells and destroy them. Note that the NK cells are not antigen- nor antibody-dependent, they function to rid the body of "foreign" cells; however the cytotoxic T cells target and destroy antigen-bearing cells by secreting cytotoxic substances.

Antibody Structure and Function

As stated previously, antibodies are protein gamma globulins formed by the lymphocytes in response to stimulation by foreign substances called antigens. Those antibodies found in the serum are called humoral antibodies or circulating antibodies.

Studies of the gamma globulin component of serum have revealed that there are five classes of antibodies. These antibodies, called immunoglobulins, have been designated IgG, IgM, IgA, IgD, and IgE. The functions of each of these classes are listed in Table 11-2.

Immunoglobulin G (IgG) is the most abundant (80%) of the serum antibodies. It binds (attaches) to antigens in the serum as well as in the lymph or intercellular fluids. Invading bacteria (antigens) are more easily destroyed by phagocytes, or lysed by complement, when antibodies are attached to them because the antibodies also bind the phagocytes or complement.

Table 11-2 Immunoglobulin Classes and Functions

Ig Class	Molecular Weight	% in Serum	Functions
IgG	150,000	80	Protects against disease; attaches to phagocytes and tissues; fixes complement; crosses placental barrier; causes certain immunological diseases; found in serum and lymph
IgM	900,000	6	Protects against early infection; bactericidal to gram-negative bacteria; fixes complement; found in serum and lymph
IgA	400,000 or 170,000	13	Protects the mucous membranes and internal cavities against infection; found as secretory antibodies in tears, saliva, colostrum, and other secretions
IgE	190,000	0.002	Causes allergies, drug sensitivity, anaphylaxis, and immediate hypersensitivity; combats parasitic diseases
IgD	185,000	1.0	Fetal antigen receptor; controls antigen stimulation of B cells; found in serum and on lymphocytes

Immunoglobulin G is the smallest of the antibodies. It can cross the placenta and move freely in the intercellular fluids as well as in the blood. It consists of four polypeptides (amino acid chains): two identical short (lightweight) chains and two longer (heavy) chains held together by disulfide (—S—S—) bonds (Fig. 11-5). This antibody is bipolar, that is, it has two ends that bind specifically to the antigen that stimulated its production. The middle section of this large molecule (macromolecule) will bind nonspecifically to complement, phagocytes, or tissue cells.

Immunoglobulin M (IgM) is the largest of the gamma globulins. This immunoglobulin consists of five IgG-type molecules held together by disulfide bonds. Because it is star shaped, it usually binds with only five identical antigens. The IgM antibodies appear to be the first antibodies formed in response to infections, especially those caused by gram-negative bacteria.

Immunoglobulin A (IgA) is designated the secretory antibody, so-called because these immunoglobulins are found in saliva, tears, colostrum, and other body secretions, as well as in the bloodstream. They consist of two IgG-sized antibodies held together by a secretory piece and serve to protect the external openings and mucous membranes from invasion by pathogens. Others, consisting of one IgG-sized molecule, are found in internal body cavity secretions.

Fig. 11-5. Structure of immunoglobulin IgG.

Immunoglobulin E (IgE) is often called P–K antibody (in honor of two scientists, Prausnitz and Küstner, who first identified it). These antibodies are present in persons with allergy, drug sensitivity, or anaphylactic shock. Most often, these antibodies are bound to target cells (basophils and mast cells) in tissues, and cause the rash or hives seen in various allergies, the "runny nose and eyes" of hay fever and asthma, the local reaction in immediate hypersensitivity skin tests, and shock reaction of anaphylaxis.

Immunoglobulin D (IgD) is a serum antibody that may function as a control mechanism for the immune response. The function of this antibody is not clearly understood, but it is probably involved in the determination of which plasma cell produces which antibody (IgG type) because it is found on the surface of B lymphocytes.

Monoclonal Antibodies   Purified monoclonal antibodies against specific antigens have been produced by a new innovative technique, in which a single plasma cell that produces only one specific type of antibody is fused with a mitosing tumor cell. The new longlived antibody-producing cell is called a hybridoma. These hybridomas are capable of producing large amounts of specific antibodies called monoclonal antibodies. Wide use has been made of these antibodies, especially in developing new diagnostic serologic tests. Because they are uniform, highly specific, and they can be produced in large quantities, they can be used routinely to bind with the antigens of particular pathogens in laboratory tests and in allergy and disease testing. Many new procedures are being developed; they may even be used for passive immunization to protect against certain diseases or to neutralize the toxins of botulism, tetanus, and perhaps snake and insect bites.

Hypersensitivity

Hypersensitivity is the defensive response gone awry. Sometimes, instead of protecting a person, the antibodies irritate and damage certain cells in the body. This can be compared to the person who builds a fire in the living room to warm the house, and burns down the house.

There are several different types of hypersensitivity reactions; some involve various antibodies and others do not. All depend on the presence of antigen and T cells sensitized to that antigen.

Hypersensitivity reactions are divided into two general categories, immediate and delayed, depending on the nature of the immune reaction and the time required for an observable reaction to occur. An *immediate reaction* occurs within a few minutes to 24 hours. There are several types of immediate reactions; type I includes the classic allergic responses of hay fever, asthma, and hives from food; allergic responses to insect stings; drug allergies; and anaphylactic shock. It involves IgE antibodies, mast cells, and basophils. Type II is the cytotoxic hypersensitivity seen in blood transfusion and Rh incompatibility reactions, and in myasthenia gravis, involving IgG or IgM antibodies and complement. Type III is the immune complex reaction of serum sickness and autoimmune diseases (systemic lupus erythematosus, rheumatoid arthritis),

Type I	II	III	IV
	Immediate		Delayed
Allergy	Cytolysis	Auto-	TB skin test
Anaphylaxis	Blood type	immunity	Transplantation
	reactions		rejection

Fig. 11-6. Types of hypersensitivity immune responses.

involving IgG or IgM antibodies, complement, and neutrophils. *Delayed hypersensitivity*, which is usually observed after 24 hours, is designated type IV. It is also referred to as cell-mediated immunity, such as occurs in tuberculin and fungal skin tests, contact dermatitis, and transplantation rejection. Delayed hypersensitivity does not involve antibodies but does depend on sensitized or primed T cells that secrete lymphokines in response to a second exposure to the sensitizing antigen (Fig. 11-6).

The Allergic Response   Immediate hypersensitivity (type I) is probably the most commonly observed type of hypersensitivity because approximately 80% of the American population is allergic to something. People who are prone to allergies produce IgE antibodies that become cell bound when they are exposed to allergens, which are the antigens that cause allergic reactions. The type and severity of an allergic reaction depend on a combination of factors, including the nature of the antigen, the amount of antigen entering the body, the route by which it enters, the length of time between exposures to the antigen, the person's ability to produce IgE antibodies, and the site of IgE attachment (Fig. 11-7).

The allergic reaction results from the presence of IgE antibodies bound to basophils in the blood or to mast cells in connective tissues, following the person's first

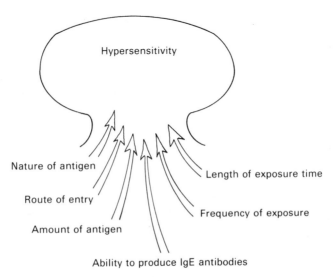

Fig. 11-7. Factors in development of hypersensitivity.

exposure to the allergen. When the cell-bound IgE binds with the allergen during the second or later exposure, the sensitized cells respond by producing and releasing irritating and damaging substances. These mediators of the allergic response include histamine, prostaglandins, serotonin, bradykinin, slow-reacting substance of anaphylaxis (SRS-A), leukotrines, and other mediating chemicals that attract eosinophils.

Localized anaphylaxis. Hay fever, asthma, and hives are localized allergic anaphylactic diseases. The symptoms depend on how the antigen enters the body and the site of IgE attachment. If the antigen (pollens, dust, fungal spores) is inhaled so that it deposits on the mucous membranes of the respiratory tract, IgE antibodies are formed and attach to the mast cells in that area. Subsequent exposure to those inhaled antigens allows the antigens (allergens) to bind to the attached IgE, causing the mast cells to release large amounts of histamine. This substance initiates the classic symptoms of hay fever. Antihistamines are quite useful in treating hay fever because they neutralize histamine. Antihistamines are not as effective in treating asthma, however, because the mediators of this lower respiratory allergy include the leukotrines in addition to histamine.

Allergens entering through the digestive tract (food and drugs) can also sensitize the host, causing hives, vomiting, and diarrhea.

Systemic anaphylactic shock. The severe allergic reaction called systemic anaphylactic shock occurs following injection of an allergen to which the host has been sensitized. Frequently these allergens are drugs or insect venom, and occasionally certain foods. With penicillin, the drug serves as a hapten, binding to host serum proteins, sensitizing the mast cells, and circulating basophils. Subsequent injections of large doses of penicillin into the sensitized host may cause the release of large amounts of histamine and other mediators of allergy into the circulatory system.

The shock reaction usually occurs immediately (within 20 minutes) following reexposure to the allergen. The first symptoms are flushing of the skin with itching, headache, facial swelling, and difficulty in breathing; this is followed by falling blood pressure, nausea, vomiting, abdominal cramps, and urination (caused by smooth muscle contractions). In many cases, acute respiratory distress, unconsciousness, and death may follow shortly. Swift treatment with epinephrine (adrenaline) and antihistamine will usually stop the reaction.

Health professionals must take particular care to ask patients if they have any allergies or sensitivities. In particular, those people with allergies to penicillin and other drugs and to insect stings should wear Medic-Alert tags so that they will not receive improper treatment during a medical crisis.

Anaphylactic reactions can be prevented by avoiding known allergens. In some cases, skin tests are used to identify the offending allergens. Then, desensitization may be accomplished by injecting small doses of allergen, repeatedly, several days apart. This treatment may be effective by causing the production of increased amounts of circulating IgG antibody instead of IgE. Thus, the IgG should bind with the allergen and block its attachment to the cell-bound IgE. These circulating IgG molecules are called *blocking antibodies.* This preventive measure usually works better for inhaled allergens than for ingested and injected allergens.

Autoimmune Diseases   An autoimmune disease is a type III hypersensitivity response that may occur when a person's immune system no longer recognizes certain body tissues as "self" and attempts to destroy those tissues as being "foreign." This may occur with certain tissues that are not exposed to the immune system during fetal development so that they are not recognized as self. Such tissues may include the lens of the eyes, the brain and spinal cord, and sperm. Subsequent exposure to this tissue (by surgery or injury) may allow antibodies (IgG or IgM) to be formed, which, with complement, could cause destruction of these tissues, resulting in blindness, allergic encephalitis, or sterility.

In some cases, cross-reacting antibodies may cause destruction of heart or kidney tissues. It is believed that antibodies (IgG and IgM) formed against group A, β-hemolytic streptococci may also bind with and destroy similar proteins found in the heart and kidney. Another theory is that the streptococcal organisms are deposited in heart tissues or glomeruli of the kidney. When the immune complex (strep antigen + IgG + C') is formed, some heart or kidney cells might also by lysed (bystander lysis). This would explain the progressive tissue damage that occurs during recurrent streptococcal sore throat infections with rheumatic fever or glomerulonephritis.

Serum sickness is probably also a cross-reacting antibody immune reaction in which the antibodies formed to globular proteins in horse serum (used for antitoxin treatments) may also bind with similar proteins in the patient's serum. The formation of these immune complexes (antigen + antibody + complement) causes the symptoms of fever, rash, kidney malfunction, and joint lesions of serum sickness.

It is also believed that certain drugs and viruses may alter the antigens on host cells, thus inducing the formation of autoantibodies or sensitized T cells to react against these altered tissue cells. This may be the underlying basis of multiple sclerosis, kuru, Hashimoto's thyroiditis, rheumatoid arthritis, systemic lupus erythematosus (SLE), and other autoimmune diseases.

Cell-mediated Hypersensitivity   The delayed hypersensitivity of type IV is characterized by sensitized T cells that secrete lymphokines in the absence of antibodies. As an example, when antigens enter and bind with tissue cells (as in tuberculosis), they may be phagocytized by macrophages, then the antigens sensitize T-cell lymphocytes. When these primed T cells are subsequently exposed to the antigen complex, they secrete a group of chemicals called lymphokines. The lymphokines then destroy the antigen directly, attract additional lymphocytes and macrophages to the area, and increase phagocytic activity. Finally, the inflamed area is walled off by scar tissue, and the tubercule of tuberculosis is formed. The action of T cells, lymphokines, and macrophages causes the localized reaction seen in tuberculosis and fungal skin tests.

The beginning of the reaction may be seen after a few hours, and the inflammation, fever, redness, and swelling remain for several days. A similar reaction occurs in contact dermatitis (poison oak and poison ivy).

The rejection of transplanted tissues containing foreign histological (tissue) antigens appears to occur in a similar manner, except that the lymphokines as well as antibodies cause the rejection of the transplant.

Antigen–Antibody Reactions and Serological Tests

By means of various clinical and research experiments it has become possible to identify the presence of various antibodies to specific antigens.

The antigens may be living microorganisms, or parts of bacteria such as flagella, capsules, or toxins. The study of antigen–antibody reactions is called *serology*. Serologic techniques are used to type blood for blood banks and transfusions, to diagnose diseases, to identify microorganisms, to type tissue for transplantation, and to detect allergy or hypersensitivity. The most common *in vitro* (in the laboratory) serologic tests are *agglutination, precipitin, complement fixation and lysis, fluorescent antibody technique, radioimmunoassay, and enzyme-immuno assays.* Sometimes it is necessary to use *opsonization, capsular swelling,* or *immobilization* to detect specific antibodies (see Fig. 11-8).

These tests are all performed in the artificial environment of the laboratory, using the patient's serum to determine if the patient has antibodies to certain antigens. The presence of specific antibodies in the patient's serum would indicate that the patient has the disease, is immune to the disease, or is allergic to the antigen. Other tests are performed *in vivo* (in living animal), such as the skin tests, in which the antigens are injected into the skin (subcutaneously) to detect the presence of antibodies. Reddening at the site of the injection would indicate that the patient either has the disease or is immune or allergic to it. Each of these serological tests is summarized in Table 11-3 and a description of them follows.

Agglutination The agglutination test is used to detect the presence and amount of humoral (serum) antibodies to particulate antigens such as those on red blood cells or bacteria. As the word suggests, particulate antigens are the antigenic sites on particles, such as cells or latex particles.

The agglutination technique is used in the Venereal Disease Research Laboratory (VDRL) and rapid plasma reagin (RPR) tests for syphilis; the Widal test for typhoid fever; the Weil–Felix test for rickettsial diseases; and a test for pregnancy. It also has many other applications.

Hemagglutination often occurs when viruses agglutinate red blood cells normally. Antibodies to these viruses would inhibit the hemagglutination reaction and could be used to positively identify the virus. This adaptation of the agglutination technique is called *hemagglutination inhibition,* and is frequently used to identify influenza viruses.

Fig. 11-8. Precipitin ring test. (*A*) A line of precipitation forms where the antigen and antiserum meet. (Volk WA, Wheeler MF: Basic Microbiology, 3rd ed. Philadelphia, JB Lippincott, 1973) (*B*) Wells 1 through 6 contain different antigenic fractions of *Yersinia pestis*. (Courtesy of Dr. Tornebene, Colorado State University, Fort Collins, Colorado)

Precipitin   In the precipitin test, the patient's serum is used to demonstrate antibodies to soluble proteins or polysaccharide antigens, such as exotoxins or serum proteins. The antigens and antibodies are suspended in agar to allow diffusion to take place, so that the correct concentration of the antigen and antibody is reached. At this point (the zone of optimal proportions) a precipitate is formed and may be seen as a white line in the agar (Fig. 11-8). This would indicate that the patient has antibodies to that specific antigen. The precipitin test is useful in detecting antibodies to the exotoxins of tetanus, diphtheria, and scarlet fever. It is also used to identify various serum proteins in blood. An interesting application is in the criminology laboratory, when it is often important to know whether a particular blood stain is from animal or human blood. Here the serum proteins are extracted and identified by the antibodies that bind specifically with them.

Other precipitation-type tests (*i.e.*, immunoelectrophoresis) are performed by separating the proteins in human serum (electrophoresis), adding known antibodies, and observing the precipitin lines (Fig. 11-9). This powerful test is often used to determine complement and antibody deficiencies in individuals.

(*Text continues on p. 204*)

Table 11-3 Serological Tests to Detect Antibodies

Reaction In vitro	Reagents			Results	
	Antigen	*Antibody*	*Other*	*+*	*−*
Agglutination	Red blood cells or bacteria	Patient's serum		Clumping	No clumping
Precipitin	Toxins, hormones, proteins	Patient's serum	Agar or solution	Precipitate	No precipitate
Lysis by Complement	Cells, bacteria	Patient's serum	Complement	Lysis	No lysis
Complement Fixation	Viruses, Toxins Foreign proteins	Patient's serum	Complement	C Fixation	No C fixation
				No free C	Free C
Add indicator system	Sheep red blood (SRB) cells	Antisheep red blood cell antiserum		No lysis of SRB cells	Lysis of SRB cells by C

Table 11-3 Serological Tests to Detect Antibodies *(continued)*

Reaction *In vitro*	Reagents			Results	
	Antigen	*Antibody*	*Other*	+	−
Fluorescent Antibody Technique	Pathogen	Patient's serum	Fluorescein	Fluorescent pathogen	No fluorescence
Opsonization	Bacteria	Patient's serum	Phagocytes	More bacteria in phagocytes	Fewer bacteria in phagocytes
Capsular Swelling (Quellung Reaction)	Encapsulated bacteria	Patient's serum		Capsule swells	No swelling
Immobilization	Motile bacteria	Patient's serum		No motility	Motility
Radio-immunoassay	Patient's serum	Rabbit antiserum	Radioactive antigen	Low radioactivity	High radioactivity
Enzyme-linked assay	Test microbe	Patient's serum	Enzyme linked antibody + Substrate	Color change	No color change

Fig. 11-9. Immunoelectrophoresis: whole human serum was placed in the well (*circle*) and subjected to electrophoresis. After 2 hours, the electric current was turned off and anti-whole human serum was placed in a trough along the length of the slide. The precipitin lines were formed where the antibodies and the antigens (separated components of whole human serum) diffused together in optimal proportions. (Volk WA, et al: Essentials of Medical Microbiology. Philadelphia, JB Lippincott, 1986)

Lysis by Complement   When the IgG and IgM antibodies are bound to antigens, the antibodies become activated and react with complement (C). This reaction in turn activates the complement. If the antigens are on cells such as red blood cells, or on pathogens such as *Vibrio cholerae*, the activated complement will lyse (destroy) the cells. An application of this reaction is in the indicator system in the complement fixation test, to be described shortly. Another use is to identify the presence of specific antibodies to a pathogen in a patient's serum, as in cholera.

Complement Fixation   Complement is bound (fixed) when antigens bind with antibodies, even if the antigens are not on a red blood cell or bacterial cell. Antigens, such as viruses or toxins, cause fixation (or binding) of complement when the specific antibodies to them are present (reaction I). Because this reaction cannot be detected visually, sheep red blood cells and antisheep red blood cell antibodies (the indicator system) are added to the serum (reaction II). If all the complement is bound in reaction I there is no unbound or free complement present to lyse the sheep red blood cells in reaction II; thus, the test results are positive because the specific antibodies to the virus or toxin were present in the patient's serum. If there were no antibodies present (if the patient were not immune) to the virus or toxin, there would be *no* antigen–antibody–complement binding in reaction I, so there would be free complement present to bind and lyse the sheep red blood cells in reaction II; therefore, the test results would be negative.

This complex reaction is used to identify certain virus infections such as smallpox, influenza, and poliomyelitis.

Fluorescent Antibody Technique   A fluorescent dye (called FITC), which is easily seen as a green glow under the ultraviolet microscope, can be attached to the antibodies from the patient's serum, which adhere to the pathogen. The pathogen might be *Treponema pallidum* (syphilis) or *Streptococcus pyogenes* ("strep" sore throat). Thus, the pathogen is beautifully outlined by the fluorescent dye when it is examined with the ultraviolet microscope if the patient's serum contains the specific antibodies for those pathogens. More often, the fluorescent dye is attached to rabbit antibodies to human gamma

Fig. 11-10. *Streptococcus pyogenes* stained with fluorescent antibody (original magnification × 200). (Volk WA, Wheeler MF: Basic Microbiology, 3rd ed. Philadelphia, JB Lippincott, 1973)

globulin, which will then outline the pathogen on the slide if the patient's gamma globulin contains antibodies to that pathogen. This test is often used for positive identification of β-hemolytic, group A *Streptococcus pyogenes* and many other pathogens (Fig. 11-10).

Radioimmunoassay   Radioimmunoassay (RIA) is a sensitive, versatile technique, using radioactively labeled antigen or antibody. It is frequently used to determine small amounts of drugs, hormones, or antigens, such as hepatitis B antigen in blood donor serum.

Enzyme-linked Immunosorbent Assays (ELISA)   These enzyme-linked assays (ELA) are sensitive techniques that use an enzyme–antibody–antigen combination adsorbed onto the sides of a test well. If the patient has antibodies or antigens for the disease agent, the linkage is formed; when the substrate for the enzyme is added a color change develops, which indicates a positive test result. If the patient does not have the serum antigen or the antibody sought, the enzyme is not linked and no color change is seen. These techniques are commonly used to test for AIDS and other diseases.

Opsonization   The opsonization test is based on the fact that phagocytes can engulf more bacteria if the specific antibodies for those bacteria are present. A control slide with bacteria and phagocytes is observed, and the number of bacteria inside each phagocyte is counted. This number is compared with the number of bacteria engulfed by phagocytes in the presence of serum from a patient with antibodies to the bacteria. This test is seldom used in a clinical laboratory; its value is as a confirming test for bacterial diseases.

Capsular Swelling (Quellung Reaction)   When serum containing antibodies to encapsulated bacteria is added to those bacteria and observed microscopically, the capsule appears to swell. The swelling is frequently referred to as the Quellung reaction.

Various capsular types of *Streptococcus pneumoniae* and other encapsulated bacteria can be identified by this test.

Immobilization If the pathogen is motile (flagellated), the immobilization test can be used. When a patient's serum is added to motile bacteria, the bacteria will be immobilized if specific antibodies to the bacterial flagella are present. Identification of cholera, salmonella, and shigella infections is more reliable using this technique; however, it is rarely used in clinical laboratories because other tests are more readily available.

Toxin Neutralization The neutralization of toxins usually is demonstrated by *in vivo* tests. These demonstrate that specific antitoxins (antibodies) neutralize the effect of a toxin.

    The animal test for diphtheria. A mouse injected with the toxin of diphtheria will die. But if the toxin is mixed with the serum of a patient who is immune to diphtheria and the combined toxin and serum is injected into a mouse, the mouse will live.

    The Schick test. Diphtheria toxin is injected under the skin (subcutaneously). The site will become reddened if the person is susceptible to diphtheria, but there will be no redness if the person is immune, because antibodies are present.

    The Dick test. The scarlet fever exotoxin is injected subcutaneously; redness will occur at the site in the susceptible person but not in one who is immune.

    The Schultz-Charlton test. The rash of scarlet fever can be positively identified by means of the Schultz-Charlton test. The antitoxin (antibodies) to the scarlet fever toxin are injected into an area of rash. If the rash clears the patient has scarlet fever, but if it does not clear the rash is due to other causes.

    Serologic reactions can provide information that is useful in the diagnosis of many infectious diseases. Most of them are extremely valuable because they can be performed quickly and easily with a high degree of specificity and sensitivity. However, some of the newer techniques may not be widely used because they are still expensive.

Problems and Questions

1. What is the immune response? Is it always a protective mechanism?
2. What types of substances are effective antigens?
3. Where in the body are antibodies formed?
4. When are antibodies formed?
5. What is the anamnestic response?
6. What is the main difference between active and passive acquired immunity?
7. Which diseases do not produce a long-lasting immunity?
8. How are vaccines prepared?
9. What is congenital immunity?

10. How are antibodies transferred in passive immunity?
11. List five classes of immunoglobulins. Where are each of these found?
12. What is the main difference between the two types of hypersensitivity ?
13. What is an allergen? Give some examples.
14. Give an example of the delayed hypersensitivity reaction.
15. Describe an example of an autoimmune disease.
16. List seven *in vitro* antigen–antibody reactions and when they are used.
17. List four *in vivo* antigen–antibody tests and when they are used.

Chapter 12

Specimen Collection, Processing, and Testing

Objectives

After studying this chapter, you should be able to
1. Discuss the role of the health worker in the collection of specimens
2. List the types of specimens that usually must be taken from patients
3. Discuss the general precautions that must be observed during the collection and handling of specimens
4. Describe the proper procedure for drawing a blood sample
5. Describe the various procedures for obtaining urine samples
6. Discuss the use of swabs in obtaining specimens
7. Understand the difference between a throat swab and a sputum sample
8. Describe how specimens should be prepared for mailing
9. Discuss the importance of quality in a microbiology laboratory

It would not be feasible in a book of this size to give a complete discussion of collection, handling, and processing of specimens. Only a few important concepts are discussed here.*

Role of Health Care Personnel

Extreme care must be taken by those involved in the collection, handling, and processing of specimens to be examined for the presence of microorganisms. The

---

*For more detailed information, refer to *Manual of Clinical Microbiology*, 3rd ed, Chap 6, American Society for Microbiology, Washington, D.C. 1980; or to *Collection, Handling, and Shipment of Microbiological Specimens*, U.S. Department of Public Health, Publication #976, Washington, D.C., 1973.

microbiological analysis can be only as reliable as the quality of the specimen allows. When specimens are improperly collected and handled, (1) the causative micro-organisms may not be found or may be destroyed, (2) overgrowth by normal flora may mask the pathogen, and (3) contaminants may interfere with the identification of the pathogens.

A close working relationship among the members of the health care team is essential for the proper identification of pathogens. When the attending physician recognizes the clinical symptoms of a possible infectious disease, he requests that specific specimens be taken and tests performed. The clinical microbiologist who will perform the laboratory microbial analysis must provide adequate collection materials and instructions for their proper use. The doctor, nurse, medical technologist, or other qualified health care worker must perform the collection procedure properly, and then the specimen must be transported quickly to the laboratory where it will be cultured, stained, analyzed, and identified. Laboratory findings must then be conveyed to the attending physician as quickly as possible to aid him in arriving at a prompt diagnosis and treatment of the disease.

Proper Collection of Specimens

When collecting specimens, these general procedures should be followed:

1. All specimens should be collected in a sterile manner. This requires that they be put into a sterile container to prevent contamination by normal flora and airborne organisms.
2. The material should be collected from the site where the suspected or-ganism is most likely to be found and where the least contamination is likely to occur.
3. Specimens should be obtained before antibotic therapy has begun. If this is not possible, the laboratory should be informed of which antibiotic is being used.
4. The acute stage of the disease is the appropriate time for the collection of most specimens. Some viruses, however, are more easily isolated during the onset stage of the disease.
5. Specimen collection should be performed with care and tact to avoid harming the patient, causing discomfort, or causing undue embarrass-ment. If the specimen, such as sputum or urine, is to be collected by the patient, clear and detailed instructions should be given.
6. A sufficient quantity of the specimen should be obtained to allow enough for all diagnostic tests that need to be performed. The amount should be indicated by the physician or laboratory microbiologist.
7. Specimens should be protected from heat and cold, and promptly deliv-ered to the laboratory so the results of the analysis will be a valid representation of the organisms present at the time of collection. If deliv-ery is delayed, some delicate pathogens will die. Anaerobes will die when

exposed to the air. Also, the normal flora may overgrow the pathogens, which will inhibit or kill them. Delay of delivery considerably decreases the chances of isolating the pathogen.

8. Dangerous specimens must be handled with even greater care to avoid contamination of the ward messenger, patients, nurses, and other hospital personnel. Such dangerous specimens are usually placed in a sealed plastic bag for immediate transport to the laboratory.

9. All specimen containers must be cleaned, sterilized, and properly stored to avoid contamination of the specimen by microbes and harmful chemicals from the container.

10. After the specimen is collected, the container must be properly labeled and accompanied by the appropriate laboratory instructions written on the requisition. The label must identify the patient and the source of the specimen (*e.g.*, throat, wound). The requisition must give the date, time of collection, doctor's name and address, and laboratory tests requested. The laboratory also should be given any additional clinical information that will aid in performing the appropriate analyses.

11. Specimens should be collected and delivered to the laboratory as early in the day as possible to allow the technicians time to process the material, especially if the hospital or clinic does not have 24-hour laboratory service.

Types of Specimens Usually Required

Special techniques in collection and handling are required to obtain specific types of specimens.

Blood Normally, the blood is sterile. Any organisms found in the blood indicate a disease condition. Therefore, extreme care must be taken to use sterile technique for drawing the blood into a sterile blood-collecting bottle containing an anticoagulant.* After locating a suitable vein, disinfect the skin with 70% ethyl alcohol, then 2% tincture of iodine, allowing it to dry. Apply a tourniquet and withdraw 10 ml to 20 ml of blood with a 21-gauge needle into a sterile container, such as the Vacutainer, containing an anticoagulant. The blood sample should be transported promptly to the laboratory and cultured in a specially prepared growth medium. If necessary, the blood sample may be refrigerated up to 2 hours before it is cultured.

In many infectious diseases, bacteremia (bacterial blood infection) may be found during certain stages. In this circumstance at least three blood samples should be taken an hour apart. These diseases include bacterial meningitis, typhoid fever and other salmonella infections, pneumococcal pneumonia, urinary infections, endocarditis, brucellosis, tularemia, plague, anthrax, syphilis, and wound infections by

*Many satisfactory blood collecting systems are available from suppliers such as Becton, Dickinson and Company, Rutherford, NJ; Hyland Laboratories, Costa Mesa, CA; Difco Laboratories, Detroit, MI; BBL-Bioquest, Cockeysville, MD; and others.

β-hemolytic streptococci, staphylococci, and bacteroids. A severe septicemia caused by gram-negative rods is frequently found in patients following gastrointestinal and urological surgery.

Urine   Urine, like blood, is normally sterile; however, it is usually contaminated by the normal flora of the urethra during urination. The contamination can be reduced by collecting a midstream "clean-catch" urine specimen. The area around the urethra is cleansed by washing with soap and rinsing with water. With the glans penis or labia folds separated, the urethra is flushed with the first portion of urine; then the middle portion of the urine is caught in a sterile container. In some circumstances the physician may prefer to collect a catheterized specimen or to use the suprapubic needle aspiration technique to obtain a sterile sample of urine.

A urinary tract infection is indicated if the number of bacteria in a midstream clean-catch urine specimen exceeds 100,000 organisms per milliliter (org/ml), as normal urine may contain less than 1000 org/ml.

Urine specimens must be processed within an hour or refrigerated at 4°C (39.2°F) to prevent continued bacterial growth until they can be analyzed (within 5 hours).

Cerebrospinal Fluid   Spinal fluid specimens must be collected into a sterile tube by a "spinal tap" under surgically aseptic conditions. This difficult procedure should be performed by a physician. Meningitis and meningoencephalitis can be caused by a variety of microbes including bacteria, fungi, protozoa, and viruses. Because the meningococci are susceptible to cold temperatures, the specimen must be cultured immediately and not refrigerated. Specimens to be further examined for viruses may be kept frozen at −20°C (−4°F).

Sputum   Sputum may be collected by allowing the patient to spit coughed-up mucus into a sterile wide-mouthed bottle with a lid, warning the patient not to contaminate the sputum with saliva from the oral cavity. If proper mouth hygiene is maintained the sputum may not be severely contaminated with oral microorganisms. If tuberculosis is suspected, extreme care in handling the specimen should be excercised because one could easily be infected with the agent. Sputum specimens usually may be refrigerated for several hours without loss of the pathogens.

However, the physician may wish to obtain a better specimen by bronchial aspiration through a bronchoscope or by inserting a needle into the trachea below the glottis. Needle biospy of the lungs may be necessary for diagnosis of *Pneumocystis carinii* (in AIDS) and for mycobacterial, fungal, and viral pathogens.

Mucous Membrane Swabs   Sterile polyester swabs are used to take specimens of exudates and secretions of the throat, nose, ear, eye, urogenital openings, rectum, wounds, operative sites, and ulcerations. Cotton swabs are no longer used because the fatty acids in the cotton inhibit the growth of some microorganisms. Handy, sterile, disposable collection units can be obtained from many supply houses. Each unit contains a sterile polyester swab in transport medium in a sterile tube. With this setup the organisms are kept alive and protected during transportation to the laboratory.

Genital swabs should be inoculated immediately into Thayer-Martin chocolate agar plates and incubated in a CO_2 (carbon dioxide) environment; or they should be inoculated into a Transgrow bottle (which contains carbon dioxide) while the bottle is held in an upright position to prevent the loss of the CO_2. These cultures should be incubated at 35°C (95°F) overnight; then the Transgrow bottles can be shipped to the public health diagnostic facility for positive identification of gonococci.

Most swabs in moist collection units may be refrigerated 2 to 3 hours before culturing without loss of the pathogens.

Shipping Specimens

Occasionally, a specimen must be sent to a laboratory in another city for identification. Such specimens should be shipped by the fastest means available. If they are sent by mail, viral cultures must be quick-frozen and shipped in dry ice. Pathogenic bacteria must be so labeled on the outside of the package. They should be cultured on solid agar in a tube, capped, with tape around the cap. The glass tube should be wrapped in cotton and placed in a metal can and then in a cardboard mailing box. These specimens should be sent by first-class mail.

Identification and Drug Sensitivity of Pathogens

After the pathogen from a specimen has been isolated, the main remaining task is to identify the organism and determine its sensitivity to antibiotic treatment.

By performing a few simple tests on a pure culture of a pathogen, the family to which the organism belongs can, at least, be determined. The Gram stain will enable the laboratory worker to describe the Gram reaction (positive or negative); morphology (cocci, bacilli, or spirilla); grouping (pairs, chains, tetrad, or cluster); and whether or not it produces spores. By observing a culture on solid agar, one can describe the shape, consistency, size, and color of the colony as well as whether it is an anaerobe or an aerobe. The use of certain selective and differential media, such as EMB (eosin methylene blue), and a few simple biochemical tests, such as those using catalase or oxidase, will substantially help determine the genus and species of the organisms. The final determination may be made by serotyping, if necessary.

Many laboratories make use of the new multiple-test systems available from Analytab Products, Inc., Roche Diagnostics, BBL-Bioquest, and many others. Each system has certain advantages and disadvantages, but, in general, they are faster, more comprehensive, and easier to use than the conventional methods. Care should be taken to evaluate each before one is adopted as the accepted analysis. Many of these identification systems are read and evaluated by computers, greatly increasing the speed and accuracy of the tests.

Fig. 12-1. An antibiotic disk dispenser. (Photograph courtesy Difco Laboratories, Detroit, Michigan)

Antibiotic Sensitivity

One of the most helpful tests for the physician is the disk antibiotic-sensitivity method described by Kirby and Bauer. In this test the pure culture of the organism in tryptose phosphate broth is streaked evenly for complete coverage on a Mueller–Hinton agar plate. The disks that have been permeated with various antibiotics are then placed on the agar plate and the plate is incubated at 37°C (98.6°F) under the proper conditions (Figs. 12-1 and 12-2).

For gram-positive bacteria, disks of tetracycline, penicillin, ampicillin, streptomycin, erythromycin, lincomycin, kanamycin, neomycin, or methicillin might be used. For gram-negative bacteria, disks of tetracycline, ampicillin, streptomycin, kanamycin, neomycin, nitrofurantoin, or colistin, as well as many other new antibiotics, might be used. Within 24 hours the diameter of the zones of inhibition around each disk should be measured in millimeters. These measurements must then be compared with the size of zone on a Kirby–Bauer table, which indicates sensitivity or resistance of the organism.

Fig. 12-2. Paper disks impregnated with various antibiotics are dropped onto the surface of inoculated plates. The antibiotic diffuses into the medium, inhibiting the growth of organisms sensitive to the antibiotic. (Volk WA, Wheeler MF: Basic Microbiology, 3rd ed. Philadelphia, JB Lippincott, 1973)

Quality Control

A quality control program is necessary in any laboratory to monitor the reliability and the quality of the work performed there. In the microbiology laboratory all media, reagents, and staining solutions should be evaluated frequently for effectiveness. Also, all equipment should be maintained and monitored for performance. Refrigerators, freezers, incubators, and water baths should be checked for accuracy of temperature control. By constant surveillance and frequent checking, the efficiency and reliability of the laboratory work can be maintained so that other members of the hospital team have confidence in the information supplied to them from the laboratory.

Problems and Questions

1. How can you be hurt by collecting and handling laboratory specimens?
2. In what ways can the specimen be contaminated?
3. Why should the nurse not locate the vein after the skin has been disinfected, when she is taking a blood specimen?
4. Which pathogens might be found in a blood sample?
5. How does one collect a "midstream clean-catch" urine specimen?

6. What is the difference between a sputum sample and a saliva sample?
7. What precautions must be taken when inoculating a Trans-grow bottle with a vaginal swab?
8. How would you prepare a pathogenic specimen for shipping to a distant laboratory?
9. How would you determine which antibiotic would be most effective against a certain pathogen?
10. How could you determine which pathogen you had isolated from a throat culture?

Chapter 13

Major Diseases of the Body Systems

Objectives

After studying this chapter you should be able to
1. Name the major organs that might become infected in each body system
2. List the most common normal microbial flora usually found in the various body systems
3. Outline the causative agent, reservoir, mode of transmission, pathogenesis, treatment and control measures for the major diseases of each system
4. For each body system, list some examples of diseases that are caused by bacteria; by viruses; by fungi; by protozoa

New Words to Pronounce and Understand

Choleragin (kal'-er-ah-gin). The exotoxin produced by *Vibrio cholerae*, that causes cholera

Cystitis (sis-ti'-tis). An infection of the urinary bladder

Cytotoxins (sigh-tow-tok'-sins). Toxic substances that injure certain cells

Dermatophytes (der-mah'-toe-fites). Fungi capable of growing on the skin surface, causing ringworm or tinea diseases

Enterotoxin (en'-ter-oh-tok'-sin). An exotoxin causing damage to intestinal cells, producing diarrhea

Exudate (eks'-oo-'date). A viscous secretion containing blood cells and cellular debris from site of inflammation

Gingivitis (gin-je-vi'-tis). An inflammation of the gingiva (gums)

Immunoglobulin (im'-you-no-glob'-you-lyn). The globulin proteins of the serum and other body secretions, including the humoral antibodies

Immunosuppression (im'-you-no-sue-presh'-un). Depression of the immune response

Malaise (mal-az'). A general feeling of illness and discomfort

Necrotoxin (neck'-row-tox'-sin). An exotoxin that destroys certain cells

Neurotoxin (new'-row-tox'-sin). An exotoxin that damages nerve tissue and interferes with nerve impulses

Oncogenic (on'-ko-jin'-ick). Capable of producing tumors

Prophylactic agent (pro'-fi-lack'-tick). An agent to ward off disease

Sebum (see'-bum). The secretion of the sebaceous (oil) glands of the skin

Tetanospasmin (tet'-ah-no-spaz'-min). The neurotoxic exotoxin produced by *Clostridium tetani,* that causes tetanus

Urethritis (you'-re-thri'-tis). An inflammation of the urethra of the urinary system

In the previous chapters you have studied the disease process, how pathogens cause disease, modes of transmission, how the body attempts to defend itself, and the chemotherapeutic agents and vaccines used to cure and prevent certain diseases. In this chapter the major infectious diseases of skin and wounds, eyes, ears, oral cavity, respiratory system, gastrointestinal tract, urogenital areas, cardiovascular and nervous systems will be discussed. Many of these infections involve several body systems, or in other types of infection, the pathogen may move from one area to another. The source of the disease-causing microbe may be opportunistic normal flora, but usually the causative agent is transmitted to the recipient from a reservoir of infection (see Chap. 7).

The early signs and symptoms of many diseases are influenza-like; usually the patient develops slight fever, headache, fatigue, malaise, gastrointestinal upset, or sneezing and coughing. Only specific characteristic signs and symptoms of the major diseases are mentioned here.

Diseases of the Skin

Normal Skin

As seen in Figure 13-1 the structure of skin is not simple. Normal healthy, intact skin serves as a formidable protective barrier for the underlying tissues. Vast numbers of microbes survive on and within the epidermal layers, in pores, and in hair follicles (see Table 5-1). Their growth is controlled by the (1) amount of moisture present, (2) pH, (3) temperature, (4) salinity of perspiration, (5) chemical wastes such as urea and fatty acids, and (6) other microbes present which secrete fatty acids and antimicrobic substances. Proper hygienic cleanliness and washing serves to flush away

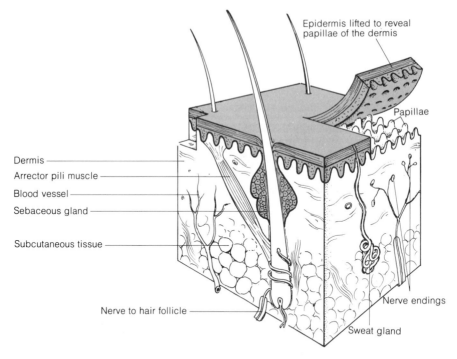

Fig. 13-1. Cross section of the skin. (Lindberg JB, Hunter ML, Kruszewski AZ: Introduction to Person-Centered Nursing. Philadelphia, JB Lippincott, 1983)

dead epithelial cells, many transient and resident microbes, and the odorous organic materials present in perspiration, sebum, and microbial secretions.

Once the skin barrier is broken (wounds, surgery, or burns) the opportunists may infect the underlying tissues, invade capillaries and lymph, and be carried by phagocytes to many regions of the body.

Opportunistic Normal Flora

Most microbes that colonize the skin are harmless, but several genera of aerobes and anaerobes may cause infections when the ecological balance of the skin environment changes chemically, physically, or microbiologically (Fig. 13-2).

Major Microbial Opportunists

Gram-positive cocci: Staphylococcus epidermidis, Staphylococcus aureus, Micrococcus species, and *Streptococcus* species are facultative anaerobes that may invade through breaks in skin to cause local, deep, or systemic infections. Many of them produce invasive enzymes and damaging exotoxins capable of causing serious diseases, such as the toxic shock syndrome caused by *S. aureus*.

Gram-positive bacilli: These pleomorphic rods, frequently referred to as diphtheroids, include *Corynebacterium, Brevibacterium,* and *Propionibacterium* species, which frequently cause hair follicle and sweat gland infections.

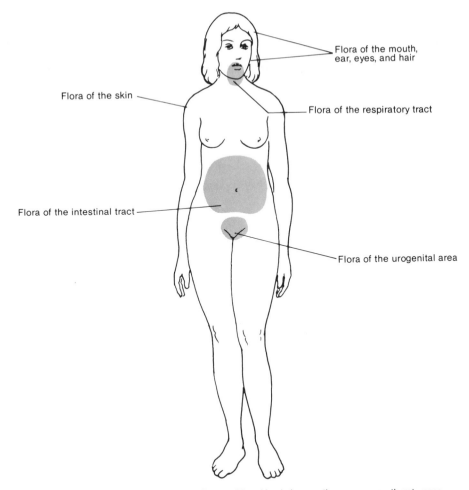

Fig. 13-2. Areas where most normal flora reside: skin, hair, mouth, ears, eyes, throat, nose, intestinal tract, and urogenital tract.

Gram-negative bacilli: In moist areas, armpits, perineum, and between toes, *Pseudomonas* and some enteric rods may be found. Microbes can grow profusely on the organic compounds in perspiration and sebum, producing malodorous fatty acids. Many deodorants contain antimicrobial agents that inhibit the growth of these bacteria.

Viral Infections of the Skin

Chickenpox, Varicella, Shingles

Characteristics Chickenpox is a respiratory infection and generalized viremia with local vesicular lesions on the skin of the face, thorax, and back that become encrusted.

Vesicles also form in mucous membranes. Usually a mild,

self-limiting disease, but can be severely damaging to fetus in pregnancy.

Reye's syndrome may follow clinical chickenpox if aspirin is given to children under 16 years of age.

Secondary bacterial infections (pneumonia, otitis media, bacteremia) frequently occur.

Shingles is a reactivation of varicella provirus in adults; inflammation of sensory ganglia of cutaneous sensory nerves producing rash and pain.

Pathogens	Varicella–zoster virus or herpes zoster virus.
Reservoir	Humans.
Transmission	Inhalation of virus, via contaminated droplets, or direct contact with vesicles, or contaminated articles.
Incubation period	15–18 days.
Epidemiology	Usually occurs in winter and early spring. Two million cases each year are estimated. Permanent immunity usually follows childhood disease.
Control	Isolation for 1 week after eruption of vesicles.
Usual treatment	No vaccine yet available. Antiviral chemotherapy (acyclovir or vidarabine) may be effective. Antibiotics to prevent secondary bacterial infections.

Measles, Rubeola

Characteristics	Upper respiratory infection, high fever, coughing, light sensitivity, Koplik's spots in mouth, maculopapular skin rash. Complications include bronchitis, pneumonia, otitis media. Autoimmune subacute sclerosing panencephalitis (SSPE) may follow a latent period.
Pathogen	Measles virus; a paramyxovirus.
Reservoir	Humans.
Transmission	Inhalation of droplets during direct contact with children.
Incubation period	8–13 days.
Epidemiology	In 1986, 6273 cases reported in the United States to CDC. Measles cases dropped 99% in the United States and Canada following immunization programs.

Control	Immunization, isolation for 4 days after rash eruption.
Usual treatment	Bed rest, fluids, preventive nursing care to prevent complications and secondary infections. Antiviral chemotherapy and antibiotics to prevent bacterial infections may be helpful.

German Measles, Rubella

Characteristics	Rash, flat pink spots spreading from face, with tender lymph nodes, low-grade fever. A milder disease than rubeola; may be subclinical. During first trimester of pregnancy may cause congenital rubella syndrome in fetus. Encephalitis is rare complication.
Pathogen	Rubella virus; a togavirus (Fig. 13-3).
Reservoir	Humans.
Transmission	Inhalation of droplets during direct contact with infected individuals; occasionally via contaminated articles.
Incubation period	14–21 days.
Epidemiology	In 1986, 502 cases in United Stated reported to CDC. Endemic worldwide, fewer epidemics in immunized communities.
Control	Immunization with live, attenuated rubella virus vaccine, especially for young women before pregnancy, and serological testing for immunity. Isolation for 7 days after onset of rash.

Fig. 13-3. Development of rubella virus in the surface and cytoplasmic membranes of infected cell cultures. (*A*) Viral particles budding from cytoplasmic membranes into vacuoles and into the cytoplasm. Numerous mature virions are present within vacuoles (original magnification × 60,000). (*B*) Viral particles budding from the surface of an infected cell (original magnification × 60,000). (Oshiro LS et al: J Gen Virol 5:205)

| Usual treatment | No chemotherapy available. |

Warts, Condyloma Acuminata

Characteristics	Fibrous superficial papules of the skin (see Fig. 13-19), and mucous membranes including genitalia.
Pathogen	Human papillomavirus, of papovavirus group.
Reservoir	Humans.
Transmission	Direct contact and sexual intercourse, fomites; spread by scratching.
Incubation period	1–20 months.
Epidemiology	Worldwide occurrence.
Control	Destroyed by freezing, acids, electrosurgery, or laser therapy.
Usual treatment	Podophyllum chemotherapy for persistent epidermal warts or idoxuridine for venereal warts. Interferon may prove to be effective for genital and laryngeal warts.

Bacterial Infections of the Skin

Impetigo, Pyoderma

| Characteristics | Skin lesions forming pustules, then amber crusts (Fig. 13-4), itching, peeling of skin. |
| Pathogens | *Staphylococcus aureus* or *Streptococcus pyogenes,* or both. Identified by culture and serologic techniques. |

Fig. 13-4. Impetigo. (Dobson RL, Abele DC: The Practice of Dermatology. Philadelphia, Harper & Row, 1985)

Pathogenicity	Spread through skin by producing hyaluronidase. Staphylococcal toxins cause scalded skin syndrome and peeling.
Reservoir	Humans.
Transmission	By direct contact, through broken skin, scratching.
Incubation period	4–10 days.
Control	Disinfectant skin lotions.
Usual treatment	Topical disinfectants and antibiotics, such as penicillin, erythromycin.

Scarlet Fever, Scarlatina, Erysipelas

Characteristics	Skin rash.
Pathogen	*Streptococcus pyogenes* (see Fig.11-10) β-hemolytic, group A, gram-positive, cocci that form chains. Identified by culture and serologic techniques.
Pathogenicity	Erythrogenic toxins; secondary complication of "strep throat" (pharyngitis) in susceptible individuals.
Reservoir	Humans.
Transmission	Person-to-person, by secretions and close contact.
Incubation period	3–5 days.
Control	Isolation until after 24 hours of antibiotic therapy.
Usual treatment	Penicillin, erythromycin, cephalosporins.

Folliculitis, Hair Follicle Infections, Furuncles (Boils), Carbuncles

Characteristics	Hair follicle pustules, small or large.
Pathogens	*Staphylococcus aureus;* gram-positive cocci in clusters. *Pseudomonas aeruginosa;* gram-negative bacilli.
Reservoir	Humans, skin and contaminated hot pools.
Transmission	Direct contact, water or fomites, poor personal hygiene, skin abrasions, cuts, contaminated hot tubs and swimming pools. *Staphylococcus aureus* may become systemic and cause recurring boils and carbuncles.
Incubation period	Variable, usually 4–10 days.

Control	Good personal hygiene, properly treated hot tubs and pools.
Usual treatment	Topical bacitracin or polymyxin B for *S. aureus*; gentamicin or carbenicillin systemically for *Pseudomonas*.

Acne

Characteristics	Inflammatory pustules, cysts and papules, infections of sebaceous glands in hair follicles on face, chest, and back.
Pathogens	Interaction of *Propionibacterium acnes*, *Staphylococcus aureus*, and *Corynebacterium* spp.
Reservoir	Humans.
Transmission	Direct contact among susceptible individuals. Usually occurs during puberty because of hormonal changes.
Incubation period	Variable, usually 4–10 days.
Control	Cleanliness, good personal hygiene, sunshine.
Usual treatment	Locally applied benzoyl peroxide, salicylic acid, or sulfur. Systemic antibiotics such as tetracycline and minocycline (Minocin), or drug therapy with isotretinoin (Accutane) for severe cases.

Anthrax, Woolsorter's Disease

Characteristics	Cutaneous blackened lesions called eschars caused by necrotoxin. Pneumonia and/or systemic infection may develop.
Pathogen	*Bacillus anthracis*, gram-positive, aerobic, endospore-forming bacillus.
Pathogenesis	Endospore germinates, bacteria produces necrotic toxins.
Reservoir	Spores in soil and on hides and skins of infected animals.
Transmission	From animal hair, wool, and hides by (1) direct contact, endospores into skin abrasions; (2) inhalation of endospores; (3) ingestion of endospores.
Incubation period	3–5 days.
Epidemiology	No cases reported in United States in 1986.
Control	Avoid contact with infected animals and soils contaminated by spores from infected animals. Vaccination of animals and humans who work with animals and animal products.
Usual treatment	Penicillin, tetracycline.

Leprosy, Hansen's Disease

Characteristics	(1) Neural, tuberculoid form; lesions on skin and peripheral nerves, loss of sensation. (2) Cutaneous, lepromatous form; progressive disfiguring nodules in skin; invades throughout body.
Pathogen	*Mycobacterium leprae;* acid-fast bacillus, cultured only in armadillos, monkeys, and mouse footpads.
Reservoir	Humans, and perhaps infected armadillos.
Transmission	(1) Prolonged exposure through skin or mucous membranes; (2) via droplets to respiratory tract.
Epidemiology	254 cases in United States reported to CDC in 1986. Worldwide prevalence.
Control	Early detection and isolation until treatment is effective.
Usual treatment	Prolonged treatment with rifampin or dapsone and clofazimine.

Fungal Infections of the Skin

Many fungi cause skin lesions and may enter the body through the skin, such as *Sporothrix* and *Candida,* but the most common are the dermatophytes that cause ringworm or superficial fungal infections of the skin, hair, and nails. The cell-mediated immune responses to fungi result in inflammation and limitation of spread of the fungus.

Dermatomycosis, Tinea, Ringworm, Dermatophytosis

Characteristics	Fungal lesions on skin (tinea corporis), scalp (tinea capitis), groin (tinea cruris or "jock itch"), foot (tinea pedis or "athlete's foot"), and nails (tinea unguium).
Pathogens	Various species of *Microsporum, Epidermophyton,* and *Trichophyton;* filamentous fungi.
Reservoir	Humans, animals, and soil.
Transmission	Direct or indirect contact with fungal spores from lesions or fomites such as shower stalls, toilet articles, and athletic supporters. Invade through breaks in skin and moist areas; germinate into filamentous growths.
Incubation period	4–14 days.
Control	Keep susceptible areas clean and dry.

Usual treatment	Topical application of miconazole (Lotrimin), clotrimazole, and other antifungal agents. Oral griseofulvin for scalp and nail infections.

Burn and Wound Infections

When the skin barrier is broken by burns, wounds, and surgical procedures, many normal flora and environmental bacteria can invade to cause local and deep-tissue infections. They may also become systemic and produce exotoxins, causing severe damage to the individual.

Burns

Many patients die following severe burns because of loss of body fluids and the presence of toxic microbial invaders, including *Staphylococcus aureus*, *Streptococcus pyogenes*, *Pseudomonas aeruginosa*, and many fungi. These organisms usually grow aerobically in the burned area, and produce many exotoxins (cytotoxins, necrotoxins, and neurotoxins) and perhaps death to the patient.

Burn victims must be treated in an aseptic environment in which the health care personnel are gloved, gowned, and masked. The burns may be left open to the air to speed healing or covered with artificial skin or film to reduce contamination and loss of fluids. Some antimicrobial topical agents (silver sulfadiazine, for example) may be used to reduce the possibility of infections during the prolonged healing period.

Wound and Surgical Infections

Most gunshot, stab, puncture, bite, and abrasive wounds are contaminated during the wounding process. The microbes introduced are frequently anaerobes from dust and normal flora that grow rapidly deep within the wound; other facultative aerobes will flourish on the surface of the wound, secreting enzymes to invade the blood and lymph. Bacterial and fungal spores may also be introduced, causing local and deep-seated infections.

Any traumatic injury must be opened and thoroughly cleansed to remove debris and inhibit the growth of microbes; then it usually is covered lightly to prevent further contamination.

Staphylococcus (see Figs.1-8 and 1-9) and *Streptococcus* (see Fig.11-10) species are the most frequent bacteria that cause focal infections. They may invade by secreting hyaluronidase and other spreading factors to cause severe toxic systemic infections of many areas including brain, spinal cord, and bone. *Pseudomonas aeruginosa*, from soil and feces, is notorious for causing deep, antibiotic-resistant infections. This gram-negative bacillus produces protease enzymes that enable it to move through tissues and an exotoxin that inhibits protein synthesis. Antibiotic sensitivity tests are essential so that the appropriate antibiotic may be administered.

The anaerobic *Clostridium* species are of grave concern in puncture wounds. Endospores of *Clostridium tetani* (see Fig. 13-28) may be introduced from soil and fecal contamination. When these spores germinate into vegetative bacteria, neurotoxins are produced that cause involuntary muscle spasms and respiratory failure. The availability of vaccines and antitoxins has greatly reduced deaths from tetanus in developed countries.

Clostridium perfringens, the major causative agent of gas gangrene, is not only of concern in accidental wounds but in surgical sites as well. The contaminating spores germinate and the vegetative pathogens produce many invasive enzymes and exotoxins, resulting in necrotic areas with gas present.

Fungal infections, such as sporotrichosis, are caused by the introduction of soil fungi and spores that invade cutaneous and lymphatic tissues through wounds that are sometimes as small as a thorn prick. This slowly progressing disease is usually localized and self-limiting, but severe cases may be treated with amphotericin or potassium iodide.

Bites

Human, insect, and animal bites introduce normal oral flora organisms, sometimes pathogenic, into the wound. Because the organisms from human bites are adapted to humans, they are more likely to produce infections than those of animal sources. Every bite should be thoroughly cleansed, disinfected, and left open to the air to prevent microbial growth. Bite wounds should not be closed tightly with stitches and bandages because this procedure would encourage the growth of anaerobic bacteria.

Human bites: Severe infections may result from anaerobic growth of *Bacteroides* and *Actinomyces,* as well as the facultative *Streptococcus* and *Staphylococcus* species and many other oral microbes. There is even some concern about the oral introduction of some viruses (*e.g.,* HIV) into the bloodstream through bites by infected individuals.

Animal bites: In general, bites of animals may introduce microbes such as staphylococci and streptococci which cause local infections in humans. The bacteria, *Pasteurella multocida* and *P. haemolytica,* are frequently found in dog- and cat-bite wounds, and may cause severe local infections and pasteurellosis. Rat-bite fever, caused by *Streptobacillus moniliformis* or *Spirillum minor,* is naturally carried by rats, mice, cats, squirrels, and weasels. The rabies virus is transmitted by the bites of infected dogs, foxes, coyotes, wolves, cats, bats, skunks, raccoons, and other rabid animals. Many other disease-causing microbes are introduced through the skin to the circulatory or nervous systems by bites of arthropod vectors (ticks, fleas, lice, mites, and mosquitoes); these diseases include encephalitis, Colorado tick fever, Rocky Mountain spotted fever, typhus, plague, tularemia, and malaria, and will be discussed elsewhere in this chapter.

Diseases of the Eye

The eye consists of tissues similar to, and contiguous with, the skin. The normal anatomy and structure of the eye are illustrated in Figure 13-5.

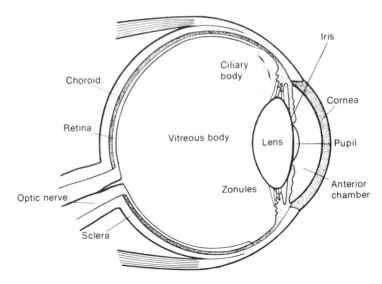

Fig. 13-5. Anatomy of the eye. (Wolf KP: Eyewise. Philadelphia, Harper & Row, 1982)

The external surface of the eye is lubricated, cleansed, and protected by tears, mucus, and sebum. Thus, continual production of tears, and the presence of lysozyme and other antimicrobial substances found in tears, greatly reduce the numbers of normal flora organisms found on the eye surfaces.

Infections of the eye caused by bacteria, chlamydias, and viruses should be differentiated from allergic conjunctivitis by microscopic examination of the exudate, culture of pathogens, or antigen–antibody laboratory tests (fluorescent antibody or enzyme-linked immunosorbent assay, ELISA).

Viral Eye Infections

Viral Conjunctivitis, Acute Hemorrhagic Conjunctivitis (AHC), Herpes Conjunctivitis

Characteristics	Viral invasion of eyelids, conjunctiva, and cornea; usually self-limiting in 1–3 weeks. Subconjunctival hemorrhages caused by adenovirus or enterovirus. Herpes lesions and occasional blindness from herpesvirus infections.
Pathogens	Picornaviruses (enterovirus 70), coxsackievirus, adenoviruses, herpes simplex, types 1 and 2.
Reservoir	Humans.
Transmission	Person-to-person, direct or indirect contact with infected eye secretions. Herpes is transmitted through saliva or genital secretions.

Incubation period	Herpes, 2–12 days; others, 1–3 days.
Control	Personal hygiene, drainage/secretion precautions. Strict asepsis in eye clinics.
Usual treatment	Herpes lesions may be treated with idoxuridine or adenine arabinoside (vidarabine; Vira-A or Ara-A) ophthalmic ointments. No recommended treatment for other self-limiting viral eye infections.

Bacterial Eye Infections

Bacterial Conjunctivitis, Pink Eye

Characteristics	Irritation, reddening of conjunctiva, edema of eyelids, mucopurulent discharge, sensitivity to light. Highly contagious.
Pathogens	*Haemophilus aegyptius, Streptococcus pneumoniae,* other streptococci, staphylococci, *Haemophilus influenzae, Moraxella lacunata, Pseudomonas aeruginosa, Corynebacterium diphtheriae* may be causative agents.
Reservoir	Humans.
Transmission	Human-to-human, through eye and respiratory discharges, fingers, clothing, eye makeup, eye medications, ophthalmic instruments, and contact lens-wetting and lens-cleaning agents.
Incubation period	1–3 days, depending on causative agent.
Control	Personal hygiene. Drainage/secretion precautions, sterilization of fomites.
Usual treatment	Ophthalmic tetracycline, erythromycin, gentamicin, or sulfonamide depending on the susceptibility of pathogen.

Chlamydial Conjunctivitis, Inclusion Conjunctivitis, Paratrachoma

Characteristics	In neonates, acute conjunctivitis with mucopurulent discharge; may result in mild scarring of conjunctivae and cornea. May be concurrent with chlamydial nasopharyngitis or pneumonia. In adults, may be concurrent with nongonococcal urethritis or cervicitis.
Pathogens	*Chlamydia trachomatis,* immunotypes B and D through K.
Reservoir	Humans.

Transmission	Genital secretions to eye, by fingers, sexual contact; to newborns, by infected birth canal; nonchlorinated swimming pools, by genitourinary exudates.
Control	Identification and treatment of chlamydial genital infections of expectant parents. Drainage/secretion precautions. Chlorination of swimming pools. Erythromycin or tetracycline ophthalmic ointments in eyes of newborns. (Chlamydias are not susceptible to silver nitrate or penicillin.)
Usual treatment	Erythromycin orally for infected pregnant women and infected neonates. Topical tetracycline, erythromycin, or sulfonamide for eye infections.

Trachoma, Chlamydia Keratoconjunctivitis

Characteristics	Highly contagious, acute or chronic conjunctival inflammation resulting in scarring of cornea and conjunctiva, deformation of eyelids, and blindness.
Pathogens	*Chlamydia trachomatis*, immunotypes C, A, and B.
Reservoir	Humans.
Transmission	Direct contact with infected ocular or nasal secretions or contaminated articles. Venereal transmission by infected cervix or urethra; to newborns through the birth canal.
Incubation period	5–12 days.
Control	Personal hygiene, improved sanitation and living conditions. Drainage/secretion precautions of hospitalized patients.
Usual treatment	Topical ophthalmic tetracycline or erythromycin, oral tetracycline or erythromycin.

Gonococcal Conjunctivitis, Ophthalmia Neonatorum

Characteristics	Acute redness and swelling of conjunctiva, purulent discharge (Fig. 13-6). Corneal ulcers, perforation, and blindness, if untreated.
Pathogens	*Neisseria gonorrhoeae*; gram-negative, kidney bean-shaped diplococci. Identified by Gram-stained smears, culture, and serologic tests.
Reservoir	Humans.
Transmission	Infection of cervix, birth canal, and secretions. To newborn,

Fig. 13-6. Purulent conjunctivitis caused by gonorrhea. (Moffett HL: Clinical Microbiology, 2nd ed. Philadelphia, JB Lippincott, 1980)

during passage through infected birth canal. To adults, through infected genital secretions.

Incubation period	1–5 days.
Control	Instill 1% silver nitrate solution or ophthalmic penicillin in eyes at birth. Ophthalmic erythromycin or tetracycline may be used to prevent chlamydial, as well as gonococcal eye infections.
Usual treatment	Penicillin, or oral cefotaxime for penicillin-resistant gonococci (penicillinase-producing *N. gonorrhoeae*, PPNG).

Diseases of the Mouth

The oral cavity is a complex ecosystem suitable for growth and interrelationships of many types of microorganisms. The actual normal microbiota living in the mouth vary greatly from person to person.

When the anatomy of the mouth (Fig. 13-7) is studied, it is obvious that there are many areas where bacteria can attach, colonize, and proliferate, even in the presence of the normal defenses. In the healthy mouth, the saliva secreted by salivary and mucous glands, helps control the growth of opportunistic normal flora. Saliva contains enzymes, immunoglobulins (IgA), and buffers to control the near-neutral *p*H, and continually flushes microbes and food particles through the mouth. Other antimicrobial secretions and phagocytes are found in the mucus that coats the oral surfaces. The hard, complex, calcium tooth enamel, bathed in protective saliva, usually resists damage by oral microbes, but when the ecological balance is upset, or not properly maintained, oral disease may result.

Normal Flora and Oral Disease

The normal flora of the mouth has been shown recently to include more than 1000 different strains of bacteria, both aerobes and anaerobes. Only a fraction of these

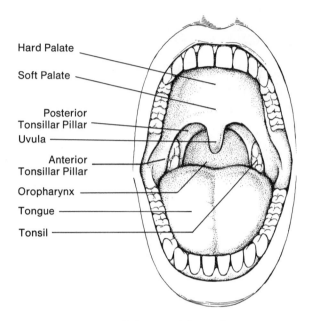

Hard Palate

Soft Palate

Posterior
Tonsillar Pillar

Uvula

Anterior
Tonsillar Pillar

Oropharynx

Tongue

Tonsil

Fig. 13-7. Anatomy of the mouth.

oral microbes have been identified. Some of them are beneficial because they produce secretions that are antagonistic to other bacteria. Several species of *Streptococcus* (*salivarius, mitis, sanguis,* and *mutans*) and *Actinomyces* species often interact to protect the oral surfaces, but in other circumstances, they are involved in oral disease.

The anaerobic condition produced by the oxidation–reduction interactions of the oral flora organisms allow certain genera of anaerobic bacteria (*Bacteroides, Fusobacterium, Lactobacillus, Actinobacillus,* and *Treponema*) to become involved in the production of oral diseases. The coating that forms on unclean teeth, called dental plaque, is a coaggregation of bacteria and their products. Many produce a slime layer or glycocalyx that enables them to attach firmly and cause damage to the tooth enamel. Certain carbohydrates are metabolized by streptococci (especially *S. mutans*) and lactobacilli, producing lactic acid, which encourages other bacteria to grow and be involved in the decay process. Calculus, a calcium phosphate material produced by some bacteria (*e.g., Actinomyces*), is a hard plaque deposit. Calcium phosphate may derive from the enamel dissolved by lactic acid-producing bacteria.

The progressive microbial activities involving formation of dental plaque, dental caries (decay), gingivitis, and periodontitis result from the unique microbial population, reduced host defenses, improper diet, and poor dental hygiene. These diseases are the consequence of at least four microbial activities: (1) formation of dextran from sugars by streptococci, (2) acid production by lactobacilli, (3) deposition of calculus by *Actinomyces,* and (4) secretion of inflammatory substances (endotoxin) by *Bacteroides* species. This combination of circumstances damages the teeth, soft tissues (gingiva), alveolar bone, and the periodontal fibers attaching teeth to bone.

Oral disease can be prevented by excellent health, good oral hygiene (brushing, flossing), adequate diet without sugars, and fluoride treatment to help control the microbial population and prevent the damaging bacterial interactions.

Bacterial Infections of the Oral Cavity

Dental Caries, Gingivitis, Periodontitis

Characteristics	Damage to teeth, gums, and alveolar bone resulting from complex interaction of bacteria with dietary sugars.
Pathogens	*Streptococcus mutans, S. mitis* (Fig. 13–8), *S. salivarius,* and *S. sanguis, Actinomyces naeslundii, A. viscosus, Lactobacillus, Bacteroides, Actinobacillus, Fusobacterium, Capnocytophaga.*
Pathogenicity	Lactic acid and endotoxin production.
Reservoir	Human oral cavity.
Transmission	Direct contact.
Incubation period	Variable.

Fig. 13-8. Electron micrograph of *Streptococcus mutans* in dental plaque.

| Control | Good oral hygiene, adequate diet without sucrose, fluoride in water, toothpaste, other preparations, and perhaps a vaccine. |
| Usual treatment | Cleaning, filling decayed tooth areas, fluoride paste, and other treatments by dentists. |

Acute Necrotizing Ulcerative Gingivitis (ANUG), Vincent's Infection, Trench Mouth

Characteristics	A noncontagious periodontitis with gingival ulcers, associated with lack of oral hygiene, nutritional deficiency, debilitating disease, stress, at least two synergistic microorganisms.
Pathogens	*Bacteroides* and *Fusobacterium* spp., anaerobic gram-negative bacilli. *Borrelia* and *Treponema* spp., anaerobic gram-variable spiral-shaped bacteria. Sometimes *Capnocytophaga, Eikenella,* and other bacteria may occur in lesions.
Pathogenicity	Lactic acid and endotoxin production.
Reservoir	Human mouth.
Transmission	Food, direct contact, lack of oral hygiene.
Incubation period	Variable.
Control	Gentle local debridement, oral hygiene, adequate nutrition, high fluid intake and rest.
Usual treatment	Penicillin, erythromycin, tetracycline, or metronidazole.

Diseases of the Ear

When the normal anatomy of the ear (Fig. 13-9) is studied, one observes that there are only three pathways for pathogens to enter: (1) through the eustachian tube, from the throat and nasopharynx, (2) from the external ear, and (3) through the blood or lymph. Usually the bacteria are trapped in the middle ear when a bacterial infection in the throat and nasopharynx causes the eustachian tube to close. The result is an anaerobic condition in the middle ear, allowing anaerobes to grow and cause pressure on the tympanum (eardrum). Swollen lymphoid (adenoid) tissues, viral infections, and allergies may also close the auditory tube, especially in young children.

Ear Infections

Otitis Media, Middle Ear Infection

| Characteristics | Pressure in middle ear, flattening of tympanum, pain, fever, production of exudate, perforation and scarring of eardrum, and loss of hearing if untreated. Most common under age 8. |

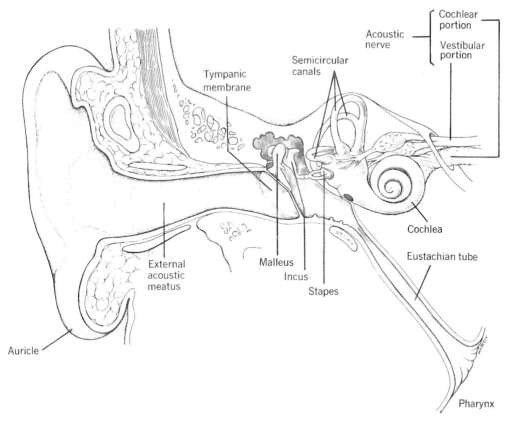

Fig. 13-9. Anatomy of the ear. (Chaffee EE, Lytle IM: Basic Physiology and Anatomy, 4th ed. Philadelphia, JB Lippincott, 1980)

Pathogens	Bacteria: *Haemophilus influenzae, Streptococcus pneumoniae, Streptococcus pyogenes, Staphylococcus aureus.* Viral: Measles virus, parainfluenza virus, respiratory syncytial virus (RSV).
Pathogenicity	Bacterial exotoxins and viral destruction of cells.
Reservoir	Human respiratory nasopharynx.
Transmission	Complication following colds, nose and throat infections, direct contact.
Incubation period	Variable.
Control	For *H. influenzae,* vaccinate to prevent meningitis. Rifampin prophylaxis is also used for prevention of meningitis. For streptococci, search for and treat carriers.
Usual treatment	Ampicillin for *H. influenzae,* amoxicillin or penicillin for streptococci, erythromycin for penicillin-resistant strains.

Enhance body defenses for viral infections. Insertion of tympanum tubes by physician to relieve pressure and the anaerobic condition.

External Otitis, External Ear Infections, Swimmer's Ear

Characteristics	Infection of ear canal with itching, pain, discharge, tenderness, redness, swelling, loss of hearing.
Pathogens	*Escherichia coli, Pseudomonas aeruginosa, Proteus vulgaris, Staphylococcus aureus;* rarely by a fungus, such as *Aspergillus.*
Reservoir	Contaminated water trapped in ear canal; also normal opportunistic flora.
Transmission	Swimming pool or bath water. Articles inserted in ear canal for cleaning out debris and wax.
Incubation period	1–3 days.
Control	Prevent contaminated water from entering and being trapped by wax in external ear canal. Allow physician to clean wax and debris from ears.
Usual treatment	Remove infected debris. Topical treatment with neomycin and polymyxin B for gram-negative rods; 1% hydrocortisone for swelling.

Diseases of the Respiratory System

The respiratory system (Fig. 13-10) is often separated into the upper respiratory tract (URT) consisting of the nose and pharynx (throat), and the lower respiratory tract (LRT) including the larynx, trachea, bronchial tubes, and alveoli, to simplify discussion of the functions, defenses, and diseases of these areas. The most common diseases are those of the upper respiratory tract (*e.g.,* colds and sore throats), which may predispose the patient to more serious infections such as sinusitis, otitis media, bronchitis, and pneumonia.

Typical normal microflora found in the mucosa of the nose and throat include bacterial species of *Streptococcus, Staphylococcus, Haemophilus, Corynebacterium, Neisseria, Bacteroides, Branhamella, Fusobacterium,* and *Actinomyces.* Many of these microorganisms may cause opportunistic diseases of the respiratory tract.

Nonspecific Respiratory Infections

Pneumonia

Characteristics	An acute nonspecific infection of the alveolar spaces and tissue of the lung, with fever, cough, acute chest pain, and respiratory

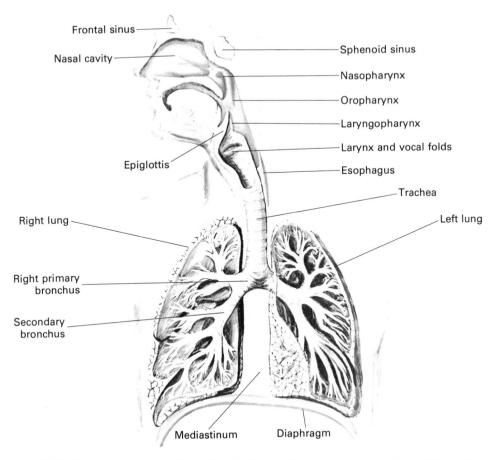

Fig. 13-10. The respiratory system. (Chaffee EE, Lytle IM: Basic Physiology and Anatomy, 4th ed. Philadelphia, JB Lippincott, 1980)

distress; identified by chest x-rays. Pneumonia is usually a secondary infection.

Pathogens   May be caused by gram-positive or gram-negative bacteria, mycoplasmas, viruses, fungi, or protozoa. The bacteria causing pneumonia include *Streptococcus pneumoniae* (see Fig. 7-4), other streptococci, *Staphylococcus aureus* (see Figs. 1-8 and 1-9), *Haemophilus influenzae, Neisseria meningitidis, Pseudomonas aeruginosa, Yersinia pestis, Klebsiella pneumonia,* and other gram-negative enteric bacilli. *Rickettsia, Chlamydia,* and *Mycoplasma* spp. may also be causative agents. Many viral respiratory infections may result in pneumonia. Especially in susceptible and immunocompromised individuals, the fungi *Histoplasma, Coccidioides, Candida, Cryptococcus,* and *Blastomyces* and the protozoan *Pneumocystis carinii* may be etiologic agents.

Reservoir	Humans.
Transmission	Direct contact, respiratory secretions, hands, and fomites.
Incubation period	Depends on pathogen involved.
Control	Depends on pathogen involved.
Usual treatment	Antibiotic therapy will depend on the causal agent identified in sputum or other LRT specimens.

Viral Respiratory Infections

Common Cold, Acute Viral Rhinitis, Acute Coryza, Upper Respiratory Infection (URI)

Characteristics	Coryza (profuse discharge from nostrils), sneezing, sore throat, bronchitis. Secondary bacterial infections frequently follow.
Pathogens	Many (>100) types of rhinovirus, adenovirus (Fig. 13-11), coronavirus, respiratory syncytial virus (RSV), influenza, parainfluenza, and other viruses.
Reservoir	Human respiratory system.
Transmission	Respiratory secretions by way of hands, direct contact, airborne droplets, soiled articles.
Incubation period	1–3 days.
Epidemiology	Most common in fall, winter, and spring.
Control	Sanitary disposal of oral and nasal discharges. Disinfect eating and drinking utensils. Avoid contact with infected individuals.

Fig. 13-11. Electron micrograph of purified type 5 adenovirus particles embedded in sodium silicotungstate (original magnification × 350,000). (Valentine RC, Pereira HG: J Mol Biol 13:13, 1965)

Oral live adenovirus vaccine is effective in the military for specific adenovirus epidemics.

Usual treatment	New antiviral agents. Antibiotics should be reserved for bacterial complications (sinusitis, otitis media, tonsillitis, bronchitis, pneumonia).

Croup, Acute Laryngotracheobronchitis

Characteristics	Acute viral inflammation of respiratory tract with subglottic swelling, respiratory distress with a high-pitched sound during inspiration.
Pathogens	Usually parainfluenza virus, less often RSV, influenza A or B, or other viruses and *Mycoplasma pneumoniae* (a bacterium)
Reservoir	Humans.
Transmission	Direct oral contact, droplets, fomites.
Incubation period	Variable.
Epidemiology	Usually seen in susceptible children 3 months to 3 years old. Symptoms are most dramatic at night, lasting 3–4 days.
Control	Usually self-limiting and not contagious.
Usual treatment	Vaporizers, humidifiers, hot shower steam may relieve symptoms. Hospitalization with oxygenation may be necessary in severe cases. Antibiotics are rarely indicated, but amantadine or other antiviral agents may help.

Influenza, "Flu"

Characteristics	A specific acute viral respiratory infection with fever, chills, headache, cough, nasal drainage; sometimes causing bronchitis, pneumonia, and death in severe cases. Rare nausea, vomiting, and diarrhea.
Pathogens	Influenza virus, types A, B, and C. Usually type A is associated with pandemics and widespread epidemics.
Reservoir	Humans.
Transmission	Respiratory secretions, direct contact, fomites, hands.
Incubation period	24–72 hours.
Epidemiology	Pandemics occurred in 1889, 1918, 1947,1957,1968. Type A epidemics occur every 1–3 years and type B every 3–4 years.

Control	Yearly immunization; prophylatic amantadine or rimantadine may be used against type A for high-risk patients. Good personal hygiene and avoiding crowds during epidemics may prevent infection.
Usual treatment	Amantadine reduces symptoms if given early in type A disease.

Bacterial Respiratory Infections

Diphtheria

Characteristics	An acute contagious respiratory disease, with fibrinous pharyngeal pseudomembrane, causing myocardial and neural tissue damage.
Pathogens	*Corynebacterium diphtheriae,* pleomorphic, gram-positive bacilli that group in palisade arrangements. Toxigenic strains are infected with a corynebacteriophage, resulting in exotoxin production that causes the heart and nerve damage. Identified by culture and serologic techniques.
Reservoir	Humans.
Transmission	Airborne droplets, direct contact, contaminated fomites, raw milk.
Incubation period	2–5 days.
Epidemiology	No cases in United States in 1986 reported to CDC. Diphtheria occurs during colder months among unimmunized children and adults. Disease has disappeared in areas with effective immunization programs.
Control	Community program of immunization of all infants and children with diphtheria–pertussis–tetanus (DPT) vaccine. Give diphtheria–tetanus booster vaccines at appropriate intervals. Patient isolation, quarantine, and disinfection of all fomites.
Usual treatment	Administer antitoxin in suspected cases, with erythromycin or penicillin in confirmed cases. Treat carriers with erythromycin or penicillin.

Legionellosis, Legionnaires' Disease, Pontiac Fever

Characteristics	An acute bacterial pneumonia with headache, high fever, dry cough, chills, diarrhea, pleural and abdominal pain.

Pathogens	*Legionella pneumophila,* a gram-negative bacillus, requiring special medium to grow *in vitro* (see Fig. 8-2). Additional species are being identified. Identification by culture, fluorescent antibody, and ELISA tests.
Reservoir	Soil, dust, and environmental water sources; lakes, creeks, hot-water and air-conditioning systems, shower heads, ultrasonic nebulizers, tap water and distilling water systems.
Transmission	Airborne from water or dust; not person-to-person.
Incubation period	2–10 days.
Epidemiology	In 1986, 833 cases reported in the United States.
Control	Search for environmental sources of infection, periodic superchlorination or superheating of water supply.
Usual treatment	Erythromycin with rifampin.

Strep Throat, Streptococcal Pharyngitis

Characteristics	An acute bacterial infection of the throat with fever, pain; inflammation of pharynx and tonsils; white patches of pus on pharyngeal epithelium. Rheumatic fever and glomerulonephritis complication may result in heart and kidney damage because of hypersensitivity reactions.
Pathogens	*Streptococcus pyogenes* (see Fig. 11-10), β-hemolytic, gram-positive cocci, catalase-negative (Fig. 13-12). The strain that produces an erythrogenic toxin causes scarlet fever rash. Identified by throat culture on blood agar plate, by susceptibility to bacitracin disks, and by fluorescent antibody serologic techniques.
Reservoir	Humans.
Transmission	Human-to-human, by direct contact, usually hands, aerosol droplets, secretions from patients, and carriers.
Incubation period	1–3 days.
Epidemiology	Over 200,000 cases/year in United States, mostly among children (5–14 years); 3% develop rheumatic fever.
Control	Throat cultures followed by antibiotic treatment; personal hygiene and cleanliness. No protective immunity following recovery; no effective vaccines.

Fig. 13-12. (*A*) Group A β-hemolytic streptococci in pneumonic lesion (rat) (original magnification × 600). (*B*) Chain formation characteristics of usual growth of streptococci in artificial media. Smear made from 24-hr culture in serum broth (original magnification × 1000). (*A*) (Glaser RJ, Wood WB Jr.: Arch Pathol 52:244, 1951. Copyright 1951, American Medical Association.) (*B*) (Davis BD, et al: Microbiology, 3rd ed. Philadelphia, Harper & Row, 1980)

Usual treatment	Penicillin, erythromycin to prevent ear infections, rheumatic fever, glomerulonephritis, and other complications.

Tuberculosis

Characteristics	An acute or chronic mycobacterial infection of the pulmonary tract; may invade lymph nodes to cause systemic disease. Infected patients show a positive hypersensitivity skin test and pulmonary tubercles may be seen on chest x-rays.
Pathogens	Primarily *Mycobacterium tuberculosis*; occasionally other *Mycobacterium* spp.; an acid-fast, nonmotile bacillus. Identified by culture techniques.
Reservoir	Humans; rarely, in diseased cattle.
Transmission	Airborne droplets, prolonged direct contact, milk, and contact with infected cattle.
Incubation period	4–12 weeks
Epidemiology	In the United States, more than 20,000 new cases a year; in 1986 there were 22,575 new cases reported to CDC.
Control	Tuberculin testing of humans and cattle. Chest x-ray of TB skin–test-positive people and prompt treatment. Vaccination or preventive treatment of close contacts of infected individuals.

| Usual treatment | A combination of antimicrobial drugs such as isoniazid (INH) with rifampin (RIF), streptomycin (SM), ethambutol (EMB), or parazinamide (PZA) is given for 9–12 months. |

Whooping Cough, Pertussis

Characteristics	An acute bacterial childhood infection. The initial catarrhal stage produces mild symptoms resembling the common cold. The second paroxysmal stage is marked by uncontrollable sieges of coughing in an attempt to expel the thick mucus in trachea and bronchi. Pneumonia may be a complication.
Pathogens	*Bordetella pertussis*, a small, encapsulated, nonmotile, gram-negative coccobacillus that produces endotoxins and exotoxins. Identified by fluorescent antibody serologic techniques.
Reservoir	Human respiratory tract.
Transmission	Airborne via droplets from coughing.
Incubation period	7–10 days usually; up to 21 days.
Epidemiology	In 1986, 4162 cases reported to CDC in United States.
Control	Vaccination of all young children with DPT (P for pertussis) containing killed *B. pertussis*.
Usual treatment	Erythromycin, tetracycline, or chloramphenicol.

Protozoan Respiratory Infections

Pneumocystosis, Pneumocystis Pneumonia, Interstitial Plasma-cell Pneumonia

Characteristics	A subacute pulmonary protozoan disease found in chronically ill children, immunosuppressed patients, and persons with AIDS. Asymptomatic in immunocompetent people; most common cause of death in AIDS patients. Patients show respiratory insufficiency with cyanosis; pulmonary infiltration of intra-alveolar tissue with frothy exudate. Usually fatal in untreated patients.
Pathogen	*Pneumocystis carinii* (Fig. 13-13), a protozoan in cyst and sporozoite form, a sporozoan.
Reservoir	Humans.
Transmission	Direct contact, transfer of pulmonary secretions from infected to susceptible persons. Perhaps airborne.

Fig. 13-13. *Pneumocystis carinii* appears as dark oval bodies when stained with special silver stain. Foamy material is also seen throughout the several alveoli in this section of the lung (original magnification × 250). (Moffett HL: Clinical Microbiology, 2nd ed. Philadelphia, JB Lippincott, 1980)

Incubation period	1–2 months or longer.
Control	Prophylaxis treatment of immunosuppressed patients with Trimethoprim-sulfamethoxazole (TMP–SMZ). Careful disinfection of respiratory therapy equipment.
Usual treatment	TMP–SMZ, or pentamidine.

Diseases of the Gastrointestinal Tract

The digestive tract consists of a long tube with many expanded areas designed for the digestion of food, absorption of nutrients, and elimination of undigested materials (Fig. 13-14). There are many transient and resident microbiota continually entering and leaving the gastrointestinal tract. Most of the microorganisms ingested with food are destroyed in the stomach and duodenum and are inhibited from growing in the lower intestines by the resident normal flora. They are then flushed from the colon during defecation, along with large numbers of indigenous microbes.

The largest number of resident microorganisms are found in the lower small intestine and colon. There, the availability of nutrients and moisture at a constant 37°C allows many facultative and obligate anaerobes to thrive. Most of these intestinal microbiota are obligate anaerobic *Bacteroides* and *Fusobacterium* species, with fewer *Clostridium* and *Veillonella* species. Facultative anaerobic bacteria occur less abundantly, but are better understood because they are easier to isolate and cultivate. Included in this group are the coliforms, the indicator organisms of fecal contamina-

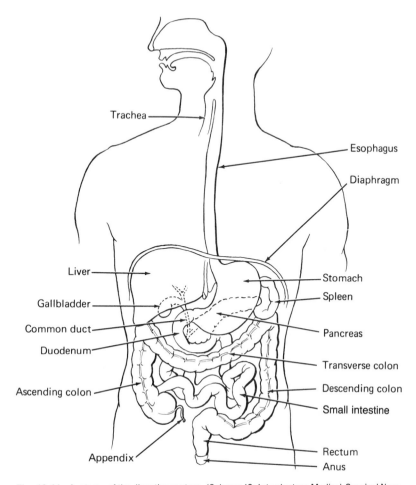

Fig. 13-14. Anatomy of the digestive system. (Scherer JC: Introductory Medical-Surgical Nursing. Philadelphia, JB Lippincott, 1982)

tion of water supplies. These enterobacteria usually include *Escherichia*, *Enterobacter*, *Proteus*, and *Klebsiella* species.

Also found in fecal material are many viruses, most of which are harmless, but some can cause gastroenteritis under certain conditions. Some may be ingested with contaminated food, such as hepatitis A virus in contaminated raw oysters.

Viral Gastrointestinal Infections

Viral Gastroenteritis, Viral Diarrhea, Epidemic Acute Infectious Nonbacterial Gastroenteropathy, "24-Hour Flu"

Characteristics   A self-limiting viral infection of the lining of the gastrointestinal tract with nausea, vomiting, diarrhea, abdominal pain, headache, malaise, and low-grade fever.

Pathogens	Norwalk virus, adenoviruses, echoviruses, rotavirus, coxsackieviruses, poliovirus, and others. Identified by serologic techniques.
Reservoir	Humans.
Transmission	Fecal–oral route, fecal contamination of food, water, and hands.
Incubation period	24–48 hours.
Control	Isolation of patient, enteric precautions.
Usual treatment	Replacement of fluids and electrolytes. Amantadine occasionally reduces symptoms.

Viral Hepatitis

Viral hepatitis includes a group of diseases involving inflammation of the liver caused by several viruses: type A (HAV), type B (HBV), non-A, non-B (NANB), and delta-type virus.

Viral Hepatitis A (HA), Type A Hepatitis, Infectious Hepatitis, Epidemic Hepatitis

Characteristics	Liver inflammation with fever, nausea, abdominal discomfort, usually jaundice. Prolonged convalescence.
Pathogen	Hepatitis A virus (HAV), a picornavirus, similar to an enterovirus; the non-A, non-B hepatitis viruses may cause similar hepatitis symptoms. Serologic and radioimmunologic identification techniques.
Reservoir	Humans.
Transmission	Fecal–oral route, person-to-person. Fecal contamination of water, food, milk, undercooked shell fish.
Incubation period	15–50 days, average 28–30 days.
Epidemiology	In 1986, 23,117 cases in United States reported to CDC.
Control	Good sanitation practices, personal hygiene. Passive immunization of exposed individuals with hyperimmune gamma globulin. Vaccination for high-risk persons. Isolation of infected patients, enteric precautions.
Usual treatment	None. Immune serum may reduce symptoms and speed recovery.

Viral Hepatitis B (HB), Type B Hepatitis, Serum Hepatitis, Australia Antigen Hepatitis

Characteristics	Viral infection and liver damage with anorexia, rash, and jaundice. May lead to chronic hepatitis or cirrhosis of liver in immunodeficient patients.
Pathogen	Hepatitis B virus (HBV), a DNA virus with several major antigenic subtypes. May also involve coinfection with delta hepatitis virus, an RNA virus. A non-A, non-B hepatitis virus causes a similar blood–liver infection. Identified by serologic tests.
Reservoir	Humans.
Transmission	Person-to-person by saliva, semen, and other body fluids; parenteral route, through contaminated syringes, needles, dialysis, and other equipment serving as vectors.
Incubation period	45–180 days, average 60–90 days.
Epidemiology	In United States, 25,867 cases reported to CDC in 1986.
Control	Vaccination against HBV. Active and passive immunization of exposed individuals. Isolation of infected persons with blood and body fluid precautions. Sterilization of all equipment.
Usual treatment	Immune globulin (IG), hyperimmune gamma globulin (HBIG), or antiviral chemotherapy when available.

Bacterial Gastrointestinal Infections

Campylobacter Gastroenteritis

Characteristics	An acute enteric disease with diarrhea, nausea, vomiting, fever, malaise, abdominal pain, usually self-limiting, lasting 1–4 days.
Pathogens	*Campylobacter jejuni* and *C. coli* of many serotypes. Rigid, helical-shaped spirilla. Identified by cultural and serologic techniques.
Reservoir	Animals, including cattle, sheep, swine, poultry, other birds, rodents, cats, dogs, other pets.
Transmission	Ingestion of bacteria in food, milk, water; contact with infected pets, wild animals, and infected infants.
Incubation period	1–10 days, average 3–5 days.

| Control | Thorough cooking of foods, especially poultry; pasteurize milk; chlorinate water supplies. Hand-washing after animal contact. Isolation of hospitalized patients, enteric precautions. |
| Usual treatment | Replacement of fluids and electrolytes. Antibiotic therapy; erythromycin, tetracycline, or aminoglycosides. |

Cholera

Characteristics	An acute enteric diarrheal disease with watery stools, vomiting, rapid dehydration, loss of blood volume, shock. Death frequently results if untreated.
Pathogens	*Vibrio cholerae* type 01, El Tor strain of *V. cholerae,* or other serotypes. A gram-negative curved rod, *C*- or *S*-shaped that secretes an enterotoxin, called choleragin. Identified by culture, morphology, and serologic techniques.
Reservoir	Humans and environmental reservoirs.
Transmission	Fecal–oral route; vomitus and feces-contaminated water and foods; soiled hands; flies. Raw or undercooked seafoods from contaminated waters. Sometimes carriers.
Incubation period	1–5 days.
Epidemiology	Occurs worldwide. Only 17 cases in United States reported in 1986.
Control	Isolation of hospitalized patients, enteric precautions. Concurrent disinfection of feces, vomitus, hands, linen, and fomites. Adequate sewage processing and water treatment. Fly control. Vaccination in some countries. Prophylactic tetracycline for exposed families, doxycycline, or furazolidone treatment.
Usual treatment	Prompt fluid and electrolyte replacement therapy; tetracycline, doxycycline, and other chemotherapy to shorten duration of disease.

Enteropathogenic *Escherichia coli* Diarrhea, "Traveler's Diarrhea"

| Characteristics | Watery diarrhea with, or without, mucus or blood, vomiting, abdominal cramping. |
| Pathogens | *E. coli,* three types; invasive, enterotoxigenic, and enteropathogenic. Gram-negative rods; some produce enterotoxin, others invade colon mucosa. Identified by cultural and serologic tests (see Fig. 2-9). |

Reservoir	Infected humans, carriers.
Transmission	Fecal–oral route, fecal contaminated water, food, hands, fomites, or direct contact.
Incubation period	12–72 hours.
Control	Proper sewage disposal, water treatment, hand-washing practices. Enteric precautions for hospitalized cases.
Usual treatment	Fluid and electrolyte replacement therapy; ampicillin or trimethoprim–sulfamethoxazole (TMP–SMZ) treatment for severe cases and carriers.

Salmonellosis and Typhoid Fever

Characteristics	A gastroenteritis, inflammation of stomach and intestines with abdominal pain, headache, nausea, usually vomiting and diarrhea. Typhoid fever, the most severe form, is a bacteremia, characterized by constipation, intestinal hemorrhage, enlarged spleen and lymph nodes, rose spots on trunk, sustained fever.
Pathogens	*Salmonella typhi* causes typhoid fever; *S. cholerae-suis, S. typhimurium*, and many other serologic types of *S. enteritidis* cause salmonellosis. Motile gram-negative bacilli with endotoxins. *Salmonella typhi* produces exotoxins and endotoxins. Identified by cultural and serologic techniques.
Reservoir	Humans, animals, wild and domestic cattle, poultry, pigs, dogs, cats, turtles, fish, and many others.
Transmission	Fecal–oral route; uncooked and undercooked feces-contaminated meat, eggs, and milk products; sewage, polluted water; hands and fingers of infected persons and carriers; flies and other flying insects.
Incubation period	1–3 weeks for typhoid fever; 1–3 days for salmonellosis.
Epidemiology	In United States only 323 cases of typhoid fever were reported in 1986.
Control	Isolation of hospitalized patients with enteric precautions. Water purification; effective sewage disposal; pasteurization of milk; thorough cooking of foods of animal and egg origin; proper hand-washing techniques; control of flies; clean food preparation area; and treatment of carriers and infected pets. Eliminate food preparation by infected persons and carriers.

Usual treatment	Fluid and electrolyte replacement therapy. Ampicillin or amoxicillin with trimethoprim–sulfamethoxazole or chloramphenicol for resistant strains.

Shigellosis, Bacillary Dysentery

Characteristics	An acute bacterial infection of lining of small and large intestine; diarrhea with blood, mucus, and pus; nausea, vomiting, cramps, fever, sometimes toxemia and convulsions.
Pathogens	Several serotypes of *Shigella dysenteriae, S. flexneri, S. boydii,* and *S. sonei.* Gram-negative bacilli, nonmotile. Plasmid associated with toxin production and virulence. Identified by cultural and biochemical techniques.
Reservoir	Humans, some primates.
Transmission	Fecal–oral route from patients or carriers. Feces-contaminated hands and fingernails, contaminated food and milk, sewage–polluted water. Flies and cockroach vectors.
Incubation period	1–7 days, average 1–3 days.
Control	Eliminate fecal contamination of food, milk, and water. Proper hand-washing and fomite cleaning. Enteric precautions with patients. Infected individuals should neither prepare nor serve food.
Usual treatment	Fluid and electrolyte replacement therapy. Trimethoprim–sulfamethoxazole, ampicillin, tetracyclines, or naldixic acid antibiotic therapy. Chloramphenicol for resistant strains.

Bacterial Food-borne Intoxications, Food Poisoning

Food-borne intoxication or food poisoning refers to diseases resulting from the ingestion of food or water contaminated with bacterial exotoxins produced by such bacteria as *Vibrio cholerae,* enterotoxigenic *E. coli, Clostridium botulinum, C. perfringens,* and *Staphylococcus aureus.*

Botulism

Characteristics	A neuromuscular disease caused by ingestion of food contaminated by *C. botulinum* spores, containing neurotoxins secreted by the pathogen. Infant botulism and wound botulism are produced by living exotoxin-producing bacteria in the gastrointestinal tract or wounds, respectively. Neurotoxins may cause nerve damage, visual difficulty, respiratory failure, flaccid

paralysis of voluntary muscles, brain damage, coma, and death within a week, if untreated.

Pathogen	*Clostridium botulinum*, a spore-forming gram-positive, anaerobic bacillus that produces several exotoxins.
Reservoir	Dust, soil, dirty foods, honey, improperly canned, neutral pH foods, lightly cured foods.
Transmission	Ingestion of food in which the pathogen has produced exotoxin; improperly cooked foods with near-neutral pH.
Incubation period	12–36 hours.
Epidemiology	Only 90 cases in United States reported in 1986.
Control	Careful washing, canning, processing, and cooking of food. Thorough cleaning of wounds. Never add raw honey to babies' milk or foods.
Usual treatment	Antitoxin and treatment of respiratory failure.

Clostridium perfringens Food Poisoning

Characteristics	A gastrointestinal toxemia with colic, diarrhea, nausea, rarely vomiting. Usually a mild disease of short duration, <24 hours, rarely fatal.
Pathogen	*Clostridium perfringens*, a gram-positive, spore-forming, enterotoxin-producing, anaerobic, thermophilic bacillus.
Reservoir	Spores in soil, gastrointestinal tract of humans and animals.
Transmission	Ingestion of food, contaminated by dirt or fecal material, kept at moderate temperatures allowing bacterial growth and exotoxin production.
Incubation period	6–24 hours.
Control	Cook food well, serve hot or cold. Train food processors in proper hand-washing and food-handling techniques.
Usual treatment	None. Usually a self-limiting disease.

Staphylococcal Food Poisoning

Characteristics	A gastroenteritis toxemia with acute onset of cramps, vomiting, nausea, occasional diarrhea, subnormal temperature and blood pressure resulting from ingested enterotoxins in foods.

Pathogens	*Staphylococcus aureus* growing in foods produces exotoxins.
Reservoir	Humans: skin, abscesses, nasal secretions; bovine-contaminated milk.
Transmission	Ingestion of *S. aureus*-contaminated foods containing staphylococcal enterotoxin; particularly starchy foods and meats.
Incubation period	1–7 hours.
Control	Training food preparers in proper personal hygiene, in cleanliness in kitchen areas, and in the need for refrigeration of starchy foods and meats. Prevent infected persons from preparing food.
Usual treatment	Fluid replacement if needed.

Protozoan Gastrointestinal Diseases

Amebiasis, Amebic Dysentery

Characteristics	A protozoan intestinal disease with dysentery, fever, chills, bloody or mucoid diarrhea or constipation, and colitis; may progress to liver, lungs, pericardium, or brain.
Pathogen	*Entamoeba histolytica,* a protozoan of Class Sarcodina; occurs in two stages: cysts (the infective stage) and the motile, reproducing trophozoite. The ameba may embed in mucous membranes of the colon, forming abscesses, or may pass with the fluid diarrhea.
Reservoir	Humans, usually asymptomatic carriers.
Transmission	Feces-contaminated warm water and vegetables, flies on food; soiled hands of infected food handlers; oral–anal sexual contact.
Incubation period	Variable days to months.
Control	Sanitary sewage disposal. Protection and treatment of water supplies. Personal hygiene and hand-washing before preparing food and eating. Eliminate fertilization of crops with human fecal material. Control flies around foods. Enteric precautions with hospitalized patients.
Usual treatment	Metronidazole (Flagyl) with iodoquinol. Fluid and electrolyte replacement.

Giardiasis, Giardial Enteritis

Characteristics	A protozoan infection of the small intestine, with nausea, gas, abdominal pain, acute malodorous diarrhea, malabsorption, and damage to mucosal membranes; may be asymptomatic.
Pathogen	*Giardia lamblia* (see Fig. 2-20), a flagellate protozoan; trophozoites attach to mucosal membranes; cysts and sometimes trophozoites are expelled in feces.
Reservoir	Humans; possibly beaver; other wild and domestic animals.
Transmission	Fecal–oral route; ingestion of cysts in fecal-contaminated cold water or foods; person-to-person by soiled hands to mouth.
Incubation period	5–25 days or longer.
Control	Proper filtration of public water supplies (chlorine does not destroy cysts); sanitary disposal of feces; boil all emergency water supplies.
Usual treatment	Quinacrine (Atabrine) or metronidazole (Flagyl)

Diseases of the Urogenital Tract

When the male and female urinary and reproductive systems are studied, it is easy to observe many areas in which infections may occur. The urinary tract is normally protected from pathogens by the frequent flushing action of urination (Fig. 13-15). The acidity of normal urine also discourages the growth of many microorganisms. Only at the opening (meatus) of the urethra will normal flora be found in the male urogenital tract and the female urinary system. These urethral bacteria include *Bacteroides, Streptococcus, Mycobacterium, Lactobacillus,* and *Neisseria,* as well as some gram-negative enteric bacteria. However, the female genital area supports the growth of many additional normal flora organisms. In the adult vagina there are many species of *Staphylococcus, Streptococcus, Lactobacillus, Neisseria, Clostridium, Actinomyces, Bacteroides,* diphtheroids, enterobacteria, and *Candida* yeasts. The balance among these microbes depends on the estrogen levels and pH of the site. The rest of the reproductive systems of both sexes should remain free of microbial life (Fig. 13-16). When any of these and other microorganisms invade further, many nonspecific infections may occur.

Sexually Transmitted Diseases

The sexually transmitted diseases (STD), formerly called venereal diseases (VD), include any of the infections transmitted by sexual activities. They are diseases of not only the reproductive and urinary tracts, but also of the skin, mucous mem-

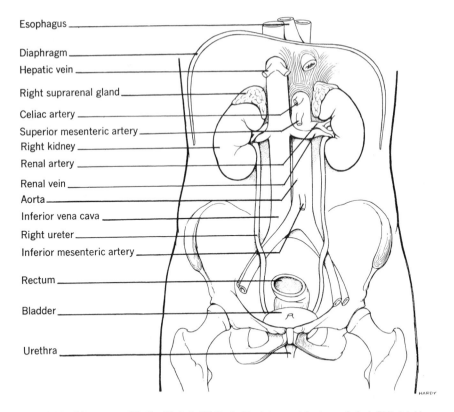

Esophagus
Diaphragm
Hepatic vein
Right suprarenal gland
Celiac artery
Superior mesenteric artery
Right kidney
Renal artery
Renal vein
Aorta
Inferior vena cava
Right ureter
Inferior mesenteric artery
Rectum
Bladder
Urethra

Fig. 13-15. Urinary tract. (Chaffee EE, Lytle IM: Basic Physiology and Anatomy, 3rd ed. Philadelphia, JB Lippincott, 1973)

branes, blood, lymphatic and digestive systems, and many other body areas. The acquired immunodeficiency syndrome (AIDS) and chlamydial infections are the epidemic STDs of the 1980s. Because the AIDS virus (HIV) primarily causes damage to the T_4 helper lymphocytes, thus inhibiting antibody production, it will be discussed with diseases of the circulatory systems. Hepatitis B, amebiasis, and giardiasis can also be considered sexually transmitted diseases.

Urinary Tract Infections

Urethritis, Cystitis, Ureteritis, Prostatitis

Characteristics   Inflammatory infections of the urethra (urethritis), the urinary bladder (cystitis), the ureters (ureteritis), or the prostate (prostatitis). May lead to kidney infections (pyelonephritis) and damage.

Pathogens   Any of the normal flora introduced by poor personal hygiene, sexual intercourse, insertion of catheters, and so forth. Most common pathogens include *E. coli, Proteus* spp., *Pseudomonas*

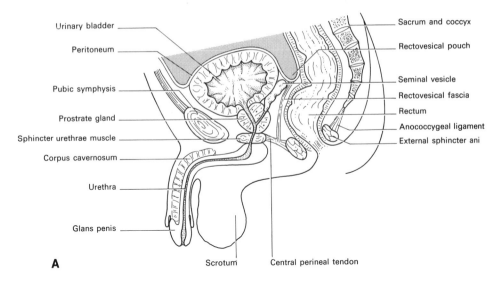

Urinary bladder

Peritoneum

Pubic symphysis

Prostrate gland

Sphincter urethrae muscle

Corpus cavernosum

Urethra

Glans penis

Scrotum

Central perineal tendon

Sacrum and coccyx

Rectovesical pouch

Seminal vesicle

Rectovesical fascia

Rectum

Anococcygeal ligament

External sphincter ani

A

Uterus

Peritoneum

Rectum

Sacrum and coccyx

Rectouterine peritoneal pouch

Urinary bladder

Pubic symphysis

Urethra

Vestibule

Vagina

Anococcygeal ligament

External anal sphincter

Central perineal tendon

B

Hymen   Sphincter urethrae muscle

Fig. 13-16. Reproductive systems. (*A*) Male; (*B*) Female. (Thompson JS: Core Textbook of Anatomy. Philadelphia, JB Lippincott, 1977)

spp., and fecal streptococci (enterococci). Nosocomial infections caused by *Serratia, Pseudomonas,* and *Klebsiella* spp. are common. Nonspecific urethritis is frequently caused by species of *Chlamydia, Ureaplasma,* and *Mycoplasma,* usually introduced by sexual contact. The gonococci may also invade the urinary tract as well as the reproductive system.

Reservoir   Humans.

Transmission   Poor personal hygiene; sexual intercourse; introduction of catheters and other instruments.

Incubation period	Variable, 1–15 days.
Control	Personal cleanliness, particularly before intercourse; use of condoms. Sterilization of catheters, cystoscopes, and other instruments and proper disinfection of the urethral area before their use.
Usual treatment	Appropriate antibiotic or chemotherapeutic agent for the identified pathogen.

Viral Urogenital Infections

Genital Herpes, Venereal Herpes

Characteristics	A herpesvirus infection of the reproductive system, producing herpetic lesions externally and/or internally with fever, headache, malaise; may become latent in nerve ganglia and asymptomatic. Progression of lesion: papule, vesicle, pustule, ulcer, crusting, healing.
Pathogen	Herpes simplex virus (HSV), type 2 usually; type 1 occasionally (Fig. 13-17).
Reservoir	Humans.
Transmission	Direct sexual contact; oral–genital, or oral–anal contact, during presence of lesions (Fig. 13-18). Mother-to-neonate during pregnancy and birth, or autoinoculation from another lesion.

A   B

Fig. 13-17. Herpes simplex virus particles embedded in phosphotungstate. (*A*) Enveloped full particle showing the thick envelope surrounding the nucleocapsid. (*B*) Naked full particle; the structure of the capsomers is plainly visible (original magnification × 200,000). (Watson DH, et al: Virology 19:250, 1963)

A   B

Fig. 13-18. (*A*) Recurrent herpes simplex of the lip. (*B*) Recurrent herpes progenitalis. (Dobson RL, Abele DC: The Practice of Dermatology. Philadelphia, Harper & Row, 1985)

Incubation period	2–28 days or longer, may remain as latent infection indefinitely.
Control	Refrain from intercourse with person with herpetic lesions; use of condoms. Cesarean delivery of infected mothers before membranes rupture. Prophylactic oral acyclovir for women of reproductive age.
Usual treatment	Acyclovir; IV, oral, or topical.

Genital Warts, Papilloma Venereum, Condyloma Acuminata

Characteristics	Viral disease with skin and mucous membrane lesions that are smooth or filiform, cauliflowerlike, fleshy or flat growths in genital areas, internally or externally (Fig. 13-19). In babies of infected mothers, laryngeal papillomas. Some infections become malignant.
Pathogen	Human papilloma virus (HPV) of genotypes 6, 11, 16, or 18. The latter two are more often involved in malignancies.
Reservoir	Humans.
Transmission	Direct contact, usually sexual; through breaks in skin or mucous membranes. From mother to neonate during birth.

Fig. 13-19. Anogenital warts (condylomata accuminata or moist warts). (Dobson RL, Abele DC: The Practice of Dermatology. Philadelphia, Harper & Row, 1985)

Incubation period	1–8 months or longer.
Control	Avoid direct contact with lesions; use of condoms. Cesarean section delivery for infected mothers.
Usual treatment	Local treatment with 25% podophyllin, 5-fluorouracil (5-FU), or other cytotoxic agents, but not in pregnant women. Cryosurgery with liquid nitrogen. Surgical removal, laser therapy, or electrocautery. Treatment repeated with recurrence.

Bacterial Urogenital Infections

Chlamydial Infections, Genital Chlamydiasis

Characteristics	The most frequent cause of nonspecific (NSU) and nongonococcal urethritis (NGU), cervicitis, vaginitis, salpingitis, epididymitis, and newborn conjunctivitis and pneumonia. Many asymptomatic carriers.
Pathogen	*Chlamydia trachomatis* serotypes D–K; tiny obligately intracellular, gram-negative bacteria in two forms, elementary body and reticulate body. Concomitant infectious agents may include

Ureaplasma ureolyticum, Mycoplasma hominis, and other sexually transmitted pathogens in 50% of cases. Identified by cell culture, staining, and serologic techniques.

Reservoir	Humans.
Transmission	Direct sexual contact or mother-to-neonate during birth.
Incubation period	2–3 weeks, may be latent.
Control	Personal cleanliness, sex education, use of condom. Prophylactic treatment of contacts and pregnant women with infection.
Usual treatment	Tetracycline or doxycycline. Erythromycin for pregnant women and resistant cases.

Gonorrhea

Characteristics	A very common acute infectious disease of urethra, anus, vagina, cervix, fallopian tubes (salpingitis), pelvic inflammatory disease (PID), and other reproductive organs. A yellow purulent urethral discharge (most commonly seen in men). Frequently asymptomatic in women and homosexual men. Also, may result in rectal gonorrhea, proctitis, conjunctivitis (see Fig. 13-6), and disseminated infections.
Pathogen	*Neisseria gonorrhoeae,* gram-negative diplococcus. Some strains have plasmids for β-lactamases (penicillinase-producing *Neisseria gonorrhoeae* or PPNG strains). Identified microscopically, culturally, and serologically.
Reservoir	Humans.
Transmission	Direct mucous-to-mucous membrane, or sexual contact; adult-to-child (may indicate sexual abuse); mother-to-neonate during birth.
Incubation period	2–7 days, or longer. Frequently asymptomatic.
Epidemiology	In United States, 913,564 new cases reported to CDC in 1986.
Control	Refrain from intercourse with infected partners. Use of condoms. Culture tests on pregnant women.
Usual treatment	Penicillin, tetracycline, ampicillin, or cephalosporin. Spectinomycin, cefoxitin, or TMP–SMZ for resistant strains. Erythromycin for pregnant women.

Syphilis, Venereal Syphilis

Characteristics   An acute and chronic treponemal disease in three stages: a primary chancre lesion (Fig. 13-20A), secondary skin rash with fever and mucous membrane lesions (Fig. 13-20B), long latent period, and tertiary stage with damage to central nervous system, cardiovascular system, visceral organs, bones, sense organs, and other sites.

Pathogen   *Treponema pallidum*, a gram-variable spirochete. Identified by dark-field microscopy and serologic tests.

Reservoir   Humans.

Transmission   Direct contact with lesions, body secretions, blood, semen, saliva, vaginal discharges; usually during sexual contact; blood transfusions; mother-to-fetus by placental transfer.

Incubation period   10 days to several weeks.

Epidemiology   In United States, 27,762 new cases reported in 1986, and 107 cases of congenital syphilis.

Control   VDRL or RPR tests with confirming serology for high-risk persons and pregnant women. Avoid sexual contact with infected persons; use of condoms.

A   B

Fig. 13-20. Syphilis. (*A*) Primary, showing a chancre of the lip with unilateral adenopathy (*arrow*). (*B*) Secondary, with mucous patches on the tongue. (Dobson RL, Abele DC: The Practice of Dermatology. Philadelphia, Harper & Row, 1985)

Usual treatment	Long-acting penicillin G (benzathine penicillin), or procaine penicillin. Tetracycline for penicillin-sensitive persons. Erythromycin for pregnant women.

Protozoan Urogenital Infections

Trichomoniasis

Characteristics	A protozoan disease causing vaginitis in women: may cause a profuse, thin, malodorous, yellowish discharge; often asymptomatic. In men, an infection of urethra, prostate, or seminal vesicles; usually asymptomatic.
Pathogen	*Trichomonas vaginalis*, a flagellate protozoan. Identified microscopically or immunologically; rarely by culture.
Reservoir	Humans.
Transmission	Direct mucous contact, sexual intercourse.
Incubation period	4–20 days.
Control	Avoid sexual relations with infected persons. Use of condoms. Concurrent treatment of sexual partners.
Usual treatment	Metronidazole (Flagyl).

Other Sexually Transmitted Diseases

Many other pathogens may be transmitted by sexual intercourse. Three, seen more often in parts of the world other than in the United States, are chancroid, granuloma inguinale, and lymphogranuloma venereum (LGV). Chancroid is caused by the bacterium *Haemophilus ducreyi* and can be treated with erythromycin or TMP–SMZ. Granuloma inguinale is a chronic infection caused by a bacterium named *Calymmatobacterium granulomatis* (*Donovania granulomatis*) and is treatable with tetracycline or TMP–SMZ. Lymphogranuloma venereum (LGV) is a chlamydial infection that invades the lymph nodes, rectum, and reproductive tract; caused by *Chlamydia trachomatis* types L-1, L-2, and L-3 (Fig. 2-14); treated with tetracyline, erythromycin, or sulfonamides. It should be noted that many sexually transmitted diseases occur and are transmitted simultaneously.

Diseases of the Circulatory System

The circulatory systems, consisting of the cardiovascular system and lymphatic system (Fig. 13-21), carry blood or lymph throughout the body. Included in these

Fig. 13-21. (*A*) The cardiovascular system. (*B*) The lymphatic system. (Tortora GJ, Anagnostakos NP: Anatomy and Physiology, 4th ed. Philadelphia, Harper & Row, 1984)

fluids are many cells: erythrocytes, leukocytes, thrombocytes, and lymphocytes. Most leukocytes and lymphocytes function to protect the body from pathogens by phagocytosis and by antibody production.

Normally, the blood is sterile; it contains no resident normal flora. When microbes invade the blood stream septicemia results if they are not quickly destroyed. In this septic condition the patient will have chills and fever; also, bacteria and their toxic products will be found in the blood stream. The lymph occasionally picks up microorganisms from the intestine, lungs, and other areas, but these transient organisms are usually quickly engulfed by phagocytic cells in the liver and lymph nodes. Frequently, transient bacteremia (temporary bacteria in the blood) results from dental extractions, wounds, bites, and damage to the intestinal, respiratory, or reproductive tract mucosa. However, when pathogenic organisms are capable of resisting or overwhelming the phagocytes and other body defenses—or when the individual is immunosuppressed or is otherwise more susceptible than normal—a systemic disease may occur.

Viruses often invade the circulatory systems and damage certain target cells, an example of which is HIV (AIDS virus), that destroys T_4 lymphocytes (helper T cells), causing the immune system to malfunction. Some cardiovascular diseases are the result of toxemia, the production of damaging exotoxins secreted by bacteria and carried to target areas by the blood stream. Toxic shock syndrome, rheumatic fever, tetanus, and botulism are examples of such diseases. Fungal and protozoan cardiovascular diseases may cause damage by actually clogging the capillaries in various regions of the body.

Viral Lymphatic and Cardiovascular Infections

AIDS, Acquired Immunodeficiency Syndrome

Characteristics	A viral infection that destroys T_4 helper lymphocytes (Fig. 13-22) of the immune system causing immunosuppression, allowing secondary infections. Viruses (CMV, herpes), protozoa (*Pneumocystis* and *Toxoplasma*), bacteria (mycobacteria), and fungi (*Candida*) may invade, usually resulting in death. Frequent complications include Kaposi's sarcoma. Symptoms include fever, fatigue, diarrhea, weight loss, enlarged lymph nodes, brain and spinal cord damage; may be asymptomatic as AIDS-related complex (ARC) for several years.
Pathogen	Human immunodeficiency virus (HIV—Fig. 13-23); formerly named human T-lymphotropic virus type III (HTLV-III) or lymphadenopathy-associated virus (LAV), and perhaps other viruses.
Reservoir	Humans.
Transmission	Direct sexual contact, homosexual or heterosexual; contaminated IV needles and syringes; blood transfusion with contaminated blood, and blood products. Transplacental and mother-to-child transfer.

Fig. 13-22. A large inclusion (*arrow*) within the cytoplasm of a peripheral blood mononuclear cell from a patient with AIDS (original magnification × 40,000). (DeVita VT, Jr, Hellman S, Rosenberg SA: AIDS. Philadelphia, JB Lippincott, 1985)

Incubation period	6 months to 5 years, or longer.
Epidemiology	Epidemic worldwide. In United States, 13,008 new cases reported in 1986 (see Fig. 8-1).
Control	Avoid sexual contact with high-risk persons: those having multiple sex partners, homosexual males, bisexuals, and those sharing drug paraphernalia (soak needles in Chlorox). Use of condoms. For hospitalized patients, blood and body fluid precautions.
Usual treatment	Azidothymidine (AZT), other derived nucleotides such as dideoxycytidine; treatment of secondary infections.

Colorado Tick Fever

Characteristics	An acute viral infection with fever, headache, fatigue, aching, and occasionally encephalitis or myocarditis, following tick bite. In western North America. Usually self-limiting.

Fig. 13-23. Extracellular HIV retrovirus particle from a lymphocyte of a patient with ARC. Note the dense cylindrical core. (DeVita VT, Jr, Hellman S, Rosenberg SA: AIDS. Philadelphia, JB Lippincott, 1985)

Pathogen	An arbovirus
Reservoir	Tick-infested small mammals.
Transmission	Bite of virus-infected tick to humans, from infected small mammals, ground squirrels, porcupines, or chipmunks.
Incubation period	4–5 days.
Control	Control of ticks and infected rodent hosts. Blood and body fluid precautions for hospitalized patients.
Usual treatment	None, but rest and nutritious diet.

Infectious Mononucleosis

Characteristics	An acute viral disease of B lymphocytes, spleen, and liver with high fever, sore throat, fatigue, weakness, and generalized lymphadenopathy; showing transformed B lymphocytes. Usually self-limiting, may be asymptomatic and latent.
Pathogen	Epstein-Barr virus (EBV), a human herpesvirus 4 which may be oncogenic. Identified by heterophil antibody and IFA (immune fluorescent antibody) tests.
Reservoir	Humans.

Transmission	Person-to-person, by direct contact and by exchange of saliva and other body fluids.
Incubation period	4–6 weeks.
Control	Limit kissing contacts. Disinfect articles contaminated with nose and throat discharges.
Usual treatment	None, but rest and nutritious diet.

Mumps, Infectious Parotitis

Characteristics	An acute viral infection of salivary glands, usually the parotid gland. Deafness, meningoencephalitis, mastitis, nephritis, thyroiditis, and pericarditis complications may occur; in adults, orchitis (inflammation of testes) or oophoritis (ovary infection).
Pathogen	Mumps virus, a paramyxovirus. Identified by serologic techniques.
Reservoir	Humans.
Transmission	Direct contact and fomites via respiratory secretions, aerosol droplets, saliva.
Incubation period	2–3 weeks, usually 18 days.
Epidemiology	In 1986, 6,807 cases reported to CDC in United States.
Control	Live-attenuated vaccine MMR (measles, mumps, rubella), for children and nonimmune adults. For hospitalized patients, respiratory isolation.
Treatment	No specific chemotherapy.

Rickettsial Cardiovascular Infections

Rocky Mountain Spotted Fever (RMSF), Tick-borne Typhus Fever

Characteristics	The most common rickettsial spotted fever. An infection of the vascular endothelial cells, with high fever, muscle pain, headache, chills, and maculopapular rash on extremities after third day; if untreated, may result in death.
Pathogen	*Rickettsia rickettsii*, a gram-negative bacteria; obligate intracellular parasite. Identified by immunofluorescent (IF) antisera, and nonspecific Weil–Felix reaction.

Reservoir	Infected ticks on dogs, rodents, and other animals.
Transmission	Bite of infected tick, from animals to humans; tick parts or feces into break in skin.
Incubation period	2–14 days after tick bite.
Epidemiology	In United States, 755 cases reported in 1986.
Control	Avoid tick-infested areas. Search for ticks on self and dogs after being in tick-infested areas. Avoid crushing ticks during removal.
Usual treatment	Tetracycline or chloramphenicol.

Endemic Murine Typhus Fever, Flea-borne Typhus

Characteristics	An acute febrile disease (similar to, but milder than, epidemic typhus) with fever, headache, and rash on body trunk.
Pathogen	*Rickettsia typhi.*
Reservoir	Infected rats with infective rat fleas.
Transmission	Rats to fleas which defecate rickettsia into bite site and skin wounds of humans. Rat→flea→human.
Incubation period	1–2 weeks.
Epidemiology	In United States, only 48 cases reported in 1986.
Control	Apply insecticide to rat-infested areas, then use rodent control measures. Avoid contact with rats.
Usual treatment	Tetracycline, doxycycline, or chloramphenicol.

Epidemic Typhus Fever, Louse-borne Typhus

Characteristics	An acute rickettsial disease with very high prolonged fever, severe headache, rash appearing on trunk by sixth day. Toxemia may involve kidneys, heart, spleen, and nerves.
Pathogen	*Rickettsia prowazekii*, a gram-negative bacteria, identified by IFA tests.
Reservoir	Humans.
Transmission	Humans to body lice (Fig. 13-24) to humans.

Fig. 13-24. Pubic louse or *Phthirus pubis* as seen with ×7.5 lens of microscope. Infected lice may transmit typhus. (Sauer GC: Manual of Skin Diseases, 5th ed. Philadelphia, JB Lippincott, 1985)

Incubation period	1–2 weeks.
Control	Use of insecticide to kill body lice. Improve personal cleanliness practices. Immunization of susceptible people.
Usual treatment	Chloramphenicol or tetracycline.

Bacterial Cardiovascular Infections

Subacute Bacterial Endocarditis (SBE)

Characteristics	A bacterial infection of heart valves damaged by rheumatic fever, syphilis, atherosclerosis, congenital heart deformities. Bacterial masses with fibrin break away to form clots that clog small blood vessels in brain, heart, kidney, spleen, liver, or other organs; resulting in death.
Pathogens	Most often species of non-group A streptococci, gram-positive cocci of low virulence. Identified by serologic techniques.
Reservoir	Humans.

Transmission	(1) Parenteral; (2) mechanical invasion of blood vessels; (3) surgery, catheterization, minor trauma, dental work.
Incubation period	Variable.
Control	Personal hygiene, sterile and aseptic techniques by dentists, physicians, and nurses.
Treatment	Bactericidal antibiotics specific for the pathogen identified.

Plague, Bubonic Plague, Septicemic Plague, Pneumonic Plague

Characteristics	An acute severe infection involving the lymph nodes (enlarging to buboes), lungs, or disseminated throughout the body, and death if untreated.
Pathogen	*Yersinia pestis*, a gram-negative, pleomorphic, nonmotile bacillus. Identified by bipolar staining of organism; culture of bubo aspirate or sputum or CSF; by FA or ELISA tests.
Reservoir	Wild rodents.
Transmission	Wild rodents to fleas to humans; from rodents directly to humans; or respiratory pathway from person to person.
Incubation period	2–6 days.
Epidemiology	In United States, only 10 human cases reported in 1986.
Control	Avoid contact with rodents and fleas from rodents. Strict isolation of pneumonic patients.
Usual treatment	Streptomycin, tetracycline, or chloramphenicol.

Tularemia, Rabbit Fever

Characteristics	An acute infection with primary local ulcer, lymph node swelling. May be systemic, pneumonic, or gastrointestinal disease.
Pathogen	*Francisella tularensis*, a small, gram-negative pleomorphic bacillus. Identified by FA and heterophil antibody tests.
Reservoir	Wild animals, such as rabbits, muskrats, beaver; some domestic animals; hard ticks.
Transmission	By handling or ingestion of contaminated meat; by drinking contaminated water, or by bites of infected animals, flies, and ticks.

Incubation period	2–10 days.
Epidemiology	In United States, only 167 human cases reported in 1986.
Control	Use impervious gloves when handling and dressing rabbits, cook wild meat well, avoid bites of insects and ticks in infected areas. Vaccinate high-risk persons.
Usual treatment	Streptomycin, gentamicin, or tobramycin.

Protozoan Cardiovascular Infections

Malaria

Characteristics	A systemic protozoan infection with fever, chills, sweats, headache, asymptomatic periods, rarely progressing to shock, renal and liver failure, and coma.
Pathogens	The sporozoans: *Plasmodium vivax*, *P. malariae*, *P. falciparum*, and *P. ovale*, that have a complex life cycle through the mosquito to the liver and erythrocytes of humans. Identified in blood smears.
Reservoir	Humans.
Transmission	Bite of infective female *Anopheles* mosquito; also by transfusion or contaminated syringes.
Incubation period	12–30 days or longer.
Epidemiology	In United States, 1089 cases reported in 1986.
Control	Insecticides and draining of breeding areas to destroy anopheline mosquitoes. Use of chemosuppressive drugs: chloroquine, amodiaquin, primaquine, Fansidar, or Maloprim (pyrimethamine and dapsone).
Usual treatment	Chloroquine, amodiaquin, Fansidar, mefloquine or primaquine (for chloroquine-resistant cases).

Toxoplasmosis

Characteristics	A systemic protozoan disease with fever, lymphadenopathy, lymphocytosis, rarely with central nervous system symptoms, pneumonia, myocarditis, rash, and death. Primary infection may be asymptomatic. Often complicates AIDS.
Pathogen	*Toxoplasma gondii*, an obligate intracellular sporozoan.

Reservoir	Rodents, cattle, sheep, pigs, goats, chickens, birds. Cats shed oocysts in fecal material.
Transmission	Humans eat infected meats, usually pork or mutton, and ingest oocysts in contaminated food and water, or inhale dust contaminated with oocysts from cat feces. Children may inhale or ingest oocysts from sandboxes containing cat feces. Transplacental infection occurs during primary infection in mother; may cause severe damage to fetus.
Incubation period	5–23 days.
Epidemiology	Estimated over 2 million people per year infected.
Control	Cook meats thoroughly. Dispose of kitty litter feces daily into toilet or bury. Pregnant women should avoid cat litter pans and cat feces-contaminated soil. Vaccinate pet cats.
Usual treatment	Pyrimethamine and sulfadiazine or triple sulfonamides with folinic acid.

Trypanosomiasis, Chagas' Disease

Characteristics	A systemic protozoan disease with chancre at site of tsetse fly or reduviid bug bite; then intense headache, lymphadenopathy, insomnia, anemia, and rash. Late stages involve CNS; "sleeping sickness," or heart failure, and frequently death.
Pathogen	*Trypanosoma gambiense, T. rhodesiense,* and *T. cruzi,* flagellate protozoa.
Reservoir	Humans and wild animals.
Transmission	To humans by bite of tsetse fly or reduviid bugs that have ingested blood of infected humans or animals.
Incubation period	3–21 days or longer.
Control	Control of tsetse fly and reduviid bugs. Treatment of infected humans.
Usual treatment	Suramin, pentamidine, or melarsoprol; none for Chagas' disease.

Diseases of the Nervous System

The central nervous system (CNS) (Fig. 13-25) is well protected; it is encased in bone, covered with the membranous three-layered meninges, bathed and cushioned in cerebrospinal fluid (CSF), and nourished by capillaries. These capillaries make up

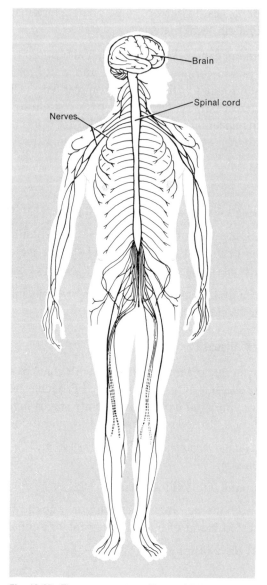

Fig. 13-25. The nervous system. (Tortora GJ, Anagnostakos NP: Anatomy and Physiology, 4th ed. Philadelphia, JB Lippincott, 1984)

the blood–brain barrier, supplying nutrients but not allowing larger particles, such as microorganisms and most antibiotics, to pass from the blood into the brain.

There are no indigenous normal flora of the nervous system. The microbes must gain access to the CNS through trauma (fracture or medical procedure), via the blood and lymph to the CSF, or along the peripheral nerves.

An infection of the meninges is called meningitis, and encephalitis is an infection of the brain itself. Several viruses may produce viral or aseptic meningitis and encephalitis. The most common are enteroviruses, coxsackieviruses, echoviruses, and mumps viruses; others include arboviruses, polioviruses, adenoviruses, measles, herpes, and varicella viruses. The arboviruses (arthropod-borne viruses) are introduced by mosquito vectors and cause several forms of viral encephalitis. The bacteria that cause almost all bacterial meningitis are *Haemophilus influenzae*, *Neisseria meningitidis*, and *Streptococcus pneumoniae* (see Fig. 7-4). Less commonly, other *Streptococcus* species, *Staphylococcus aureus*, *Listeria monocytogenes*, *Escherichia coli*, *Pseudomonas aeruginosa*, *Salmonella*, *Klebsiella*, and other enterobacteria are found. Some free-living amebae that may cause meningoencephalitis are of the genera *Naegleria* and *Acanthamoeba*. Other protozoa that may invade the meninges are the *Toxoplasma* and *Trypanosoma*. Occasionally fungal pathogens, especially *Cryptococcus neoformans*, are seen in meningitis patients.

Early symptoms of meningitis are similar to those of colds. Later, fever, severe headache, pain, and stiffness of neck and back develop. Then neurological symptoms of dizziness, convulsions, minor paralysis, coma, and death within a few hours may occur.

Diagnosis is usually by symptoms, examination, and culture of the cerebrospinal fluid obtained by a lumbar puncture (spinal tap). The treatment of meningitis is supportive, and chemotherapeutic agents may be administered depending on the causal agent involved.

Several central nervous system diseases are caused by toxins. Some examples of bacterial neurotoxins are botulin, the exotoxin of botulism; neurotoxins of *Staphylococcus aureus* in toxic shock syndrome, and the tetanospasmin of tetanus. Fungal toxins include ergot from grain molds and mushroom poisoning. *Gonyaulax* is an alga found in algal blooms; it produces neurotoxins, which may concentrate in bivalve shell fish and cause paralytic symptoms following ingestion of the contaminated shell fish.

Viral Nervous System Infections

Poliomyelitis, Infantile Paralysis

Characteristics	An acute viral infection of the medulla, spinal cord, and nerves, with fever, headache, nausea, vomiting, sore throat, muscle pain and spasms, neck and back stiffness, with or without paralysis. Usually asymptomatic, or mild disease similar to influenza. Most often infects young children, occasionally further damage occurs many years later.
Pathogen	Poliovirus types 1, 2, and 3; small RNA enteroviruses (Fig. 13-26). Type 1 (wild type) most often causes paralysis. Types 2 and 3 are frequently vaccine-associated. Identified by tissue culture, cytopathic effects, and neutralizing antibody tests.
Reservoir	Human gastrointestinal tract.

Fig. 13-26. Development of poliovirus particles in pieces of cytoplasmic matrix of artificially disrupted cells. Particles in various stages of assembly from empty shells (*s*) to complete virions (*v*) can be seen (original magnification ×200,000). (Horne RW, Nagington J: J Mol Biol 1:333, 1959. Copyright by Academic Press, Inc., Ltd.)

Transmission	By direct contact or fecal–oral route in areas with poor sanitation. Virus is inhaled or ingested, carried by lymph to lymph nodes, to blood, to CNS, damaging motor nerve impulses to muscles. During infection and following vaccination with attenuated live vaccine, viruses are transmitted by pharyngeal secretions and fecal material.
Incubation period	3–35 days, usually 7–14 days.
Epidemiology	In United States, only 2 paralytic polio cases were reported in 1986.
Control	Immunize all infants and children with a series of Salk inactivated polio vaccine (IPV) or Sabin oral attenuated live poliovirus vaccine (OPV). In hospitalized patients, isolate with enteric precautions. Adequate sewage and water treatment precautions. Adequate sewage and water treatment.

Usual treatment	None. Provide therapy and assistance for paralytic patients.

Rabies

Characteristics	A fatal acute viral encephalomyelitis (CNS infection) of mammals, with depression, headache, fever, malaise, paralysis, hydrophobia (fear of water), salivation, spasms of throat muscles, convulsions, and death caused by respiratory failure.
Pathogen	Rabies virus (Fig. 13-27), a rhabdovirus; a large, complex, enveloped RNA virus. Identified by virus isolation and FA antibody tests to confirm direct observation of Negri inclusion bodies in animal brain tissue.
Reservoir	Many wild and domestic mammals: dogs, foxes, coyotes, cats, skunks, raccoons, and bats.
Transmission	Rabid animal bites introducing virus-laden saliva; airborne transmission from bats in caves; person-to-person by saliva.

Fig. 13-27. Intact rabies virus particle embedded in phosphotungstate and viewed in negative contrast. On the left are well-resolved surface projections 6–7 nm long (*arrow*) (original magnification × 400,000). (Hummeler K, et al: J Virol 1:152, 1967)

Incubation period	2–8 weeks or longer.
Epidemiology	In United States, no human cases, but 5297 animal cases reported in 1986.
Control	Vaccinate all pets (dogs, cats, raccoons, skunks, monkeys). Avoid all sick, aggressive, or friendly, wild animals. Prophylactic immunization of high-risk persons with human diploid cell rabies vaccine (HDCV). Isolation of hospitalized patients.
Usual treatment	Prompt treatment of bite wounds with soap and water and local infusion of rabies immune globulin (RIG) antiserum. Vaccinate patient with HDCV.

Bacterial Nervous System Infections

Tetanus

Characteristics	An acute infectious neuromuscular disease induced by the exotoxin, tetanospasmin, with convulsions and intermittent spasms of the voluntary muscles, especially masseter and neck; exhaustion, respiratory failure, and death may result.
Pathogen	*Clostridium tetani* (Fig. 13-28), a motile, gram-positive, anaerobic, spore-forming bacillus that produces a potent neurotoxin, tetanospasmin.

Fig. 13-28. Cells of *Clostridium tetani* after 24 hours on a cooked meat–glucose medium. Note spherical terminal endospores (original magnification × 4500). (Volk WA, et al: Essentials of Medical Microbiology, 3rd ed. Philadelphia, JB Lippincott, 1986)

Reservoir	Soil contaminated with feces; intestines of humans and animals.
Transmission	Spores of *C. tetani* are introduced into a puncture wound, burn, or needle prick by contamination with soil, dust, or feces. Spores anaerobically germinate within the wound into vegetative *C. tetani* producing the exotoxin.
Incubation period	3–21 days or longer.
Epidemiology	In United States, 61 cases reported in 1986.
Control	Active immunization of all children with DPT, a combined diphtheria–tetanus–pertussis vaccine, containing tetanus toxoid. Boosters of DT should be given at 10-year intervals and after a wound or accident with no booster for 5 years. Unimmunized persons may be given human tetanus immune globulin (TIG) following a puncture wound.
Usual treatment	Dirty wounds should be cleaned and left open, when feasible, to inhibit the anaerobic growth. Administer penicillin to destroy wound organisms, antitoxin (TIG) to neutralize the exotoxin, and vaccinate with DT.

Problems and Questions

1. Name six factors that control the number of microbes on the skin. How may opportunists invade through the skin?
2. Which bacteria cause most burn, wound, and bite infections? What types of toxins do they produce?
3. How do oral bacteria interact to cause dental caries? How can you prevent dental caries?
4. By what pathways may microbes invade to cause ear infections? Which bacteria are usually found in ear infections?
5. Why is pneumonia called a nonspecific disease? Name several pathogens that might cause pneumonia.
6. Differentiate between food-borne infections and food-borne intoxications. Name some examples of each.
7. Which protozoa cause gastrointestinal infections? How do they get there?
8. How are urinary tract infections transmitted? Why might *E. coli* be found more often in female cystitis than in male cystitis?
9. How may sexually transmitted infections be prevented? List the genital infections that may cause congenital and neonatal infections. How could transmission to the fetus and newborn be prevented?

10. Differentiate between typhus fever and typhoid fever. How are they transmitted and controlled?

11. By what means might children be exposed to plague, tularemia, toxoplasmosis, and rabies? After exposure, how should the children be treated to prevent or reduce the symptoms of these diseases?

12. List several areas, systems, or organs where there are no indigenous normal flora. Why might this be so?

13. What are the usual symptoms of disease in the nervous system? Define meningitis and encephalitis.

14. List several diseases caused by neurotoxins. List several nonspecific diseases discussed in this chapter.

Appendix

Classification of Bacteria According to *Bergey's Manual of Systematic Bacteriology*

Kingdom Procaryotae

divided into four divisions:

Division I. Gracilicutes;

procaryotes with thin cell walls, implying a gram-negative type of cell wall.

Division II. Firmicutes;

procaryotes with thick and strong skin, indicating a gram-positive type of cell wall.

Division III. Tenericutes;

procaryotes of a pliable and soft nature, indicating the lack of a rigid cell wall.

Division IV. Mendosicutes;

procaryotes with faulty cell walls, suggesting the lack of conventional peptidoglycan.

Volume 1

Section 1
The Spirochetes
Order I. *Spirochaetales*
  Family I. *Spirochaetaceae*
    Genus I. *Spirochaeta*
    Genus II. *Cristispira*
    Genus III. *Treponema*
    Genus IV. *Borrelia*
  Family II. *Leptospiraceae*
    Genus I. *Leptospira*

Other organisms: Hindgut spirochetes of termites and *Cryptocercus punctulatus* (wood-eating cockroach).

Section 2
Aerobic/Microaerophilic, Motile, Helical/Vibrioid Gram-Negative Bacteria
Genus I. *Aquaspirillum*
Genus II. *Spirillum*
Genus III. *Azospirillum*

Genus IV. *Oceanospirillum*
Genus V. *Campylobacter*
Genus VI. *Bdellovibrio*
Genus VII. *Vampirovibrio*

Section 3
Nonmotile (or rarely motile), Gram-Negative Curved Bacteria
Family I. *Spirosomaceae*
  Genus I. *Spirosoma*
  Genus II. *Runella*
  Genus III. *Flectobacillus*
Other genera:
  Genus *Microcyclus*
  Genus *Meniscus*
  Genus *Brachyarcus*
  Genus *Pelosigma*

Section 4
Gram-Negative Aerobic Rods and Cocci
Family I. *Pseudomonadaceae*
  Genus I. *Pseudomonas*
  Genus II. *Xanthomonas*
  Genus III. *Frateuria*
  Genus IV. *Zoogloea*
Family II. *Azotobacteraceae*
  Genus I. *Azotobacter*
  Genus II. *Azomonas*
Family III. *Rhizobiaceae*
  Genus I. *Rhizobium*
  Genus II. *Bradyrhizobium*
  Genus III. *Agrobacterium*
  Genus IV. *Phyllobacterium*
Family IV. *Methylococcaceae*
  Genus I. *Methylococcus*
  Genus II. *Methylomonas*
Family V. *Halobacteriaceae*
  Genus I. *Halobacterium**
  Genus II. *Halococcus**
Family VI. *Acetobacteraceae*
  Genus I. *Acetobacter*
  Genus II. *Gluconobacter*
Family VII. *Legionellaceae*
  Genus I. *Legionella*
Family VIII. *Neisseriaceae*
  Genus I. *Neisseria*
  Genus II. *Moraxella*
  Genus III. *Acinetobacter*
  Genus IV. *Kingella*

Other genera:
  Genus *Beijerinckia*
  Genus *Derxia*
  Genus *Xanthobacter*
  Genus *Thermus*
  Genus *Thermomicrobium*
  Genus *Halomonas*
  Genus *Alteromonas*
  Genus *Flavobacterium*
  Genus *Alcaligenes*
  Genus *Serpens*
  Genus *Janthinobacterium*
  Genus *Brucella*
  Genus *Bordetella*
  Genus *Francisella*
  Genus *Paracoccus*
  Genus *Lampropedia*

Section 5
Facultatively Anaerobic Gram-Negative Rods
Family I. *Enterobacteriaceae*
  Genus I. *Escherichia*
  Genus II. *Shigella*
  Genus III. *Salmonella*
  Genus IV. *Citrobacter*
  Genus V. *Klebsiella*
  Genus VI. *Enterobacter*
  Genus VII. *Erwinia*
  Genus VIII. *Serratia*
  Genus IX. *Hafnia*
  Genus X. *Edwardsiella*
  Genus XI. *Proteus*
  Genus XII. *Providencia*
  Genus XIII. *Morganella*
  Genus XIX. *Yersinia*
Other genera of the family
Enterobacteriaceae:
  Genus *Obesumbacterium*
  Genus *Xenorhabdus*
  Genus *Kluyvera*
  Genus *Rahnella*
  Genus *Cedecea*
  Genus *Tatumella*
Family II. *Vibrionaceae*
  Genus I. *Vibrio*
  Genus II. *Photobacterium*
  Genus III. *Aeromonas*
  Genus IV. *Plesiomonas*
Family III. *Pasteurellaceae*
  Genus I. *Pasteurella*

Genus II. *Haemophilus*
Genus III. *Actinobacillus*
Other genera:
Genus *Zymomonas*
Genus *Chromobacterium*
Genus *Cardiobacterium*
Genus *Calymmatobacterium*
Genus *Gardnerella**
Genus *Eikenella*
Genus *Streptobacillus*

Section 6
Anaerobic Gram-Negative Straight, Curved, and Helical Rods

Family I. *Bacteroidaceae*
Genus I. *Bacteroides*
Genus II. *Fusobacterium*
Genus III. *Leptotrichia*
Genus IV. *Butyrivibrio**
Genus V. *Succinimonas*
Genus VI. *Succinivibrio*
Genus VII. *Anaerobiospirillum*
Genus VIII. *Wolinella*
Genus IX. *Selenomonas*
Genus X. *Anaerovibrio*
Genus XI. *Pectinatus*
Genus XII. *Acetivibrio*
Genus XIII. *Lachnospira**

Section 7
Dissimilatory Sulfate- or Sulfur-Reducing Bacteria

Genus *Desulfuromonas*
Genus *Desulfovibrio*
Genus *Desulfomonas*
Genus *Desulfococcus*
Genus *Desulfobacter*
Genus *Desulfobulbus*
Genus *Desulfosarcina*

Section 8
Anaerobic Gram-Negative Cocci

Family I. *Veillonellaceae*
Genus I. *Veillonella*
Genus II. *Acidaminococcus*
Genus III. *Megasphaera*

Section 9
The Rickettsias and Chlamydias

Order I. *Rickettsiales*
Family I. *Rickettsiaceae*
Tribe I. *Rickettsieae*

Genus I. *Rickettsia*
Genus II. *Rochalimaea*
Genus III. *Coxiella*
Tribe II. *Ehrlichieae*
Genus IV. *Ehrlichia*
Genus V. *Cowdria*
Genus VI. *Neorickettsia*
Tribe III. *Wolbachieae*
Genus VII. *Wolbachia*
Genus VIII. *Rickettsiella*
Family II. *Bartonellaceae*
Genus I. *Bartonella*
Genus II. *Grahamella*
Family III. *Anaplasmataceae*
Genus I. *Anaplasma*
Genus II. *Aegyptianella*
Genus III. *Haemobartonella*
Genus IV. *Eperythrozoon*
Order II. *Chlamydiales*
Family I. *Chlamydiaceae*
Genus I. *Chlamydia*

Section 10
The Mycoplasmas

Order I. *Mycoplasmatales*
Family I. *Mycoplasmataceae*
Genus I. *Mycoplasma*
Genus II. *Ureaplasma*
Family II. *Acholeplasmataceae*
Genus I. *Acholeplasma*
Family III. *Spiroplasmataceae*
Genus I. *Spiroplasma*
Other genera:
Genus *Anaeroplasma*
Genus *Thermoplasma**
Mycoplasmalike organisms of plants and invertebrates

Section 11
Endosymbionts

A. Endosymbionts of protozoa
Genus I. *Holospora*
Genus II. *Caedibacter*
Genus III. *Pseudocaedibacter*
Genus IV. *Lyticum*
Genus V. *Tectibacter*
B. Endosymbionts of insects
Genus I. *Blattabacterium*
C. Endosymbionts of fungi and invertebrates other than arthropods

Volume 2

Section 12
Gram-Positive Cocci
Family I. *Micrococcaceae*
  Genus I. *Micrococcus*
  Genus II. *Stomatococcus*
  Genus III. *Planococcus*
  Genus IV. *Staphylococcus*
Family II. *Deinococcaceae*
  Genus I. *Deinococcus*
Other organisms: "Pyogenic" streptococci,
"Oral" streptococci, "Lactic" streptococci
and enterococci
  Genus *Leuconostoc*
  Genus *Pediococcus*
  Genus *Aerococcus*
  Genus *Gemella*
  Genus *Peptococcus*
  Genus *Peptostreptococcus*
  Genus *Ruminococcus*
  Genus *Coprococcus*
  Genus *Sarcina*

Section 13
Endospore-Forming Gram-Positive Rods and Cocci
Genus *Bacillus*
Genus *Sporolactobacillus*
Genus *Clostridium*
Genus *Desulfotomaculum*
Genus *Sporosarcina*
Genus *Oscillospira*

Section 14
Regular, Nonsporing, Gram-Positive Rods
Genus *Lactobacillus*
Genus *Listeria*
Genus *Erysipelothrix*
Genus *Brochothrix*
Genus *Renibacterium*
Genus *Kurthia*
Genus *Caryophanon*

Section 15
Irregular, Nonsporing, Gram-Positive Rods
Animal and saprophytic corynebacteria
(*Corynebacterium*)
Plant corynebacteria

Genus *Gardnerella**
Genus *Arcanobacterium*
Genus *Arthrobacter*
Genus *Brevibacterium*
Genus *Curtobacterium*
Genus *Caseobacter*
Genus *Microbacterium*
Genus *Aureobacterium*
Genus *Cellulomonas*
Genus *Agromyces*
Genus *Arachnia*
Genus *Rothia*
Genus *Propionibacterium*
Genus *Eubacterium*
Genus *Acetobacterium*
Genus *Lachnospira**
Genus *Butyrivibrio**
Genus *Thermoanaerobacter*
Genus *Actinomyces*
Genus *Bifidobacterium*

Section 16
Mycobacteria
Family I. *Mycobacteriaceae*
  Genus I. *Mycobacteria*

Section 17
Nocardioforms
Genus *Nocardia*
Genus *Rhodococcus*
Genus *Nocardioides*
Genus *Pseudonocardia*
Genus *Oerskovia*
Genus *Saccharopolyspora*
Genus *Micropolyspora*
Genus *Promicromonospora*
Genus *Intrasporangium*

Volume 3

Section 18
Gliding, Nonfruiting Bacteria
Order I. *Cytophagales*
  Family I. *Cytophagaceae*
    Genus I. *Cytophaga*
    Genus II. *Sporocytophaga*
    Genus III. *Capnocytophaga*
    Genus IV. *Flexithrix*
    Genus V. *Flexibacter*
    Genus VI. *Microscilla*
    Genus VII. *Saprospira*
    Genus VIII. *Herpetosiphon*

Order II. *Lysobacterales*
  Family I. *Lysobacteraceae*
    Genus *Lysobacter*
Order III. *Beggiatoales*
  Family I. *Beggiatoaceae*
    Genus I. *Beggiatoa*
    Genus II. *Thioploca*
    Genus III. *Thiospirillopsis*
    Genus IV. *Thiothrix*
    Genus V. *Achromatium*
  Family II. *Simonsiellaceae*
    Genus I. *Simonsiella*
    Genus II. *Alysiella*
  Family III. *Leucotrichaceae*
    Genus *Leucothrix*
Families and genera *incertae sedis* (status of species questionable):
    Genus *Toxothrix*
    Genus *Vitreoscilla*
    Genus *Chitinophagen*
    Genus *Desulfonema*
  Family IV. *Pelonemataceae*
    Genus *Pelonema*
    Genus *Achroonema*
    Genus *Peloploca*
    Genus *Desmanthus*

Section 19
Anoxygenic Phototrophic Bacteria
Purple Bacteria

Family I. *Chromatiaceae*
  Genus I. *Chromatium*
  Genus II. *Thiocystis*
  Genus III. *Thiospirillum*
  Genus IV. *Thiocapsa*
  Genus V. *Amoebobacter*
  Genus VI. *Lamprobacter*
  Genus VII. *Lamprocystis*
  Genus VIII. *Thiodictyon*
  Genus IX. *Thiopedia*
Family II. *Ectothiorhodospiraceae*
  Genus *Ectothiorhodospira*
Purple nonsulfur bacteria
  Genus *Rhodospirillum*
  Genus *Rhodopseudomonas*
  Genus *Rhodobacter*
  Genus *Rhodomicrobium*
  Genus *Rhodopila*
  Genus *Rhodocyclus*

Green Bacteria

Green sulfur bacteria
  Genus *Chlorobium*
  Genus *Prosthecochloris*
  Genus *Anacalochloris*
  Genus *Pelodictyon*
  Genus *Chloroherpeton*
Multicellular filamentous green bacteria
  Genus *Chloroflexus*
  Genus *Heliothrix*
  Genus *Oscillochloris*
  Genus *Chloronema*
Genera *incertae sedis*
  Genus *Heliobacterium*
  Genus *Erythrobacter*

Section 20
Budding and/or Appendaged Bacteria
Prosthecate Bacteria

Budding bacteria
  Genus *Hyphomicrobium*
  Genus *Hyphomonas*
  Genus *Pedomicrobium*
  Genus *"Filomicrobium"*
  Genus *"Dicotomicrobium"*
  Genus *"Tetramicrobium"*
  Genus *Stella*
  Genus *Ancalomicrobium*
  Genus *Prosthecomicrobium*
Nonbudding bacteria
  Genus *Caulobacter*
  Genus *Asticcacaulis*
  Genus *Prosthecobacter*
  Genus *Thiodendron*

Nonprosthecate Bacteria

Budding bacteria
  Genus *Planctomyces*
  Genus *Pasteuria*
  Genus *Blastobacter*
  Genus *Angulomicrobium*
  Genus *Gemmiger*
  Genus *Ensifer*
  Genus *Isophaera*
Nonbudding stalked bacteria
  Genus *Gallionella*
  Genus *Nevskia*
Morphologically unusual budding bacteria involved in iron and manganese deposition
  Genus *Seliberia*
  Genus *Metallogenium*
  Genus *Caulococcus*
  Genus *Kuznezovia*
Others: Spinate bacteria

Section 21
Archaeobacteria
Methanogenic Bacteria
Genus *Methanobacterium*
Genus *Methanobrevibacter*
Genus *Methanococcus*
Genus *Methanomicrobium*
Genus *Methanospirillum*
Genus *Methanosarcina*
Genus *Methanococcoides*
Genus *Methanothermus*
Genus *Methanolobus*
Genus *Methanoplanus*
Genus *Methanogenium*
Genus *Methanothrix*

Extreme Halophilic Bacteria
Genus *Halobacterium**
Genus *Halococcus**

Extreme Thermophilic Bacteria
Genus *Thermoplasma**
Genus *Sulfolobus*
Genus *Thermoproteus*
Genus *Thermofilum*
Genus *Thermococcus*
Genus *Desulfurococcus*
Genus *Thermodiscus*
Genus *Pyrodictium*

Section 22
Sheathed Bacteria
Genus *Sphaerotilus*
Genus *Leptothrix*
Genus *Haliscominobacter*
Genus *Lieskeella*
Genus *Phragmidiothrix*
Genus *Crenothrix*
Genus *Clonothrix*

Section 23
Gliding, Fruiting Bacteria
Order I. *Myxobacterales*
  Family I. *Myxococcaceae*
    Genus *Myxococcus*
  Family II. *Archangiaceae*
    Genus *Archangium*
  Family III. *Cystobacteraceae*
    Genus I. *Cystobacter*
    Genus II. *Melittangium*
    Genus III. *Stigmatella*

  Family IV. *Polyangiaceae*
    Genus I. *Polyangium*
    Genus II. *Nannocystis*
    Genus III. *Chondromyces*
  Genus *incerta sedis*
    Genus *Angiococcus*

Section 24
Chemolithotrophic Bacteria
Nitrifiers
Family I. *Nitrobacteraceae*
  Genus I. *Nitrobacter*
  Genus II. *Nitrospina*
  Genus III. *Nitrococcus*
  Genus IV. *Nitrosomonas*
  Genus V. *Nitrospira*
  Genus VI. *Nitrosococcus*
  Genus VII. *Nitrosolobus*

Sulfur Oxidizers
Genus *Thiobacillus*
Genus *Thiomicrospira*
Genus *Thiobacterium*
Genus *Thiospira*
Genus *Macromonas*

Obligate Hydrogen Oxidizers
Genus *Hydrogenbacter*

Metal Oxidizers and Depositors
Family I. *Siderocapsaceae*
  Genus I. *Siderocapsa*
  Genus II. *Naumaniella*
  Genus III. *Ochrobium*
  Genus IV. *Siderococcus*

Other Magnetotactic Bacteria

Section 25
Cyanobacteria
Others
Order I. *Prochlorales*
  Family I. *Prochloraceae*
    Genus *Prochloron*

Volume 4

Section 26
Actinomycetes that Divide in More
Than One Plane
Genus *Geodermatophilus*

Genus *Dermatophilus*
Genus *Frankia*
Genus *Tonsilophilus*

Section 27
Sporangiate *Actinomycetes*
Genus *Actinoplanes* (including
  Amorphosporangium)
Genus *Streptosporangium*
Genus *Ampullariella*
Genus *Spirillospora*
Genus *Pilimelia*
Genus *Dactylosporangium*
Genus *Planomonospora*
Genus *Planobispora*

Section 28
Streptomycetes and Their Allies
Genus *Streptomyces*
Genus *Streptovertillium*
Genus *Actinopycnidium*
Genus *Actinosporangium*
Genus *Chainia*
Genus *Elytrosporangium*
Genus *Microellobosporia*
(The last five genera may be merged with
Streptomyces)

Section 29
Other Conidiate Genera
Genus *Actinopolyspora*
Genus *Actinosynnema*
Genus *Kineospora*
Genus *Kitasatospora*
Genus *Microbispora*
Genus *Micromonospora*
Genus *Microtetrospora*
Genus *Saccharomonospora*
Genus *Sporichthya*
Genus *Streptoalloteichus*
Genus *Thermomonospora*
Genus *Actinomadura*
Genus *Nocardiopsis*
Genus *Excellospora*
Genus *Thermoactinomyces*

*Genera that have been placed in more
than one volume: *Gardnerella*, *Lachnospira*,
and *Butyrivibrio* have thin, gram-positive
walls but stain as gram-negatives. *Halobacterium*, *Halococcus*, and *Thermoplasma* are
Archaeobacteria that are also included among
the GRAM-NEGATIVE RODS AND COCCI
or THE MYCOPLASMAS.

Glossary

Adenosine triphosphate (ATP) (add-den'-o-sin tri'-fos-fate). High–energy-rich organic molecule

Agglutination (uh-glue-ten-ay'-shun). The clumping of cells following reaction with antibodies

Algae (al'-gee). Plants with chlorophyll (capable of producing their own food)

Allergen (al'-ur-jen). An antigen that causes an allergic reaction

Allergy (al'-ur-gee). A disease resulting from exposure to an antigen

Amebiasis (a-me-bi'-ah-sis). A disease caused by a protozoan, *Entamoeba histolytica*

Amphitrichous (am-fit'-ri-kus). Bacteria with flagella on both ends

Anabolism (an-ab'-bow-liz-em). Metabolic reactions that result in the biosynthesis of complex cellular materials

Anamnestic response (an-am-nest'-tick). Memory response following antigen exposure in sensitized individuals

Anaphylactic shock (an-na-fill-lack'-tick). A severe allergic reaction that may result in death

Antibiosis (an-tea-buy-oh'-sis). An antagonistic relationship

Antiobiotic (an-tea-buy-ot'-tick). Substance produced by microorganisms that inhibit or destroy pathogens during the disease process

Antibody (an'-tea-body). Protein produced by the body in response to foreign antigens

Antigen (an'-ti-gin). A foreign substance that stimulates the production of antibodies

Antiseptic (an-ti-sep'-tick). Chemical disinfectants that are safe to use on living tissues

Antitoxin (an-tie-tox'-sin). An antibody that neutralizes a toxin

Arthropod (ar'-throw-pod). A phylum classification of animals including insects, mites, lice, ticks, and fleas

Arthus reaction (ar'-thus). A complex immune skin reaction at the site of repeated injections

Asepsis (a-sep'-sis). Absence of infectious microorganisms on living tissue

Attenuated (uh-ten'-you-ate-ted). A weakened, less pathogenic organism

Autogenous vaccine (awe-tah'-gin-us). A vaccine prepared from a local infection, injected back into the same person

Autoimmune disease (awe-toe-im-mune'). A disease in which the body produces antibodies to its own tissues

Autotrophs (awe'-toe-trophs). Organisms that obtain carbon from inorganic sources, as from carbon dioxide

Bacillus (buh-sill'-us), *pl* bacilli (buh-sill'-eye). A rod-shaped bacterium; also, *Bacillus* is a genus of aerobic spore-forming rods

Bacteria (back-tier'-ee-uh). Procaryotic, mostly unicellular cells; most primitive organisms

Bactericidal (back-tear-i-side'-all). Bacteria-killing action

Bactericide (back-tear'-i-side). An agent that kills bacteria

Bacteriolytic (back-tear-ee-oh-lit'-tick). A substance that lyses or breaks apart bacteria

Catabolism (ca-tab'-bow-liz-em). Metabolic reactions that break down organic materials into simple molecules

Catalyst (cat'-uh-list). A chemical agents that speeds up a reaction

Catalyze (cat'-uh-lyz). To speed up a reaction

Centrosome (sen'-trow-soam). A eucaryotic cytoplasmic organelle containing two centrioles

Chemolithotrophs (key-moe-lith'-oh-trophs). Organisms that use a chemical source of energy and an inorganic source of nutrients

Chemoorganotrophs (key-moe-or-gan'-oh-trophs). Organisms that use a chemical source of energy and an organic source of nutrients

Chemotaxis (keem-oh-tacks'-sis). Movement of organisms in response to a chemical substance; the attraction of leukocytes to an area of injury is probably due to the release of a chemical substance from the injured tissue

Chemotherapy (key-mow-ther'-uh-pea). The treatment of diseases and infection using chemicals

Chemotrophs (chem'-oh-trophs). Organisms that obtain their energy from chemical sources

Choleragin (kol'-er-ah-gin). The exotoxin produced by *Vibrio cholerae* which causes cholera

Chromosome (crow'-mow-soam). The genetic material carrying the genes of heredity, containing DNA

Cilia (sill'-ee-uh). Short, hairlike structures that provide for movement; characteristic of Protozoa, Class Ciliata

Coagulase (co-ag'-you-laze). An enzyme that clots plasma around the bacteria

Coccus (cock'-cuss), *pl* cocci (cock'-sigh). Spherical or ball-shaped bacterium

Collagenase (co-lodge'-in-aze). An enzyme that breaks down collagen in connective tissue

Commensalism (co-men'-sal-is-um). A relationship in which one member benefits and the other is unaffected in any way

Complement (com'-ple-ment). A blood serum protein group involved in certain antibody–antigen reactions

Cystitis (sis-ti'-tis). An infection of the urinary bladder

Cytology (sigh-tol'-oh-gee). The study of cells

Cytoplasm (sigh'-tow-plaz-um). The protoplasm outside the nucleus of the cell

Cytotoxins (sigh-tow-tok'-sins). Toxic substances that injure certain cells

Dermatophytes (der-mah'-toe-fites). Fungi capable of growing on the skin surface, causing ringworm or tinea diseases

Disinfectant (dis-in-feck'-tant). A chemical agent used to destroy pathogens on or within nonliving materials

DNA, deoxyribonucleic acid (dee-ox'-ee-rye'-bow-nu-clay'-ick). The genetic material in the chromosomes

Encapsulate (en-cap'-sue-late). To surround by a capsule

Encephalitis (en-seff-fall-eye'-tis). A disease involving inflammation of the brain

Endemic (en-dem'-ick). A disease present in normal numbers in a community

Endoplasmic reticulum (end-oh-plasz'-mick re-tick'-you-lum). A eucaryotic cell organelle for transport and support

Enterotoxin (en'-ter-oh-tok'-sin). An exotoxin causing damage to intestinal cells, producing diarrhea

Enzyme (en'-zym). An organic catalyst

Epidemic (ep-i-dem'-ick). More than the normal number of cases of a disease in a community at a particular time

Epidemiology (ep-i-dem-ee-ol'-oh-gee). The systematic study of epidemics

Eucaryon (you-care'-ree-on). A cell with a true nucleus

Exotoxin (ek'-so-tock-sin). A toxic substance secreted by a living organism

Exudate (x'-you-date). A viscous secretion containing blood cells and cellular debris from site of inflammation

Facultative anaerobe (fack'-ul-tay-tive an'-air-robe). A microorganism that prefers to live in the absence of free oxygen, but survives in an oxygen environment

Fecal (fee'-cull). Referring to feces or bowel movement

Fibrinolysin (fy-bri-nol'-i-sin). An enzyme that breaks down fibrin clots

Filamentous (fil-uh-men'-tus). Having many threads or filaments

Flagella (fluh-gel'-uh). Protein strands used for movement

Fomes (fo'-meez) or **fomite** (fo'-mite), *pl* fomites (fo'-mi-teez). An object, such as a book or an item of clothing, that is not in itself harmful but that is able to harbor pathogenic organisms and thus serve as an agent for transmission of an infection

Fungi (fun'-ji). Microorganisms that are incapable of producing their own food and that live on decaying organic material; primitive plants

Fungicide (fun'-juh-side). A substance that kills fungi

Germicide (germ'-uh-side). A substance that kills microorganisms

Gene (jean). The genetic material coding for one polypeptide

Glycolysis (gly-col'-eh-sis). The anaerobic breakdown of glucose to pyruvic acid or lactic acid with the production of energy

Golgi (goal'-gee). A eucaryotic cell organelle involved in secretion

Haloduric (hey-low-dur'-ick). Surviving in a salty environment

Hapten (hap-ten'). A nonantigenic small molecule that becomes antigenic when combined with a large molecule

Hemolysin (heem-moll'-uh-sin). An enzyme that breaks down red blood cells

Hepatitis (hep-uh-tight'-us). A disease of the liver, usually caused by a virus

Herpes (her'-peas). A viral disease, cold sores, caused by *Herpesvirus hominis*

Heterotrophs (het'-ter-oh-trophs). Organisms that obtain carbon from organic sources

Histamine (hiss'-tuh-mean). Potent chemical released from cells during some immune reactions, causing swelling and inflammation

Hyaluronic acid (high-al-your-ahn'-ick). A chemical in connective tissue

Hyaluronidase (high-al-your-ahn'-uh-daze). An enzyme that breaks down connective tissue

Hypersensitivity (hi-purr-sense-uh-tive'-it-tea). An antigen–antibody reaction to foreign proteins in which cell-bound antibodies cause tissue destruction or inflammation

Hypertonic (hi-per-tahn'-ick). Having a greater osmotic pressure outside the cell membrane than inside the cell

Hypotonic (hi-po-tahn-'-ick). Having less osmotic pressure outside the cell membrane than inside the cell

Immunity (im-mu'-nit-tea). Resistance to disease imparted by the presence of antibodies

Immunoglobulin (im'-you-no-glob'-you-lyn). The globulin proteins of the serum and other body secretions, including the humoral antibodies

Immunology (im-mew-noll'-oh-gee). The science that deals with immunity from disease and the production of immunity

Immunosuppression (im'-you-no-sue-presh'-un). Depression of the immune response

Infection (in-feck'-shun). The growth of parasitic microorganisms in a host

Innate (in-ate'). Present in an individual at birth

Interferon (in-ter-fear'-ahn). Antiviral, soluble protein substances produced by cells infected with almost any animal virus; interferon is cell-specific and species-specific, but not virus-specific

In vitro (in vee'-trow). In the laboratory, in an artificial environment

In vivo (in vee'-vo). In the living organism

Isotonic (i-so-tahn'-ick). Having the same osmotic pressure inside and outside a cell membrane

Leukocidin (lew-co-side'-in). An enzyme that destroys white blood cells

Lipopolysaccharide (lip'-o-pol-ee-sack'-car-ride). A macromolecule of combined lipid and polysaccharide, often found in gram-negative bacterial cell walls

Logarithm (log'-uh-rhi-thm). Mathematically, the power to which a number must be raised to produce a given number

Lysozyme (lie'-so-zime). The cellular digestive enzyme in lysosomes

Lymphokines (lim'-fo-kines). T-cell secretions following antigenic stimulation

Malaise (mal-az'). A general feeling of illness and discomfort

Mesophilic (mess-so-fill'-ick). Thriving at 30° to 45°C (86° to 113°F)

Mesosome (me'-so-soam). A procaryotic cell organelle involved in cellular respiration

Metabolism (mu-tab'-bow-liz-em). The sum of all the chemical reactions in living cells

Microbial (my-crow'-bee-al). Pertaining to microbes

Microbicide (my-crow'-bi-side). An agent that kills microbes

Microbistasis (my-crow-bi-stay'-sis). The inhibition of growth and reproduction of microorganisms

Microorganism (my-kro-or'-gan-iz-em). Microscopic organisms, usually single cells; sometimes called microbes

Microtubules (my-crow-tube'-yules). Eucaryotic cell organelle involved in support and secretion

Mitochondria (my-tow-con'-dree-uh). Eucaryotic organelles involved in cellular respiration for the production of energy

Monoclonal antibodies (mon-o-clone'-al). Antibodies for a single antigenic determinant produced by hybridoma cells (lymphocytes fused with tumor cells) *in vitro*

Monotrichous (mon-ot'-trick-us). Bacteria with one flagellum

Motile (mow'-till). Having the ability to move

Mutagenic (mu-tuh-jen'-ick). An agent that produces mutations or genetic changes in organisms

Mutant (mu'-tant). An organism that has survived mutation

Mutation (mew-tay'-shun). A change in genetic material and traits that is inherited by offspring

Mutualism (mew'-chew-al-is-um). A relationship in which both organisms benefit

Necrotoxin (neck'-row-tox'-sin). An exotoxin that destroys certain cells

Neurotoxin (new'-row-tox-sin). An exotoxin that damages nerve tissue

Nosocomial (no-so-com'-ee-ul). An infection acquired during hospitalization

Nucleoid (new'-klee-oid). The nuclear area of procaryotic cells

Nucleolus (new-klee'-oh-lus). The dense portion of the nucleus, containing RNA

Nucleoplasm (new'-klee-oh-plaz-um). The protoplasm inside the nucleus

Oncogenic (on-ko-jen'-ick). Capable of producing tumors

Opportunist (op-poor-tune'-ist). A microbe that causes disease in susceptible individuals

Opsonization (op-son-a-zay'-shun). The engulfment of cells or bacteria by phagocytes, owing to the presence of specific antibodies

Organelles (or-gan-ells'). Discrete structures inside the cell

Osmotic pressure (oz-mah'-tic). The pressure exerted on the cell membrane by the solution inside the cell

Pandemic (pan-dem'-ick). A worldwide epidemic

Parasitism (par'-uh-sit-ism). A relationship in which an organism benefits at the expense of the host organism

Pasteurization (pass-tur-uh-zay'-shun). A process by which heat is used to kill pathogens in foods

Pathogen (path'-o-jen). Disease-causing microorganism

Pathogenicity (path-oh-gin-iss'-city). The ability of an organism to cause disease

Peptidoglycan (pep-tid-o-gly'-can). The rigid component of bacterial cell walls, consisting of polysaccharide chains linked together by peptide chains

Peristalsis (pear-uh-stall'-siss). Waves of contraction passing along tubular organs, particularly the intestine, mixing contents and moving them along

Peritrichous (pear-ri'-trick-us). Covered by flagella

Phagocyte (faj'-oh-site). White blood cells capable of ingesting foreign particles, including microorganisms

Photolithotrophs (foe-toe-lith'-oh-trophs). Organisms that use light for energy and inorganic chemicals for nutrients

Photoorganotrophs (foe-toe-or-gan'-oh-trophs). Organisms that use light for energy and organic chemicals for nutrients

Phototrophs (foe'-toe-trophs). Organisms that use light as their source of energy

Plasmolysis (plaz-moll'-uh-sis). The shrinking of the cell membrane and cytoplasm from the cell wall, causing the cell to shrink

Plasmoptysis (plaz-mop'-ti-sis). A process in which water enters a cell through the cell walls

Poliomyelitis (pole-ee-oh-my-oh-light'-us). A viral disease

Polymer (pol'-e-mer). Long-chain molecule consisting of repeated subunits

Precipitin (pre-sip'-it-tin). An antibody to soluble antigen that forms a visible precipitate

Primordial (pry-mor'-dee-al). Early or first in time

Procaryon (pro-kar'-ee-on). Primitive cells without a true nucleus

Protoplasm (pro'-tow-plaz-um). The semifluid material inside cells

Protoplasts (pro'-toe-plasts). A bacterial cell with no cell wall

Protozoa (pro-toe-zoe'-uh). Single-celled microscopic animals found in water and soil

Psychroduric (sigh-crow-dur'-ick). Having the ability to endure temperatures of −20° to 5°C (−5° to 40°F)

Purine (pure'-reen). A DNA base; adenine or guanine

Pyogenic (pie-oh-jen'-ick). Pus producing

Pyrimidine (perr'-rim-uh-dean). A nucleic acid base; thymine, cytosine, or uracil

Resident flora (flur'-uh). Microorganisms usually found in an area of the human body

Ribosomes (rye'-bow-soams). Organelles necessary for protein synthesis

RNA, ribonucleic acid (rye'-bow-new-clay'-ick). Nucleic acid necessary for protein synthesis

Saprophyte (sap'-row-fight). An organism that obtains its nutrients from dead, decaying organic matter

Sebum (see'-bum). The secretion of the sebaceous (oil) glands of the skin

Serological tests (ser-o-lodge'-eh-cal). Antigen–antibody tests used for diagnostic purposes

Spirochetes (spy'-row-keets). Spiral-shaped bacteria

Sporicidal (spor-uh-sigh'-dull). Having the ability to kill spores

Streptokinase (strep-tow-kine'-ase). An enzyme that helps streptococci to invade the body

Symbionts (sim'-bee-yonts). Organisms living together

Symbiosis (sim'-bee-oh'-sis). A constant relationship between two or more unlike species of organisms

Synergism (sin'-er-jiz-um). A mutualistic relationship in which organisms accomplish together what neither could do alone

Taxonomy (tax-ah'-no-me). A systematic classification of organisms

Teichoic acid (tie-ko'-ick). A chemical in the cell wall of gram-positive bacteria

Tetanospasmin (tet'-ah-no-spaz'-min). The neurotoxic exotoxin that causes tetanus produced by *Clostridium tetani*

Thermoduric (ther-mow-dur'-ick). Having the ability to survive boiling

Toxigenicity (tox-uh-gen-iss'-city). The ability of a pathogen to produce a toxin, causing damage to the host

Toxin (tok'-sin). A toxic or damaging substance

Toxoid (tok'-soid). An inactivated toxin that can stimulate antitoxin production but not cause disease

Transient flora (flur'-uh). Microorganisms temporarily found in certain area of the body

Tuberculocidal (too-bur-cue-low-sigh'-doll). Killing the bacteria that cause tuberculosis (*Mycobacterium tuberculosis*)

Tyndallization (tin-dull-uh-zay'-shun). A process of boiling and cooling in which spores are allowed to germinate and then are killed

Urethritis (you'-re-thri'-tis). An inflammation of the urethra of the urinary system

Vaccine (vack-scene'). An inactivated agent used to cause the production of antibodies to protect against disease

Vacuoles (vack'-you-oles). Membrane-bound storage spaces in the cell

Vector (veck'-tore). A carrier of pathogenic organisms from one host to another

Virology (vi-rol'-oh-gee). The study of viruses and the diseases they cause

Virucide (vi'-ruh-side). A substance that kills viruses

Virulence (veer'-you-lence). The properties of an organism that make it pathogenic

Virulent (veer'-you-lent). Able to produce disease

Virus (vi'-rus). An infective agent smaller than a bacterium

Selected References for Suggested Reading

Books

Alexander M: Introduction to Soil Microbiology, 3rd ed. New York, John Wiley & Sons, 1982

American Hospital Association: Infection Control in the Hospital, 4th ed. Chicago, American Hospital Association, 1980

Ayliffe GA, Taylor LJ: Hospital-Acquired Infections: Principles and Prevention. Littleton, John Wright-PSG, 1982

Beaver PC, Jung RC: Animal Agents and Vectors of Human Disease, 5th ed. Philadelphia, Lea & Febiger, 1985

Block SS (ed): Disinfection, Sterilization and Preservation, 3rd ed. Philadelphia, Lea & Febiger, 1983

Boyd HC, Payne MJ: Introduction to the Algae, 2nd ed. Englewood Cliffs, NJ, Prentice-Hall, 1985

Boyd RF, Hoerl BG: Basic Medical Microbiology, 2nd ed. Boston, Little, Brown & Co, 1980

Brock TD (ed): Milestones in Microbiology. Washington, DC, American Society for Microbiology, 1974

Bryan LE (ed): Antimicrobial Drug Resistance. New York, Academic Press, 1984

Carr NG, Whitton BA: The Biology of Cyanobacteria. Botanical Monographs, vol. 19. Berkeley, University of California Press, 1982

Castle M: Hospital Infection Control, New York, John Wiley & Sons, 1980

Clayton RK, Sistrom WR (eds): The Photosynthetic Bacteria. New York, Plenum Press, 1978

Davis BD, et al: Microbiology, 4th ed. New York, Harper & Row, 1987

Difco Manual: Dehydrated Culture Media and Reagents for Microbiology, 10th ed. Detroit, Difco Laboratories, 1984

Faust EC, Beaver PC, Jung RC: Animal Agents and Vectors of Human Diseases, 4th ed. Philadelphia, Lea & Febiger, 1975

Fenner F, et al: The Biology of Animal Viruses, 2nd ed. New York, Academic Press, 1974

Finegold SM, Martin WJ: Diagnostic Microbiology, 6th ed. St. Louis, CV Mosby, 1982

Freeman BA: Burrows' Textbook of Microbiology, 22nd ed. Philadelphia, WB Saunders, 1985

Friedman RM: Interferons: A Primer. New York, Academic Press, 1981

Gauri KK: Antiviral Chemotherapy: Design of Inhibitors of Viral Functions. New York, Academic Press, 1981

Gerhardt P, et al (eds): Manual of Methods for General Bacteriology. Washington, DC, American Society for Microbiology, 1981

Goodfellow M, Mordarski M, Williams S: Biology of the Actinomycetes. New York, Academic Press, 1984

Gottschalk G: Bacterial Metabolism. New York, Springer-Verlag, 1979

Holt JG (ed): Bergey's Manual of Systematic Bacteriology, 1st ed., vol. 1. Baltimore, Williams & Wilkins, 1984; vol. 2 (1985); vol. 3 (1986); vol. 4 (1987)

Hood LE, Weissman IL, Wood WB, Wilson JH: Immunology, 2nd ed. Menlo Park, Benjamin/Cummings, 1984

Hurst A, Gould GW: The Bacterial Spore. New York, Academic Press, 1984

Ingraham JL, Maaloe O, Neidhardt FC: Growth of the Bacterial Cell. Sunderland, Sinauer Associates, 1983

Jawetz E: Review of Medical Microbiology, 16th ed. Los Altos, Appleton and Lange, 1984

Joklik WK, et al: Zinsser's Microbiology, 18th ed. New York, Appleton and Lange, 1984

Lennette EH, et al (eds): Manual of Clinical Microbiology, 4th ed. Washington, DC, American Society for Microbiology, 1985

Margulis L: Early Life. Boston, Science Books International, 1982

Mausner JS, Kramer S: Mausner and Bahn Epidemiology. Philadelphia, WB Saunders, 1984

Mitchell R (ed): Water Pollution Microbiology, vol. 2. New York, John Wiley & Sons, 1978

Myrvik QN, Weiser RS: Fundamentals of Immunology. Philadelphia, Lea & Febiger, 1984

Nester EW, et al: Microbiology, 3rd ed. New York, Holt, Rinehart & Winston, 1983

Nolte WA (ed): Oral Microbiology, 4th ed. St. Louis, CV Mosby, 1982

Pelczar MJ, Chan ECS, Krieg NR: Microbiology, 5th ed. New York, McGraw-Hill, 1986

Perkins JJ: Principles and Methods of Sterilization in Health Sciences, 2nd ed. Springfield, Charles C Thomas, 1982

Rippon JW: Medical Mycology, 2nd ed. Philadelphia, WB Saunders, 1982

Rose NR, Fahey JL, Friedman H: Manual of Clinical Immunology, 3rd ed. American Society for Microbiology, 1986

Smith L deS: The Pathogenic Anaerobic Bacteria, 3rd ed. Springfield, Charles C Thomas, 1984

Standard Methods for the Examination of Water and Wastewater, 15th ed. Washington, DC, American Public Health Association, 1981

Stryer L: Biochemistry, 2nd ed. San Francisco, WH Freeman, 1981

Sutter V, et al: Wadsworth Anaerobic Bacteriology Manual, 3rd ed. St. Louis, CV Mosby, 1980

Tortora GJ, Funke BR, Case CL: Microbiology, 2nd ed. Menlo Park, Benjamin/Cummings Publishing Co, 1986

Volk WA: Essentials of Medical Microbiology, 3rd ed. Philadelphia, JB Lippincott Co, 1986

Watson JD: The Double Helix. Stent GS (ed). New York, WW Norton, 1980

Watson JD, Tooze J, Kurtz DT: Recombinant DNA: A Short Course. New York, WH Freeman, 1983

Webster J: Introduction to Fungi, 2nd ed. New York, Cambridge Univeristy Press, 1980

Wehrle PF, Top FH (eds): Communicable and Infectious Diseases, 9th ed. St. Louis, CV Mosby, 1981

Wilson ME, Mizer HE, Morello JA: Microbiology in Patient Care, 4th ed. New York, Macmillan, 1984

Wistreich GA, Lechtman MD: Microbiology, 4th ed. New York, Glencoe Press, 1984

Youmans GP, Paterson PY, Sommers HM: The Biologic and Clinical Basis of Infectious Diseases, 3rd ed. Philadelphia, WB Saunders, 1985

Journal Publications

Abraham EP: The beta-lactam antibiotics. Sci Am 244:76–86, June 1981

Bishop JM: Oncogenes. Sci Am 246:80–92; March 1982

Brill WJ: Biologic nitrogen fixation. Sci Am 236:68–74, 1977

Buisseret PD. Allergy. Sci Am 247:86–95, Aug 1982

Collier RJ, Kaplan DA: Immunotoxins. Sci Am 251:56–64, July 1984

Cohen SN, Shapiro SA: Transposable genetic elements. Sci Am 242:40, 1980

Cooper MD, Lawson AR: The development of the immune system. Sci Am 231:58–70, 1974

Edelson RL, Fink JM: The immunologic function of skin. Sci Am 256:46–53, June 1985

Ferris FG, Beveridge TJ: Functions of bacterial cell surface structures. BioScience 35:172–177, 1985

Frankel–Conrat H, Kimball P: Virology, 1982

Fraser DW, McDade JE: Legionellosis. Sci Am 241:82–99, Oct 1979

Friedman MJ, Trager W: The biochemistry of resistance to malaria. Sci Am 244(3):154, 1981

Godson GN: Molecular approaches to malaria vaccines. Sci Am 252:52–59, May 1985

Karpas A: Viruses and leukemia. Am Sci 70:277–285, 1982

Leder P: The genetics of antibody diversity. Sci Am 246:102, 1982

Lerner RA: Synthetic vaccines. Sci Am 248:66–74, Feb 1983

Marrack P, Kappler J: The T-cell and its receptor. Sci Am Feb 1986

Novick RP: Plasmids. Sci Am 243(6):102, 1980

Prusiner SB. Prions. Sci Am 251:50–59, Oct 1984

Simons K, Garoff J, Helenius A: How an animal virus gets into and out of its host cell. Sci Am 246:58–66, Feb 1982

Stark A-A: Mutagenicity and carcinogenicity of mycotoxins. Ann Rev Microbiol 34:235, 1980

Yelton DE, Scharff MD: Monoclonal antibodies. Am Sci 68:510–516, 1980

Index

Page numbers followed by *t* and *f* indicate tables and figures, respectively. Page numbers in italics indicate major discussions.